NURSES' HANDBOOK OF FLUID BALANCE

SECOND EDITION

NURSES' HANDBOOK OF FLUID BALANCE

Norma Milligan Metheny, R.N., M.S.

Assistant Professor of Nursing, Meramec Community College, St. Louis, Missouri.

W. D. Snively, Jr., M.D., F.A.C.P.

Professor of Life Sciences, School of Nursing, University of Evansville, Evansville, Indiana; Visiting Professor of Continuing Medical Education, University of Alabama Medical Center, Birmingham, Alabama; Clinical Professor of Pediatrics, Indiana University School of Medicine, Bloomington, Indiana.

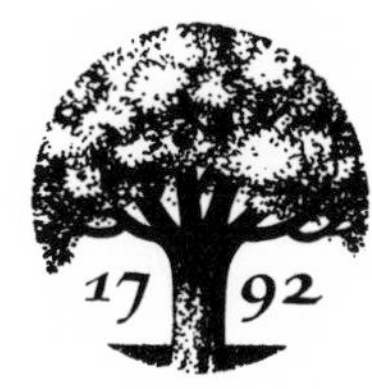

J.B. Lippincott Company | Philadelphia and Toronto

SECOND EDITION

Original illustrations by Robert Wiethop

ISBN-0-397-54155-4
Library of Congress Catalog Card Number 73-22393
PRINTED IN THE UNITED STATES OF AMERICA

9 8

Distributed in Great Britain by
Blackwell Scientific Publications, London, Oxford, and Edinburgh

Library of Congress Cataloging in Publication Data
Metheny, Norma Milligan.
Nurses' handbook of fluid balance.
Includes bibliographical references.
1. Body fluids. 2. Body fluid disorders. 3. Fluid therapy. 4. Nurses and nursing. I. Snively, W. D., joint author. II. Title.
[DNLM: 1. Body fluids—Nursing texts. 2. Nursing care. 3. Water-Electrolyte Balance–Nursing texts. WY156 M592n 1974]
RT69.M4 1974 612'.01522 73-22393

"Water . . . is the image of the ungraspable phantom of life; and this is the key to it all."

Herman Melville in *Moby Dick*

CONTENTS

PREFACE to the Second Edition

The reception of the *NURSES' HANDBOOK OF FLUID BALANCE* has been most gratifying. Because of the burgeoning involvement of the nursing profession in areas of diagnosis and therapy, in addition to the traditional routine care of patients with body fluid disturbances, both publisher and authors decided on a thorough-going revision of the text.

Chapters dealing with the fundamentals of body fluid disturbances were both rewritten and expanded. Recently acquired knowledge concerning the basics of body fluid disturbances was incorporated. Especially noteworthy are the additions to the material on acid-base disturbances. New information concerning the use of blood gases was incorporated.

Just as searching and comprehensive were the changes in the chapters dealing with the nurse's practical application of knowledge of body fluid disturbances. For example, the chapter on the formulation of the nursing diagnosis was completely rewritten and greatly expanded. The same could be said for the chapter on the nurse's role in preventing imbalances of water, electrolytes, and other nutrients. Material dealing with the nursing implications of parenteral fluid administration was considerably enlarged. Especial emphasis was laid on the body's reaction to stress in the chapter dealing with the body's response to surgical trauma. Fluid balance in the badly burned patient was thoughtfully brought up to date. In addition to incorporation of the latest methods of treatment, a patient-care study was included.

Fluid balance in the patient with digestive tract disease incorporates numerous additions. So do the chapters dealing with urologic disease and cardiac disease. In the latter, due attention is paid to recent knowledge on the effects of potassium, calcium, magnesium, and pH. The sections on the electrocardiograph and on diuretics were rewritten.

Many additions, particularly relating to the management of diabetic acidosis, were incorporated in the chapter on endocrine disease. New additions in the area of neurologic disease include recent information on diabetes insipidus. Fluid balance in the patient with respiratory disease presents new sections on hypoventilation, hypoxemia, oxygen administration, and dyspnea. Hyperventilation received additional emphasis, as did respiratory implications of blood gas concentrations. Water balance in prolonged mechanical ventilation is emphasized. Increased emphasis is laid on the need for potassium for prevention of heat stress disease. In the chapter on fluid balance disturbances in infants and children, new emphasis is placed on determination of body surface area, factors influencing fluid intake, tube feedings, and parenteral hyperalimentation.

The new chapter on fluid balance in pregnancy presents the dramatic new cautions concerning sodium restriction.

Most of the illustrations were redone. Particularly important in this connection are the new "clinical pictures" of body fluid disturbances. Not only were most of the drawings redone, fifteen new photographs were incorporated in the book.

The authors take pleasure in expressing their appreciation to Donna R. Beshear for significant editorial services and counsel and to Robert Wiethop for his artistic contributions. David Miller, Vice President, J. B. Lippincott Company, provided invaluable advice in this revision, as in the initial publication of the book.

N. M. M.
W. D. S., Jr.

PREFACE to the First Edition

The authors' goal for this textbook is to provide the nurse, student and graduate alike, with an *inviting, clear, comprehensive* and—above all—*practical* handbook on body fluid disturbances. With this goal ever in mind, we have first presented general information concerning body fluid disturbances—their nature, pathogenesis, clinical manifestations and diagnosis, and the principles of medical therapy. Our approach is *systematic,* for only such an approach can bring order from the apparent chaos that is so often synonymous with the subject. Sir William Osler might well have been speaking of body fluid disturbances (although he was not) when he said: "System, or as I shall term it, the virtue of method, is the harness without which only the horses of genius travel."

After laying the foundation, we have built on it the nurse's management in the eminently practical matters of observation, interpretation and intervention. We have dealt with the more important clinical areas in which body fluid disturbances play such a cogent role. Always, we have laid great emphasis on the *how,* as well as the *why,* and with generous use of illustrations. The surgical patient, the badly burned patient, the patient with digestive, urologic, cardiac, endocrine, respiratory disease—each has his day in court. Problems associated with drowning and with excessive exposure to heat are not forgotten, nor is the child, with his peculiar proneness to body fluid disturbances.

To avoid cluttering the text, we have used a minimum of footnotes; but following Chapter 27 the reader will find a comprehensive list of references for looking up moot points as well as for additional reading.

Our tack cannot but reveal our conviction that the nurse's role in the management of patients is becoming an increasingly complex and crucial one, especially so for the patient with a body fluid disturbance, whose status changes from hour to hour. The unique contribution of the nurse, who is with the patient around the clock, includes not only the physical care of the patient, but also her intelligent observations and judgments—knowing *what* to look for and *how* to look for it. The careful recording of fluid intake and output, and the understanding of the purely nursing problems posed by the patient's condition and treatment are also part of her comprehensive care plan. All this is essential not only to the patient, but also to the physician, who bears the primary responsibility for management. Clearly, the nurse's contributions will be infinitely greater if she has more than a casual familiarity with body fluid disturbances.

We hope our book might be epitomized by something Oliver Wendell Holmes said: "Science is a first-rate piece of furniture for a man's upper chamber, if he has common sense on the ground floor." We have tried to provide the nurse both with science for her upper chamber, and with the practical information that will enable her to exercise common sense on the ground floor, as she goes about her work with patients suffering from body fluid disturbances.

This book, like the proper care of the patient with a body fluid disturbance, represents the joint efforts of a nurse and a physician. It could not have been written without both contributors; nor can the hospitalized patient with a fluid imbalance receive optimal care without such a team effort.

N. M. M.
W. D. S., Jr.

INTRODUCTION

Much Ado About Something

Although Thomas Latta treated cholera "by the copious injection of aqueous and saline fluids into the veins" in 1832, it has been only during the past quarter century that disturbances of water and electrolytes have been accorded the attention their importance deserves. Especially in the decade beginning in 1950 did interest reach a high intensity. The realization had dawned at last that body fluid disturbances represent the common denominator of a host of illnesses; that every seriously ill patient is a candidate for one or more of these disturbances; that many patients with moderate or even mild illnesses can develop them; that whether many patients live or die depends upon how their medical attendants solve the problems posed by body fluid disturbances. It has become clear that a working knowledge of body fluids is required for the intelligent management of most of the diseases listed in the diagnostic nomenclature.

The list of clinical problems in which body fluid disturbances tend to be especially important is a long one. It includes the seriously burned patient, the patient with ulcerative colitis, the diabetic patient, the patient with congestive heart failure, the patient undergoing surgery, the patient with hypertension and the patient taking potent diuretics. Indeed, in many respects medical progress has *increased* the potential number of body fluid disturbances. For example, sulfonamide diuretics, such as the thiazides, cause a dangerously increased excretion of potassium in nearly half the patients taking these diuretics for a prolonged period. The resultant body fluid disturbance, potassium deficit, can cause permanent damage to the heart muscle and to the kidney tubules. However, this is only one of some 50 important causes of potassium deficit. Therapy involving several hormones of the adrenal cortex represents a great triumph for medicine, yet it has brought in its train a significant increase in body fluid disturbances.

Because many hospitalized patients are seriously ill, the incidence of body fluid disturbances in hospitals is often high. Surveys of 2 hospitals revealed that more than 20 per cent of the patients were suffering from potassium deficit that was largely undiagnosed by the attending physician! In these studies, other imbalances were not sought out. It is interesting to speculate what the incidence of *other* fluid imbalances would have been, had they been investigated. Since the early diagnosis of body fluid disturbances depends upon close observation of the patient, the nurse carries a heavy responsibility. She must be alert to untoward events in the patient's progress and must understand the significance of those events.

Observations that might once have been regarded as of little or no importance now rank with TPR as vital signs. At one time, sweating called only for the application of nursing comfort measures; now its potentially serious clinical result has to be considered. The same statement applies to losses of body fluids from whatever source. The nurse is the on-the-spot observer not only of the patient's output of fluids, but also of his intake. All this clearly means that the nurse must know what the various body fluid disturbances are, how they develop and what characterizes them. This knowledge is required so that she can take the proper action, which includes the accurate reporting of significant facts to the physician.

The nursing profession has been prompt to respond to the challenge of the new knowledge of body fluid disturbances. Splendid courses in body fluids are being taught in schools all over the land. Numerous articles on the various aspects of body fluid disturbances are appearing in the nursing literature. Certainly the subject deserves the increased interest, which represents *much ado about something*—something of vital importance to every nurse, every physician, and every patient who entrusts himself to their professional care.

TERMINOLOGY

The old bugbear of terminology plagues everyone who writes a book on a technical subject. The problem is at least as formidable in the medical field as in any other. All too frequently, identical entities are described by entirely different terms. Sometimes a term that has one meaning for one group of workers has exactly the opposite meaning for another. Inconsistency of terminology appears at times to mount into a 20th century Tower of Babel.

Of all the fields of medicine, none has suffered more confusion in terminology than fluid balance. For years we desperately needed a classification that was at once *systematic, clear, logical, clinical, all-inclusive,* and perhaps most important of all, *not susceptible to misinterpretation.* The ideal classification had to be eminently practical, having to serve as a useful basis for understanding, diagnosis and treatment.

A classification meeting many of these criteria was introduced by Moyer in 1952 in his classic *Fluid Balance: A Clinical Manual.* It was modified and extended considerably by Snively and Sweeney in 1956, in their book *Fluid Balance Handbook For Practitioners.* This classification has since been further modified by Snively, and that modification is employed in this text, with its rationale being described in detail in Chapter 5. In Chapter 10 is presented a comparative table showing, in parallel columns, body fluid disturbances described by our terminology under the heading of *physico-clinical imbalance*; the less realistic and more confusing *conventional terminology*; and, in the third column, *closely related clinical states.*

There are lesser problems caused by the fact that several perfectly correct terms may be used interchangeably. For example, the ubiquitous term *glucose* is usually referred to as *dextrose* when it occurs as part of the name of a parenteral solution, because it is the U.S.P. designation for glucose of requisite purity. *Solution of sodium chloride* is usually designated by the shorter term *saline*; but when used as part of a solution description, it is described by the longer term. The old term *uremia* has been replaced—in part, at least—by the more modern term *azotemia.* Roughly equivalent to the term *plasma* are *intravascular extracellular fluid, serum,* and *intravascular space,* and the term *interstitial fluid* is approximated by the terms *extravascular extracellular fluid* and *interstitial space.* Yet, in the strictly technical sense, *plasma* has had an anticoagulant added, at least as it occurs when prepared for intravenous administration; *serum,* upon which laboratory determinations are performed, has not. And certainly, if one wants to be technical, a fluid is not a *space,* nor a space a fluid. Throughout the book we have endeavored to use these roughly synonymous terms in the natural way in which they would be employed by nurses and physicians in the hospital.

Now let us plunge boldly into our subject, with the consideration of body fluid, our heritage from the sea.

1 Body Fluid, Our Heritage From the Sea

Life on earth began in the ocean about two billion years ago. Scientists are far from certain as to the exact nature of that first form of life, but it may have been the single-celled organism that we know as the protozoan. Whether the protozoan was first or not, it most certainly appeared quite early in the development of life.

The ocean water surrounding that first microorganism and its infinite progeny contained everything necessary to maintain life. Dissolved in the sea water were oxygen and other gases besides various nutrients. The physical characteristics of the ocean—its ability to maintain a constant temperature, its volume, and its surface tension, among others—all suited the minuscule organism's needs.

The sea was a kind mother to the primitive organism that is the most ancient ancestor of our body cells. To this day every one of us contains within his body a tight little pond that we might think of as a tiny, personal portion of the sea. We call it *body fluid.* Body fluid accounts for 60, 70, perhaps 80 per cent of our total body weight, depending upon age, sex, and body fat content. In general, the younger the individual, the higher his percentage of body fluid. Women have a lower body water content than men, and a fat person contains less fluid than a thin person, since fat has little water associated with it.

But how did this sea water get into our bodies? Scientists explain it thus: over the course of millions of years, the single-celled organisms were joined to each other, forming many-celled metazoa. The metazoa were just as dependent on their physicochemical bath water, the ocean, for the maintenance of life as were the protozoa. Eons later certain sea creatures began to develop physical characteristics that would eventually enable them to exist on the continental land masses. An essential step in this evolutionary process occurred when some of the sea water was enclosed within their bodies. These creatures could never have left the ocean without some means of carrying their oceanic bath water along with them. James Gamble, a great physiologist, described the step in these words:

> Before our extremely remote ancestors could come ashore to enjoy their Eocene Eden or their Paleozoic Palm Beach, it was necessary for them to establish an enclosed aqueous medium which would carry on the role of sea water.

These early animals contained two types of body fluid—the fluid within the individual cells, or *cellular fluid,* and an additional fluid that served to surround and bathe the cells, the *extracellular fluid.* These two types of fluid also occur in man. They are our heritage from the sea.

2 Cellular and Extracellular Fluid, Secretions and Excretions

The body fluid is divided into two major compartments. The first compartment, *the cellular fluid,* comprises the fluid contained within the billions of body cells and accounts for about three-fourths of the total body fluid. We might think of it as a vast multitude of tiny, encapsulated droplets suspended in another type of fluid, the *extracellular fluid.* Extracellular fluid constitutes about one-fourth of the total body fluid.

During the evolutionary process, the extracellular fluid was further divided into two subdivisions. Once the sea water became enclosed within the body it had to be circulated to carry nutrients and other substances to the cells and waste materials away from them. A heart and a circulatory system evolved, and part of the extracellular fluid—about a fourth of it—was appropriated for circulation through the system. This intravascular extracellular fluid is the *plasma*—the liquid fraction of the blood. The other three-fourths of the extracellular fluid lies outside the blood vessels in the interstitial spaces between the body cells. This extravascular portion of the extracellular fluid is called *interstitial fluid.* Lymph and cerebrospinal fluid, while they have highly specialized and unique functions, are usually regarded as interstitial fluid.

In addition to the two major divisions of body fluid, the cellular and extracellular fluid, there are other essential fluids—the *secretions and excretions.* The secretions include the juices manufactured in the stomach, pancreas, liver, and intestine. Urine and feces are excretions. Perspiration is also regarded as an excretion, although its purpose is not to rid the body of wastes but rather to aid in body heat regulation.

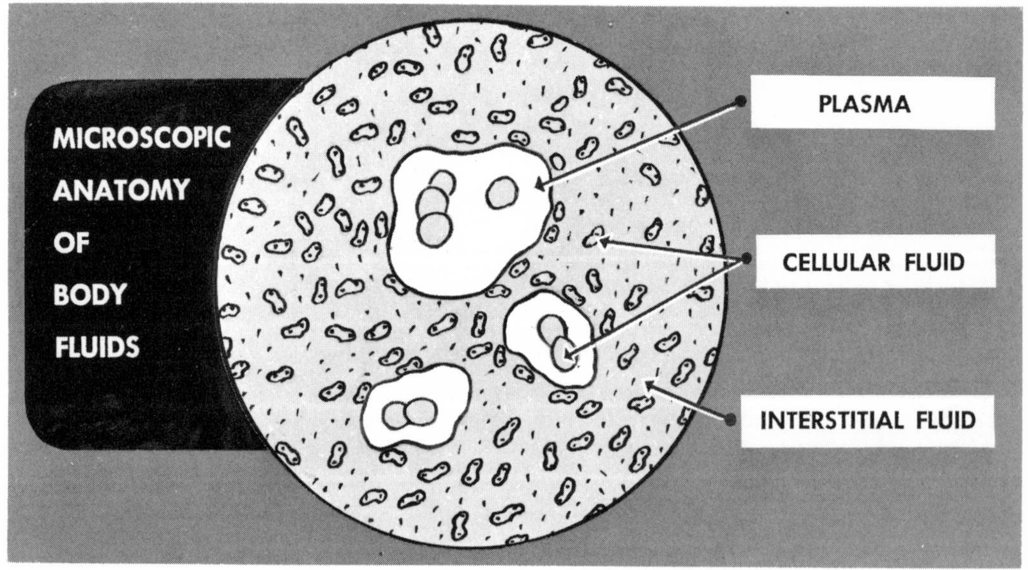

Fig. 2-1. Microscopic anatomy of body fluids.

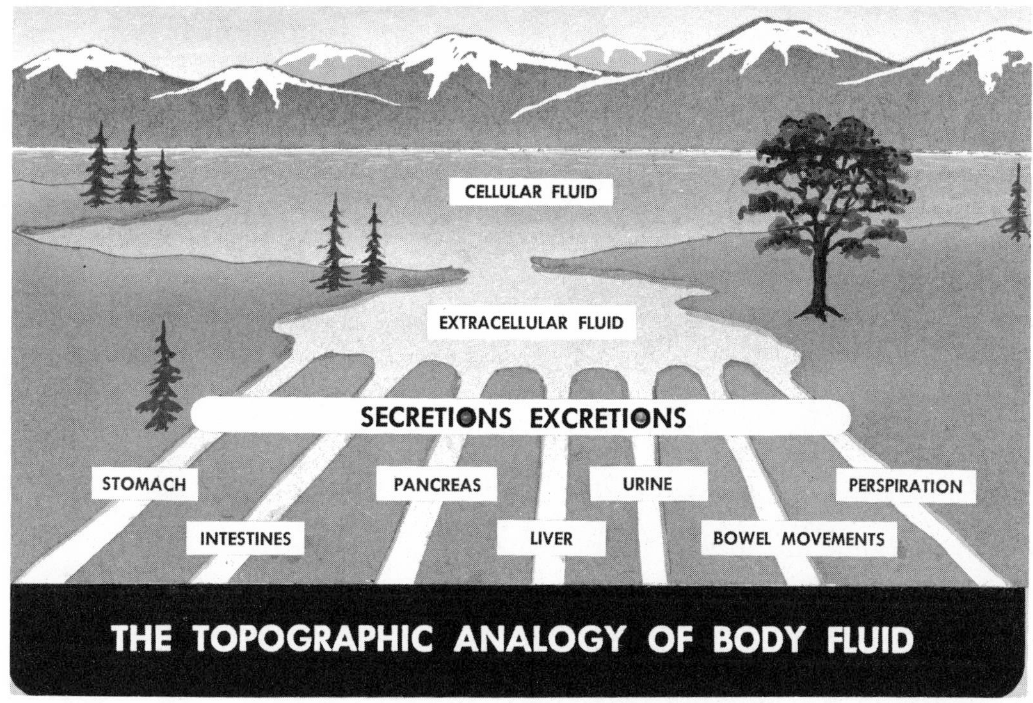

Fig. 2-2. The topographic analogy of body fluid.

Even though secretions and excretions are derived from extracellular fluid, they are not actually extracellular fluid.

By the use of a topographic analogy, we can visualize the relationships between cellular fluid, extracellular fluid, and the secretions and excretions. Cellular fluid can be regarded as a vast ocean that holds three-fourths of the body fluid. It is fed by the extracellular fluid, which is pictured as a great river. The secretions and excretions represent streams and rivulets flowing from the extracellular fluid, which supplies them with all needed materials.

COMPOSITION OF BODY FLUIDS

Body fluid consists chiefly of *water* and certain dissolved substances sometimes referred to as salts, minerals, or crystalloids, but more correctly called *electrolytes*.

Water is the most essential nutrient to life. No known form of plant or animal life can exist for very long without it. Indeed, humans can live a long time without other nutrients, but only for a few days without water. Water possesses unique chemical and physical characteristics and there is no substitute for it in the living cycle. Water's boiling point (100° C.) and its freezing point (0° C.) enable the human body to withstand all but the most drastic changes in heat or cold. Water is the closest substance known to a universal solvent. Since the adult body is from 60 to 70 per cent water, each one of us is, in a real sense, a bag of more or less solid materials dissolved in water. Water is required for the countless chemical reactions of the body; no major physiologic function can proceed without it.

Electrolytes are so named because they ionize—develop electrical charges—when they are dissolved in water. Some electrolytes, including sodium, potassium, calcium, and magnesium, develop positive charges; some, including chloride, bicarbonate, sulfate, phosphate, proteinate, carbonic acid, and other organic acids, develop negative charges.

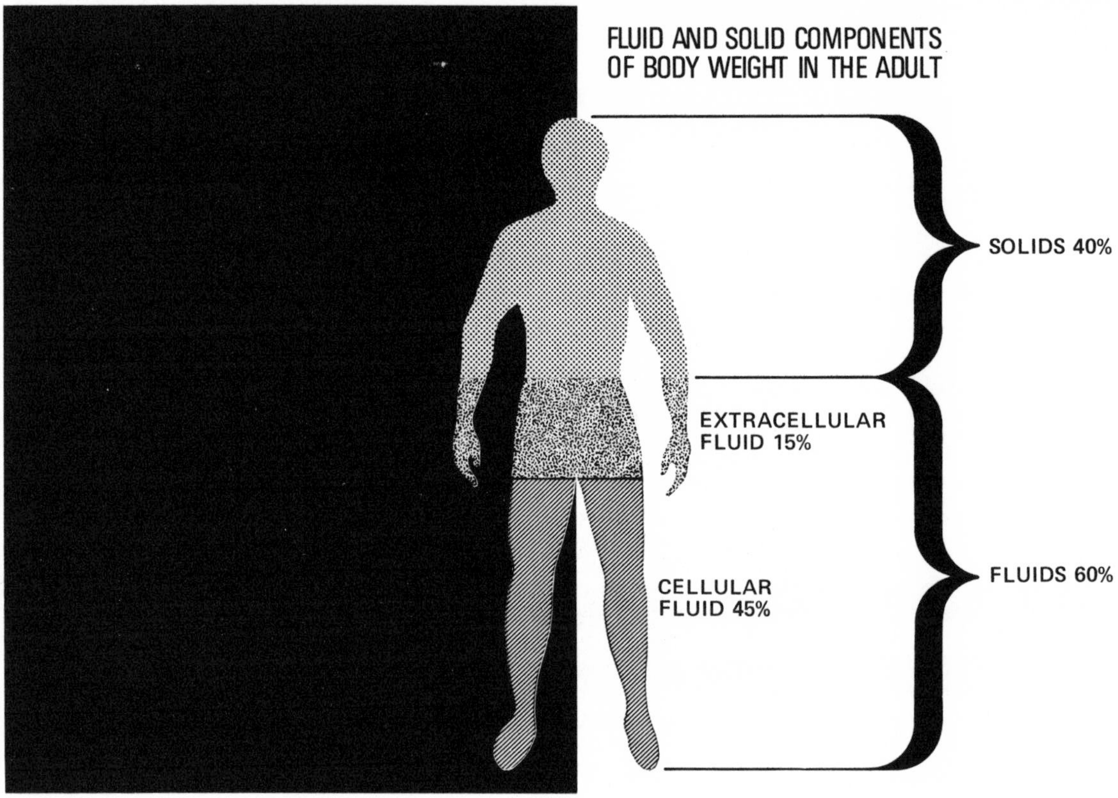

FLUID AND SOLID COMPONENTS OF BODY WEIGHT IN THE ADULT

SOLIDS 40%

EXTRACELLULAR FLUID 15%

CELLULAR FLUID 45%

FLUIDS 60%

Fig. 2-3. Fluid and solid components of body weight in the adult.

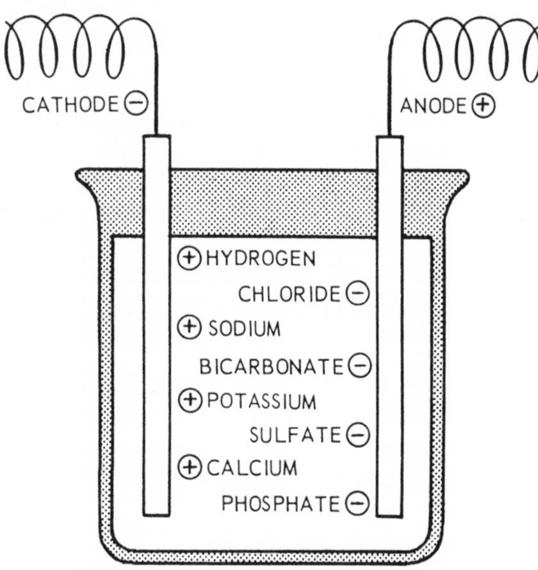

Fig. 2-4. In a wet electric cell cations go to the negative pole or cathode, anions to the positive pole or anode.

One can determine which electrolytes carry positive charges and which carry negative charges by placing the electrolyte in question in a wet electric cell through which an electric current is conducted. Such a cell has a negative pole called a *cathode* and a positive pole called an *anode*. Since unlikes attract, positively charged particles travel to the negative pole, or cathode. Such particles are therefore designated as *cations*. Negatively charged particles, called *anions*, migrate to the positive pole, or anode. The term *ion* refers to both cation and anion. In all electrical systems, positive charges and negative charges balance each other. Cations and anions exist in equal strength and numbers when measured according to their chemical activity or ability to unite with other ions to form molecules.

Each body fluid has its own normal composition of water and electrolytes. Cellular fluid contains large amounts of potassium, magnesium, and phosphate, and only small amounts of other electrolytes. Its composition, geologists explain, is not unlike that of the seas of two billion years ago. Extracellular fluid reflects the composition of the Cambrian seas of some 350 million years ago, in that it contains large amounts of sodium, calcium, and chloride. The composition of sea water has changed over the years as the continental land masses have gradually dissolved and washed into it; hence, the two types of body fluid vary greatly in composition since they were enclosed within the body during two different geologic periods. Electrolytes in present-day sea water are several times as concentrated as they are in either of our body fluids, which explains why we are unable to drink it.

The chief difference between the plasma and the interstitial fluid is that plasma contains a much greater amount of proteinate, which acts as a sponge to prevent excess plasma from seeping into the interstitial fluid.

The composition of secretions and excretions varies considerably, particularly in illness. Therefore, the quantities of electrolyte per unit volume must be related to a constant, which consists of the levels of sodium, potassium, chloride, and bicarbonate in plasma. On this basis, we find that gastric secretions have about half the sodium concentration of plasma, about the same potassium, about half again as much chloride, and a fraction of the bicarbonate. Pancreatic secretions have about the same sodium and potassium, about a third the chloride, and about three times the bicarbonate. Perspiration, a dilute secretion, has more than half the sodium and chloride and about the same potassium. Diarrheal stools in children have a fraction of the sodium, several times as much potassium, a fraction of the chloride, and probably much more bicarbonate.

FUNCTIONS OF BODY FLUIDS

The main function of body fluids is to maintain healthy living conditions for the body cells. For although we may regard ourselves as highly complex, highly civilized organisms, the cells remain the basic units of life. A living body could no more exist without cells than could a brick building exist without bricks. Unlike bricks, however, our cells are live, dynamic, working units that

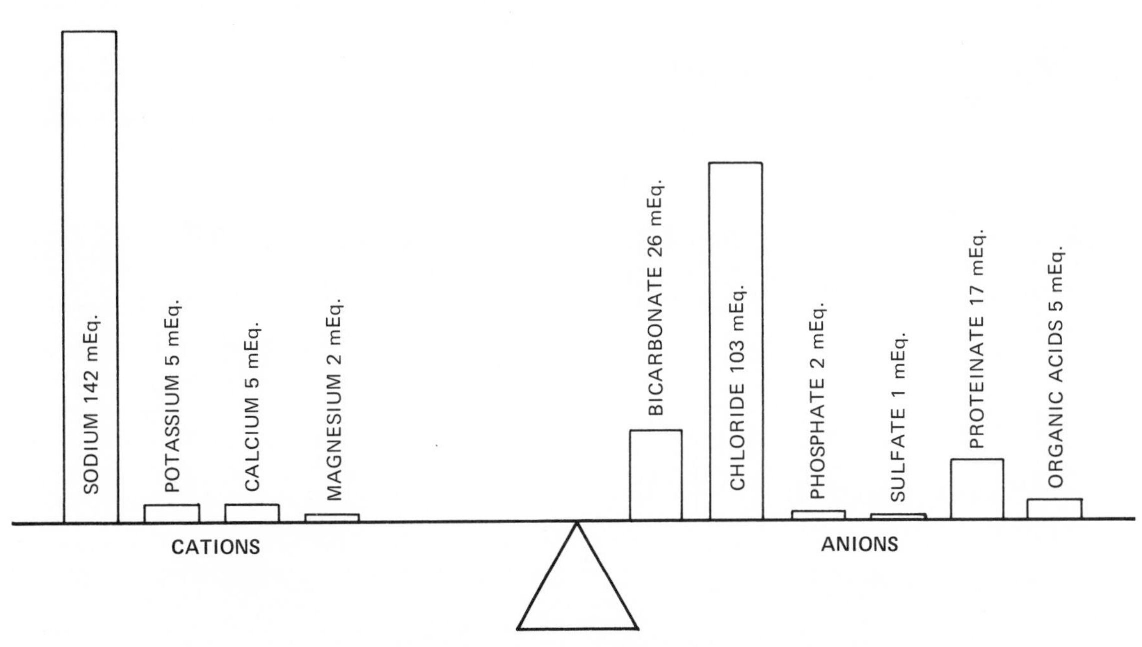

Fig. 2-5. The cations and anions of the extracellular fluid balance each other when expressed in milliequivalents.

must be nourished. The cellular fluid, which normally contains all the nutrients the cells need, serves as the supply source to replenish nutrients as they are used up. In addition, the cellular fluid must be cleared of wastes, such as carbon dioxide and breakdown products of protein; the extracellular fluid performs these services. Nutrients and other materials seep from the plasma into the interstitial fluid at the arterial end of the capillary beds, which exist in every part of the body, and are carried to the cells via the interstitial fluid. Waste materials pass from the cellular fluid into the interstitial fluid and back to the plasma via the venous capillaries. The plasma then sorts the waste products for storage or excretion and carries them to their proper destinations.

In addition to transporting nutrients and wastes, extracellular fluid transmits enzymes and hormones, plus many additional substances. It carries red blood cells through the body and white blood cells to attack bacteria.

3 Routes of Transport

Materials are transported between cellular and extracellular fluid via several routes, including osmosis, diffusion, filtration, active transport, pinocytosis, and phagocytosis, of which *osmosis* is the most important.

OSMOSIS A quick way of describing osmosis is to say, "Water goes where salt is." This means that if there are two solutions separated by a semipermeable membrane, the solution with the greatest concentration of electrolyte draws water from the solution with the lesser concentration of electrolyte. It is almost as if there were an effort on the part of each electrolyte particle to surround itself with its fair share of the available water.

Osmosis is highly important in the body. If pure water not containing electrolytes were injected directly into the bloodstream, the red blood cells would absorb water, swell and burst. If an extremely salty solution were injected into a vein, the red blood cells would lose water to their salty environment and would shrink, just as your fingers do if they have been in water too long. Osmosis occurs when the extracellular fluid develops an electrolyte content lower or higher than normal, because of disease or an accident such as drowning.

Osmotic pressure refers to the drawing power for water, and depends on the number of molecules in solution. Electrolytes and substances such as mannitol with their low molecular weights exert ordinary osmotic pressure. Albumin and other substances with high molecular weights exert a special kind of osmotic pressure known as *colloid osmotic pressure* or *oncotic pressure.* Colloids possess special importance since they cannot pass through the capillary wall, the barrier between

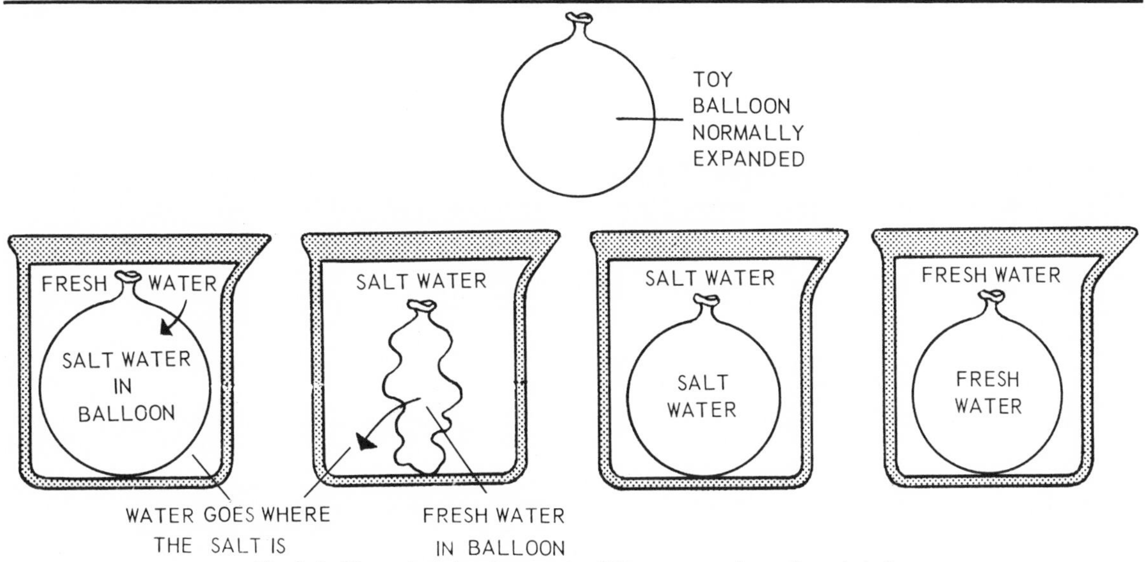

Fig. 3-1. The principle of osmosis: "Water goes where the salt is."

plasma and interstitial fluid. Mannitol, with its low molecular weight, raises the osmotic pressure of plasma when given intravenously, whereas human albumin, having an extremely high molecular weight, exerts an oncotic pressure.

DIFFUSION The physical process, called diffusion, occurs through the random movement of ions and molecules, which tend to become equally concentrated in all parts of a vessel. The molecules move incessantly, bump into each other, and bounce away. They scatter from regions where their concentration is high and pass to regions where the concentration is low. Exchanges of oxygen and carbon dioxide by the lung alveoli and capillaries occur through diffusion.

ACTIVE TRANSPORT When it is necessary for ions to move from areas of lesser concentration to areas of greater concentration, active transport occurs, whereby adenosine triphosphate (ATP) is released from a cell to enable certain substances to acquire the energy needed to pass through the cell membrane. This method of transfer, still not fully understood, may involve carrier systems located within cell membranes. Sodium ions, potassium ions, and amino acids are probably carried through all cell membranes by active transport, which also occurs in the transfer of chloride ions, hydrogen ions, phosphate ions, calcium ions, magnesium ions, creatinine, and uric acid through some cell membranes.

FILTRATION The transfer of water and dissolved substances through a permeable membrane from a region of high pressure to a region of low pressure is called filtration. The force behind filtration is *hydrostatic pressure,* produced by the pumping action of the heart. Examples of filtration include the passage of water and electrolytes from the arterial end of the capillary beds to the interstitial fluid and the passage of water and small molecules from the glomerular capillaries of the kidneys into the tubules. Opposing the hydrostatic pressure, which tends to force water and electrolytes out of the capillaries, is the oncotic pressure of the plasma proteins, which tends to hold them back.

PINOCYTOSIS AND PHAGOCYTOSIS A form of movement by which large molecular weight substances, such as protein, enter body cells is pinocytosis, by which protein molecules are taken into the cell by invagination of the cell membrane. In phagocytosis, the microorganisms, cells, or foreign particles are engulfed or digested by phagocytes. Leukocytes employ phagocytosis in attacking bacteria.

COMMENT It is via these methods of exchange that the body cells are nourished and excrete wastes, which greatly alters the composition of extracellular fluid. The effects would be catastrophic were it not for chemical regulatory activities that are carried out by the body. This enables the pond within the skin to maintain its compositional integrity and, at the same time, to keep the body cells just as healthy as if they were still floating in the wide blue sea, under the towering Cambrian clouds.

4 Organs of Homeostasis

For the maintenance of health, the body must maintain homeostasis—the normal state of the body fluids. The volume and electrolyte composition of extracellular fluid must be held very close to normal, in view of the many possible abnormalities involving water or electrolytes. Body cells constantly pour the results of chemical reactions into the extracellular fluid; they constantly withdraw from it substances needed for specific organ or cell activities. We eat and drink a wide variety of materials not needed by our body, and the digestive tract indiscriminately absorbs most of the substances offered it.

The volume of the liquids we drink would overcome us if there were no mechanism for maintaining a constant extracellular fluid volume. These problems in health are multiplied in disease, and this adds to the already gigantic task of maintaining homeostasis.

THE HOMEOSTATIC MECHANISM

Fortunately, nature has provided each of us with a system of automation, which demonstrates the wisdom of the body. In its handling of a complex task, this system, called the *homeostatic mechanism*, puts man-made automation to shame.

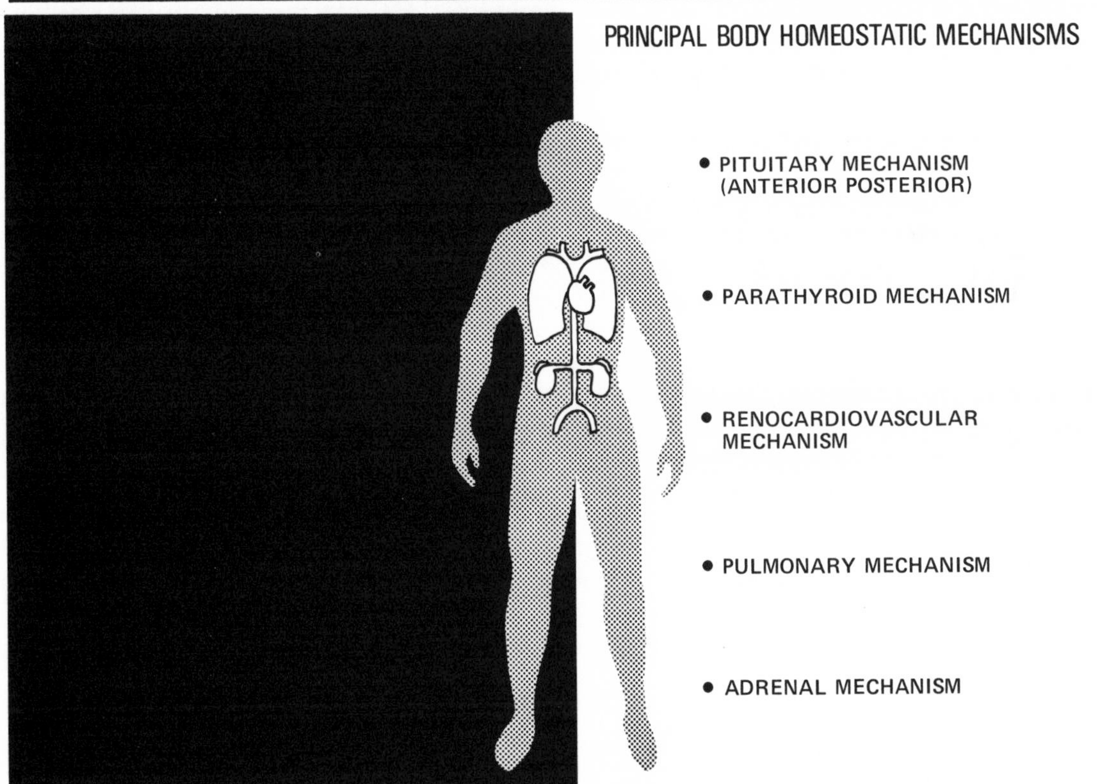

Fig. 4-1. Principal body homeostatic mechanisms.

The homeostatic mechanism utilizes every body system and every body organ, with the possible exception of the reproductive organs. The lungs, kidneys, heart, adrenal glands, pituitary gland, and parathyroid glands are particularly involved, and because these organs are so important, we call them the *organs of homeostasis.*

The lungs serve to regulate the oxygen level and carbon dioxide level of blood. Since carbon dioxide stems from the carbonic acid in the blood, the lungs help maintain the extremely important balance between acids and alkalies in extracellular fluid.

Other organs play a somewhat different role. The kidneys are most influential in maintaining homeostasis. They might be called the master chemists of our body fluids, for it is not what we eat and drink, but how the kidneys function that determines the volume and chemical composition of extracellular fluid. They excrete chemical wastes and remove from the extracellular fluid a great variety of foreign substances indiscriminately absorbed by the digestive tract. The kidneys further sort out electrolytes as they pass from the blood through their filtering beds, excreting all but those that the body needs. We can exist for hours, days, or even longer without the use of our bones, muscles, digestive organs, nerves, endocrine glands, and even the cerebrum, but if the kidneys totally cease their chemical regulation of the extracellular fluid for an hour, physiologic deterioration promptly commences.

The kidneys are completely dependent on the heart, which pumps about 1,700 L. of blood to the kidneys for cleansing every day. Some 180 L. of this amount is filtered through the kidneys, and approximately 1.5 L. of this daily filtrate passes out as urine—the rest is reabsorbed.

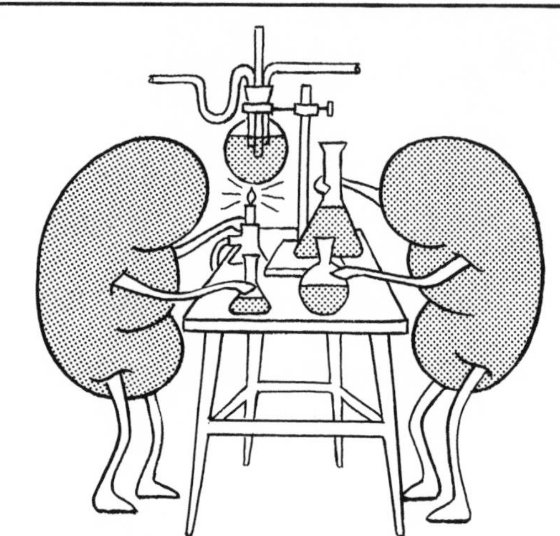

Fig. 4-2. The kidneys are the master chemists of our *sea within.*

The adrenal glands, located above the kidneys, secrete numerous hormones that influence the body in many ways, both in health and in disease. These glands function in the retention and excretion of water and electrolytes, especially sodium, chloride, and potassium.

The pituitary gland, located within the brain, directly affects the body's conservation of water via its secretion of antidiuretic hormone (ADH).

The parathyroid glands are the last of the major organs of homeostasis. Located near or embedded in the thyroid gland, these pea-sized glands regulate the level of calcium in the extracellular fluid.

The organs of body automation usually function efficiently; nevertheless, when any of the organs of homeostasis does malfunction, those persons caring for the patient face a formidable task.

5 Disturbances of Water and Electrolytes

If the volume and chemical composition of the body fluid deviates even slightly from the safe bounds of normal, disease results. Diseases involving body fluids are called *body fluid disturbances* or *body fluid imbalances*. Such disturbances may be primary, or they may occur secondarily to other conditions. Indeed, every patient with a serious illness is a potential candidate for body fluid disturbance, and even the patient who is only moderately or mildly ill may be stricken with one imbalance or a combination of two or more.

Despite the frequency and the importance of body fluid disturbances, probably no group of clinical problems has been so poorly understood.

Much of the early knowledge concerning imbalances of the body fluids originated with teachers who were biochemists first and clinicians second—if, indeed, they were clinicians at all. Quite naturally, they presented body fluid disturbances in the light of their own research. As a result, muc of the early teaching about body fluid disturbances was concerned with detailed descriptions of all the possible imbalances that could occur in the one or two diseases on which the teacher had concentrated. Body fluid disturbances began to be regarded as *biochemical appendages* of disease states, rather than as a broad group of problems representing the common denominator of many ailments. No over-all view of these disturbances was presented. The subject as taught was so complex, so specialized, and so sophisticated that most members of the medical and nursing professions came to regard the subject as difficult, if not impossible. One student in the class of a famous pediatrician-biochemist described the subject: "as clear as if written backwards by Gertrude Stein in Sanskirt."

A completely different and enlightened approach to the study of body fluid disturbances might be termed the *clinical picture approach*; first introduced by Carl Moyer, it was enlarged upon considerably by Snively and Sweeney. Its basic breakthrough involved understanding that disturbances of water and electrolytes are produced by a fairly small number of mechanisms, most of which are simple and readily comprehensible.

Essential to the application of the clinical picture approach is a simple diagnostic classification, which divides body fluid disturbances into some 16 basic imbalances or clinical pictures. Each has its own set of causative mechanisms; its own symptoms, subjective and objective; its own laboratory findings.

There is nothing new to this pedagogic technique for studying disease. When ailments such as rheumatic fever, appendicitis, lobar pneumonia, or the contagious diseases are presented to nursing students, they are presented as clinical pictures, and the students analyze them as clinical pictures. Each picture includes the history, the symptoms—both subjective and objective—and the laboratory data. When the student studies body fluid disturbances by this method, she analyzes the underlying mechanisms responsible for the disturbances through clinical pictures.

Sometimes one of these disturbances exists by itself; at other times, it occurs in combination with one or more additional imbalances. Frequently, body fluid disturbances are associated with other disease states and, indeed, interact intimately with them. Sometimes a succession of body fluid disturbances occurs, one after another. Clearly, one must understand single imbalances if one is to understand the combinations.

6 Units of Measure

A long time ago, a gentleman named John Selden said,

> . . . if they should make the standard for the measure we call a "foot" a Chancellor's foot; what an uncertain measure would this be! One Chancellor has a long foot, another a short foot, a third an indifferent foot . . .

Master Selden was pointing out, quite correctly, that without standard, invariable units of measure, we are severely limited. In the same light, we could never understand, diagnose and treat body fluid disturbances without simple, accurate units of measure.

MEASUREMENT OF EXTRACELLULAR FLUID

Because of the constant exchanges between cellular and extracellular fluid, changes in either are reflected in the other. Therefore, imbalances in the extracellular fluid ultimately cause imbalances in the cellular fluid, and vice versa. Since cellular fluid is divided among the billions of body cells, it is not readily available for examination.

However, the extracellular fluid is easily accessible; disturbances in this fluid are accurately reflected in the symptoms and findings shown in illness. For this reason, we focus our chief attention upon the extracellular portion of the body fluid when we study imbalances of water and electrolytes.

MEASUREMENT OF VOLUME One of the most essential units of measure is the measurement of volume. The European system of weights and measures is used increasingly in science; it uses the *liter* (L.) for volume measurement. The liter is broken down into 1,000 parts or milliliters (ml.), each milliliter representing 1/1,000 of a liter. A milliliter is virtually identical to the cubic centimeter (cc.), but the milliliter is preferred, because the centimeter is a linear rather than a volumetric unit of measure. Expressed in terms of weight rather than volume, a liter of water weighs 1,000 grams (Gm.), or about 2.2 lbs.

MEASUREMENT OF CHEMICAL ACTIVITY The electrolytes of the body fluid are active, dynamic chemicals. Since we are interested in their activity, we must have a unit that expresses *chemical activity,* or *chemical combining ability,* or the power of cations to unite with anions to form molecules. Virtually any cation can unite with any anion. The cation sodium, for example, combines with the anion chloride to form the molecule sodium chloride. Sodium united with proteinate forms the molecule sodium proteinate. Or, it may combine with nitrate, forming sodium nitrate. Similarly, the cations potassium, magnesium, and calcium can unite with any of the anions. Therefore, why could we not merely use as our unit of measure the weight of the ions in which we are interested? Unfortunately, this does not solve our problem, since the *weight* of a chemical bears no relation to its *chemical activity.* *One* mg. of sodium unites chemically with *180* mg. of proteinate to form the compound sodium proteinate, for example.

In searching for a unit of chemical activity, chemists have discovered the *milliequivalent* (mEq.). A traditional measurement of physical power in our civilization is the power of an imaginary average horse; our unit of chemical power, the milliequivalent, is *equivalent* to the activity of 1 mg. of hydrogen. In other words our

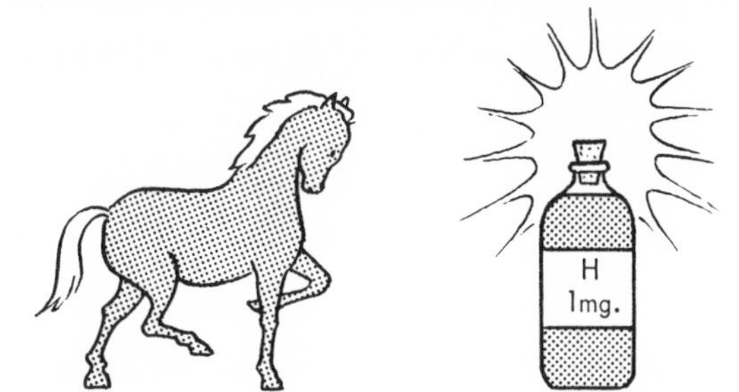

Fig. 6-1. One milligram of hydrogen represents the unit for chemical combining power: it is the electrolyte horsepower.

chemical horse is 1 mg. of hydrogen (Figure 6-1). One milligram of hydrogen exerts 1 mEq. of chemical activity; so do 23 mg. of sodium, 39 mg. of potassium, 40 mg. of calcium, 35 mg. of chloride, or 4,140 mg. of proteinate. Each of these weights represents 1 mEq. of the ion in question, whether it is cation or anion.

When electrolytes are measured in milliequivalents, cations and anions always balance each other, and a given number of milliequivalents of a cation always reacts with exactly the same number of milliequivalents of an anion. Here is something useful to memorize:

One Milliequivalent of Any
Cation Is Equivalent
Chemically to One Milliequivalent
of Any Anion

It matters not a bit whether the cation is sodium, potassium, calcium, or magnesium, or whether the anion is chloride, bicarbonate, phosphate, sulfate, or proteinate.

The milliequivalent value of an element or molecule is determined by taking the millimole (mM.)—the atomic or molecular weight of the element or compound in milligrams—and dividing by the *valence*—the numerical measure of combining power for one atom of a chemical element. Valence also reflects the number of hydrogen atoms which can be held in combination or displaced in a reaction by one atom of an element. If a substance is *univalent* (e.g. chloride), *1 mM. equals 1 mEq.* If a substance is *bivalent* (e.g. calcium), *1 mM. equals 2 mEq.* Therefore, *2 mM.* (2 mEq.) of a *univalent* substance reacts chemically with only *1 mM.* (2 mEq.) of a *bivalent* substance.

MEASUREMENT OF OSMOTIC PRESSURE

The milliequivalent is also a *rough* unit of measure for the osmotic pressure, or drawing power, of a solution. However, since not all substances that exert osmotic pressure can be measured in milliequivalents, a more accurate measure of osmotic pressure is the *milliosmole* (mOsm.). To determine the number of milliosmoles in a solution, we again refer to the millimole. *One millimole of a substance that does not dissociate into ions* (e.g. glucose) *equals 1 mOsm.* However, *a millimole of a compound that does dissociate into ions equals two or more milliosmoles,* depending on how many ions it dissociates into. Sodium chloride (NaCl), for example, dissociates into one sodium ion and one chloride ion, so 1 mM. of this salt equals 2 mOsm. A millimole of a more complex salt such as disodium phosphate (Na_2HPO_4) dissociates into two sodium ions and one phosphate ion, so it equals 3 mOsm. The osmotic pressure of a solution, therefore, is calculated by adding up all the ions, or milliosmoles, it contains.

The milliequivalents per liter and the milliosmoles per liter of plasma, interstitial fluid, and cellular fluid are as follows:

	mEq./L.	mOsm./L.
Plasma	308	296.50
Interstitial fluid	311	300.75
Cellular fluid	364	305.00

MEASUREMENT OF CHEMICAL REACTION

The final unit of measure with which we shall concern ourselves is *pH,* which tells us whether the chemical reaction of a fluid is acid, neutral, or alkaline. Basically, the reaction of a fluid is determined by the number of hydrogen ions it contains. Hydrogen is present in the body fluid in only tiny amounts, between .0000001 and .00000001 gm./L. of extracellular fluid. As a convenient way of expressing such minute hydrogen ion concentrations without resorting to decimals, the symbol pH was devised.

pH represents the reciprocal of the logarithm of the hydrogen ion concentration. Put more simply, pH is the power of 1/10, and it tells us the grams of hydrogen per liter of extracellular fluid. For example, pH $3 = 1/10^3$. As you probably recall from elementary arithmetic, power represents the product arising from the continued multiplication of a number by itself. Therefore, pH $3 = 1/10 \times 1/10 \times 1/10$, or 1/1,000 gm. hydrogen per liter of extracellular fluid. Similarly, pH $7 = 1/10^7$, which, when multiplied, equals 1/10,000,000 gm. hydrogen per liter of extracellular fluid.

It is not really necessary to do all that multiplying, however. All one has to do is put down 1/1 and add zeroes equal to the number of the pH. For example, if the pH is 3, you simply write down 1/1 and add three zeroes, and you see immediately that pH 3 = 1/1,000 gm. hydrogen per liter of extracellular fluid.

The more zeroes we have, of course, the smaller the amount of hydrogen. Since it is the amount of hydrogen in a fluid that determines its acidity, *as pH goes up, the fluid becomes less acid, and as pH goes down, the fluid becomes more acid.* pH 7, for example, is ten times more acid than pH 8; pH 6 is ten times more acid than pH 7, and 100 times more acid than pH 8. The normal pH of extracellular fluid is between 7.35 and 7.45.

This unit of measure is extremely important in understanding acid-base (or acid-alkali) balance, which we shall discuss in a later chapter.

7 Gains and Losses of Water and Electrolytes

Whether they be primary or secondary to other conditions, all body fluid disturbances are caused by abnormal differences between gains and losses of water and electrolytes.

The body gains water and electrolytes in various ways: water alone is gained by drinking distilled water and by oxidation of foodstuffs and body tissues; softened water, well water, mineral water, and most city water supplies provide both water and electrolytes. Food also supplies both, for although it consists largely of water, it is rich in electrolytes and other nutrients, such as protein, fat, carbohydrate, and vitamins. Hospitalized patients frequently gain water and electrolytes, as well as other materials, via nasogastric tube, intravenous needle, or rectal tube.

Normal losses of both water and electrolytes occur through the lungs in breath, through the eyes in tears, through the kidneys in urine, through the skin in perspiration, and through the intestines in feces. In addition, water alone is lost through the skin in insensible perspiration, which goes on constantly. Abnormal losses can occur during illness or injury, as in burn or

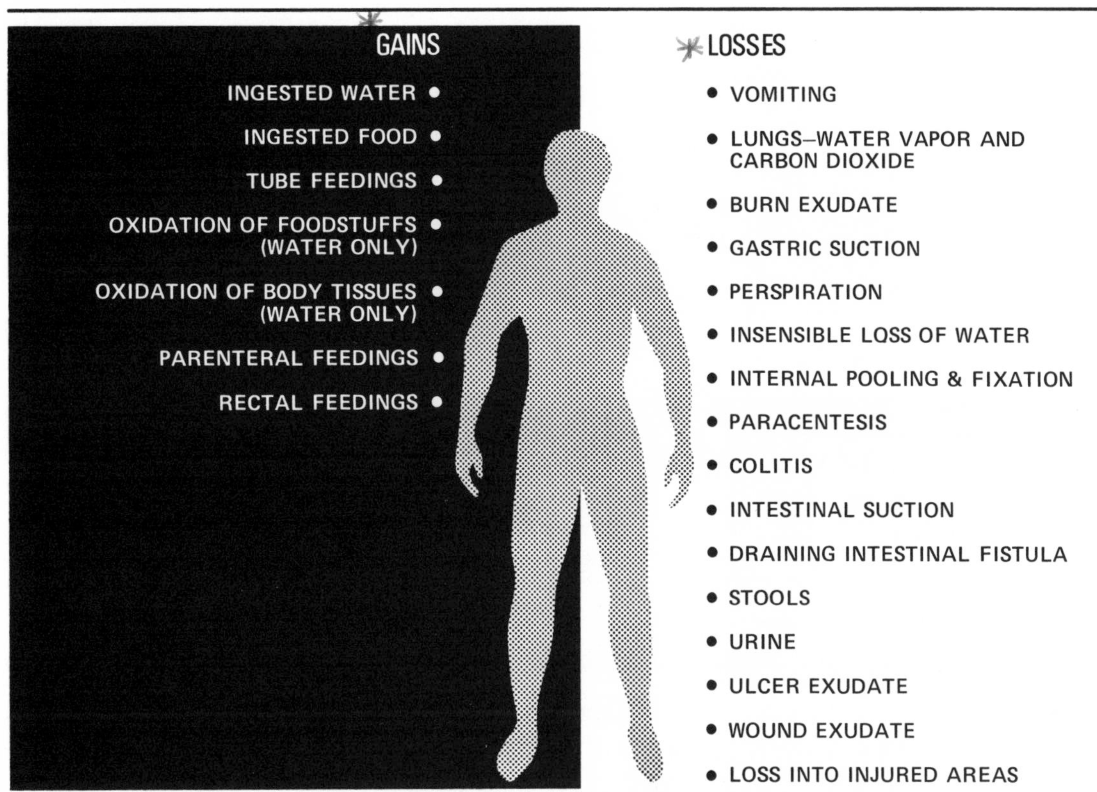

Fig. 7-1. Gains and losses of water.

wound exudate, hemorrhage, vomiting, and diarrhea. Rapid breathing, suction via gastric or intestinal tube, enterostomy, colostomy, and cecostomy also cause great losses of water and electrolytes. Drainage from sites of surgical operations or from abscesses contains both water and electrolytes, as does fluid extracted via paracentesis. Fluids surrounding the brain and spinal cord can be lost if there is an abnormal opening to the outside. Indeed, fluids may be lost even inside the body, since when abnormal closed collections of fluid develop, as in intestinal obstruction, these fluids are just as useless to the body economy as if they were outside the body.

In the healthy adult, the volume of urine excreted is approximately equal to the volume of fluid ingested as fluid; and water derived from solid food and from chemical oxidation in the body approximately equals the normal losses of water through the lungs and skin and in the stool. Thus, in health gains approximately equal losses, whereas during illness gains and losses are not always equal. Intake of food and fluids may cease or diminish, while the normal losses continue, and the losses may outweigh the gains by as much as one half liter or more a day. The daily losses are cumulative, so a serious deficit can develop in a short time. If abnormal losses are occurring in addition, as in vomiting or diarrhea, the patient may become gravely ill within a matter of hours. The type of imbalance caused depends upon the kind of fluid lost, since body secretions and excretions vary greatly in electrolyte compositions and concentrations.

Serious imbalances also occur when the gains are greater than the losses, as when the kidneys are not functioning properly. Excesses are just as dangerous as deficits and can prove fatal in a short period of time.

Thus, abnormal differences between gains and losses cause all of the 16 basic imbalances in our diagnostic classification; these imbalances involve changes in volume, composition, and position of the extracellular fluid.

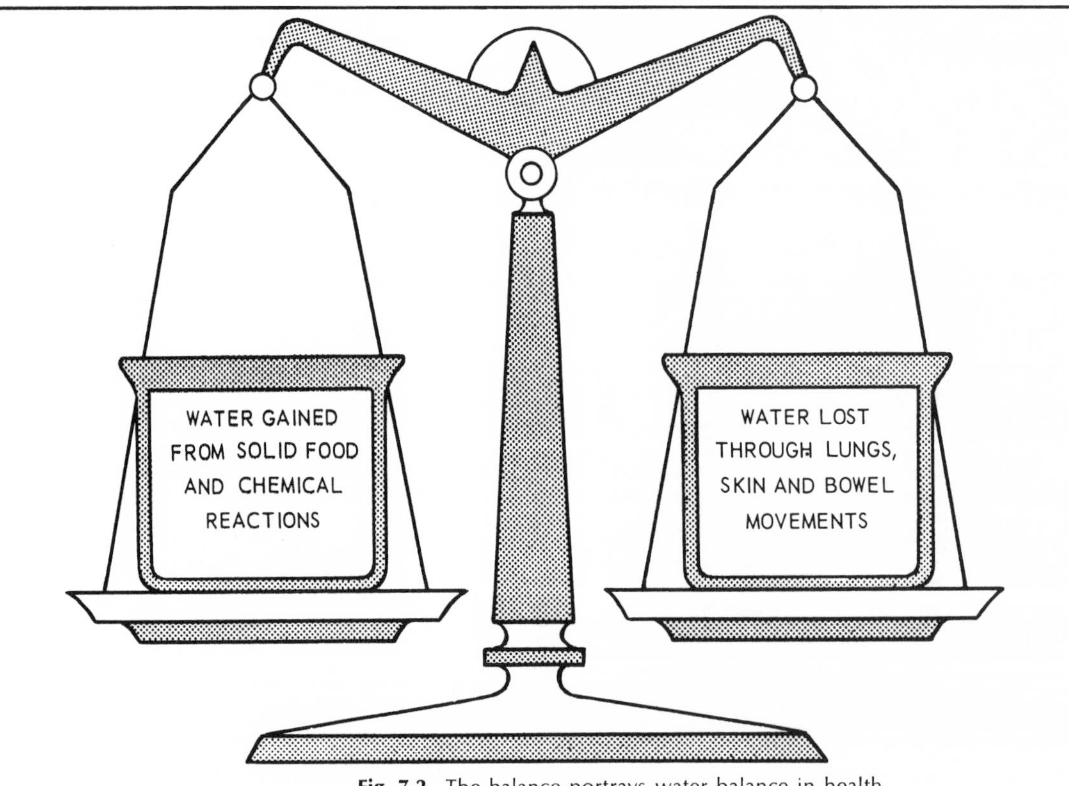

Fig. 7-2. The balance portrays water balance in health.

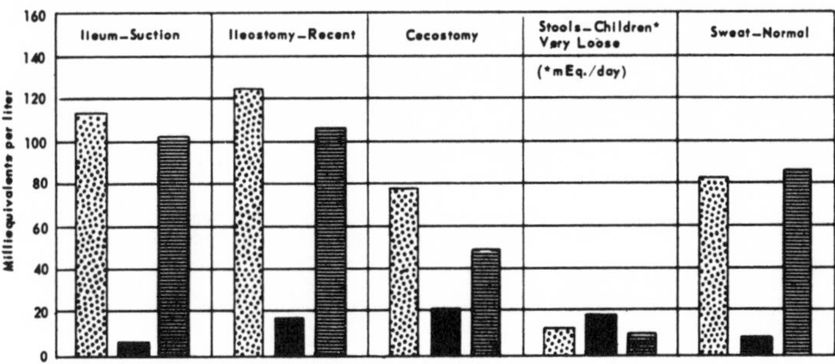

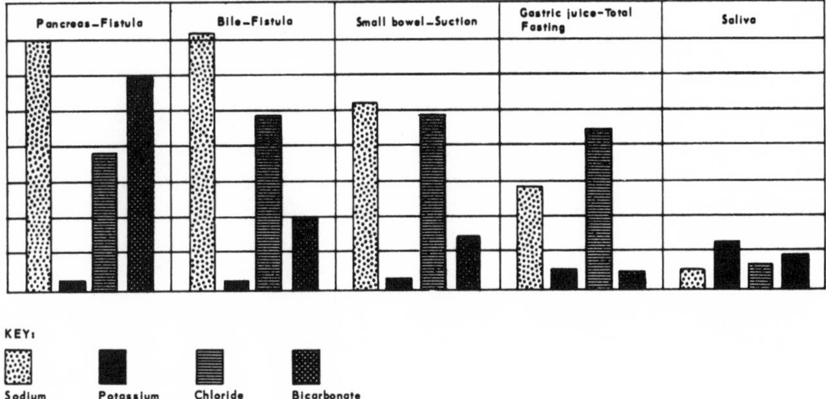

KEY:
Sodium
Potassium
Chloride
Bicarbonate

Fig. 7-3. Electrolyte composition of various body secretions or excretions.

8 Volume Changes in Extracellular Fluid

Both extracellular fluid volume deficit and extracellular fluid volume excess are particularly fascinating to study. One of them (volume deficit) has caused more death than all the wars in history. Even today, it is a massive problem for countries without modern medical facilities.

Volume disturbances of the extracellular fluid represent either deficits or excesses of both water and electrolytes—not water alone—in approximately the same proportions as would be found in the normal state. Thus, although the extracellular fluid changes in volume, the percentages of water and electrolytes remain about the same. It is also important to note that when volume changes occur in the extracellular fluid, there are corresponding changes in the cellular fluid. An uncorrected volume deficit of extracellular fluid, for example, will ultimately cause a volume deficit of cellular fluid as well.

EXTRACELLULAR FLUID VOLUME DEFICIT

Among the terms frequently used to describe this imbalance are fluid deficit, hypovolemia, and dehydration. The term dehydration is incorrect, however, since it involves the loss of water only.

Volume deficit results from an abrupt decrease in fluid intake, from an acute loss of secretions and excretions, or from a combination of decreased intake and increased loss. It usually begins with one of the following: a loss of secretions and excretions, as occurs in vomiting; diarrhea; fistulous drainage; a systemic infection, with its attendant fever and increased utilization of water and electrolytes; intestinal obstruction. As secretions and excretions are depleted, they are replenished by water and electrolytes of the extracellular fluid, thus reducing the volume of the extracellular fluid. With continued depletion of the extracellular fluid, water and electrolytes are drawn from the cells, thus causing a deficit in the cellular fluid as well, although not immediately.

A volume deficit can develop slowly or with great rapidity, in which case it may cause death within hours after onset. In epidemics of Asiatic cholera, thousands upon thousands died of an extracellular fluid volume deficit produced by the severe vomiting and purging associated with the disease. Fortunately, increased knowledge concerning body fluids has virtually eliminated deaths caused by cholera, and today's cholera victim usually survives with no aftereffects if given prompt treatment for the extracellular fluid volume deficit that occurs during the initial period.

Diagnosis of Extracellular Fluid Volume Deficit

Extracellular fluid volume deficit is frequently difficult to diagnose since so many of its clinical symptoms appear in any seriously ill patient. In the infant, depression of the anterior fontanel is diagnostic. In others, observations that are generally useful include longitudinal wrinkles in the tongue—one of the most valuable; dry skin and mucous membranes; fatigue; a urine flow rate of less than 20 to 40 ml./hr. in an adult, and materially lower in children. A systolic blood pressure of 10 mm. Hg less for the patient in the standing position than in the supine is also indicative. Characteristically, the pulse is rapid, the temperature is normal—unless infection is present, as it often is—the respiratory rate is elevated, and the venous pressure—which can be measured either centrally or peripherally—is de-

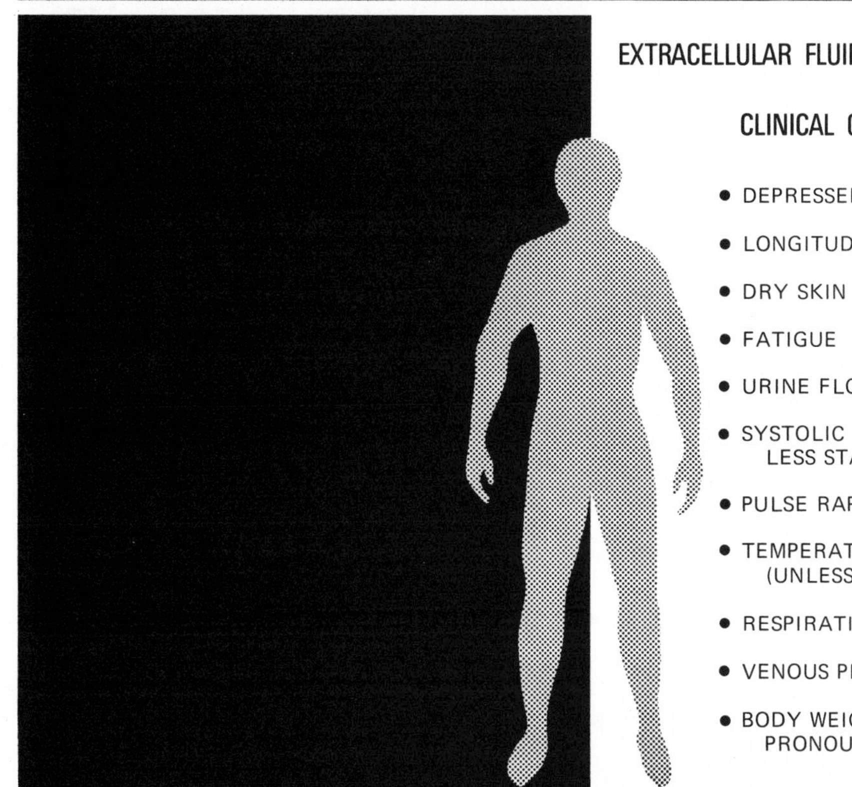

EXTRACELLULAR FLUID VOLUME DEFICIT

CLINICAL OBSERVATIONS

- DEPRESSED FONTANEL (INFANT)
- LONGITUDINAL WRINKLES IN TONGUE
- DRY SKIN AND MUCOUS MEMBRANES
- FATIGUE
- URINE FLOW RATE UNDER 20–40 ml./hr.
- SYSTOLIC BLOOD PRESSURE 10 mm. Hg. LESS STANDING THAN WHEN SUPINE
- PULSE RAPID
- TEMPERATURE SUBNORMAL (UNLESS INFECTION)
- RESPIRATION ELEVATED
- VENOUS PRESSURE DECREASED
- BODY WEIGHT LOSS (MILD DEFICIT, 2%; PRONOUNCED, 5%; SEVERE, 8%)

Fig. 8-1. Extracellular fluid volume deficit.

creased. Acute body weight loss is enormously helpful in diagnosis; for a mild deficit, weight loss might be 2 per cent, for a pronounced deficit, 5 per cent, and for a severe deficit, 8 per cent or more. Unfortunately, the patient often does not know his pre-illness weight.

The laboratory offers us little help in diagnosing volume deficit, although findings of hemoconcentration may be present in a severe deficit.

One of the great hazards of a severe extracellular fluid volume deficit is inadequate perfusion of the kidney, since there is not enough extracellular fluid to bring the requisite amount of plasma to the glomeruli.

Extracellular fluid volume deficit is frequently followed by other body fluid disturbances, including bicarbonate deficit and potassium deficit. If excessive water is lost in watery stools or with rapid breathing, sodium excess also may develop.

The goal of therapy for extracellular fluid volume deficit is to restore the volume to normal without altering the electrolyte composition of the fluid. This is accomplished by oral or parenteral administration of a solution formulated to provide electrolytes in quantities balanced between the patient's minimal needs and maximal tolerances. It also provides free water to form urine and to carry out metabolic functions. Such a solution is called a *balanced solution*, or a *Butler-type solution*. When this type of solution is used, the homeostatic mechanisms selectively retain or excrete water and electrolytes according to the patient's individual needs.

Clinical Example. An 18-month-old baby was admitted to the hospital with a history of severe diarrhea and vomiting for the preceding 24 hours. The infant had been well prior to that time. The mother stated that following onset, he had had an almost continuous running off of the bowels with frequent spells of vomiting. The baby took a few sips of water, but refused food. On examination, the infant was found to have lost approximately 6 per cent of his pre-illness body weight, and his skin and mucous membranes appeared dry. The skin was inelastic, body temperature was 98°F, the diaper was not wet, and the mother felt there had been a definite decrease in urination. A red blood cell count revealed 6,500,000 cells, and the hemoglobin was found to be 14 Gm.

EXTRACELLUAR FLUID VOLUME EXCESS

This imbalance is frequently called *fluid excess* or *overhydration*, but the latter term is incorrect since it represents an excess of water only.

A volume excess develops when the kidneys are unable to rid the body of unneeded water and electrolytes. This inability may result from simple overloading of the body by oral or parenteral administration of excessive quantities of an isotonic solution of sodium chloride. Somewhat paradoxically, it is the quantity of sodium in the body that determines the volume of the extracellular fluid; therefore, excess sodium from any cause may well precede extracellular fluid volume excess. The imbalance may occur in diseases that affect the function of the homeostatic mechanisms, such as chronic kidney disease, chronic liver disease with portal hypertension, congestive heart failure, and malnutrition. In all of these conditions, there is abnormal retention of water and sodium, and whether the volume excess is caused by simple overloading or by diminished function of the homeostatic mechanisms, the result is the same: the extracellular fluid becomes excessively salty. Therefore, in an attempt to maintain its normal composition, the extracellular fluid draws water from the cells.

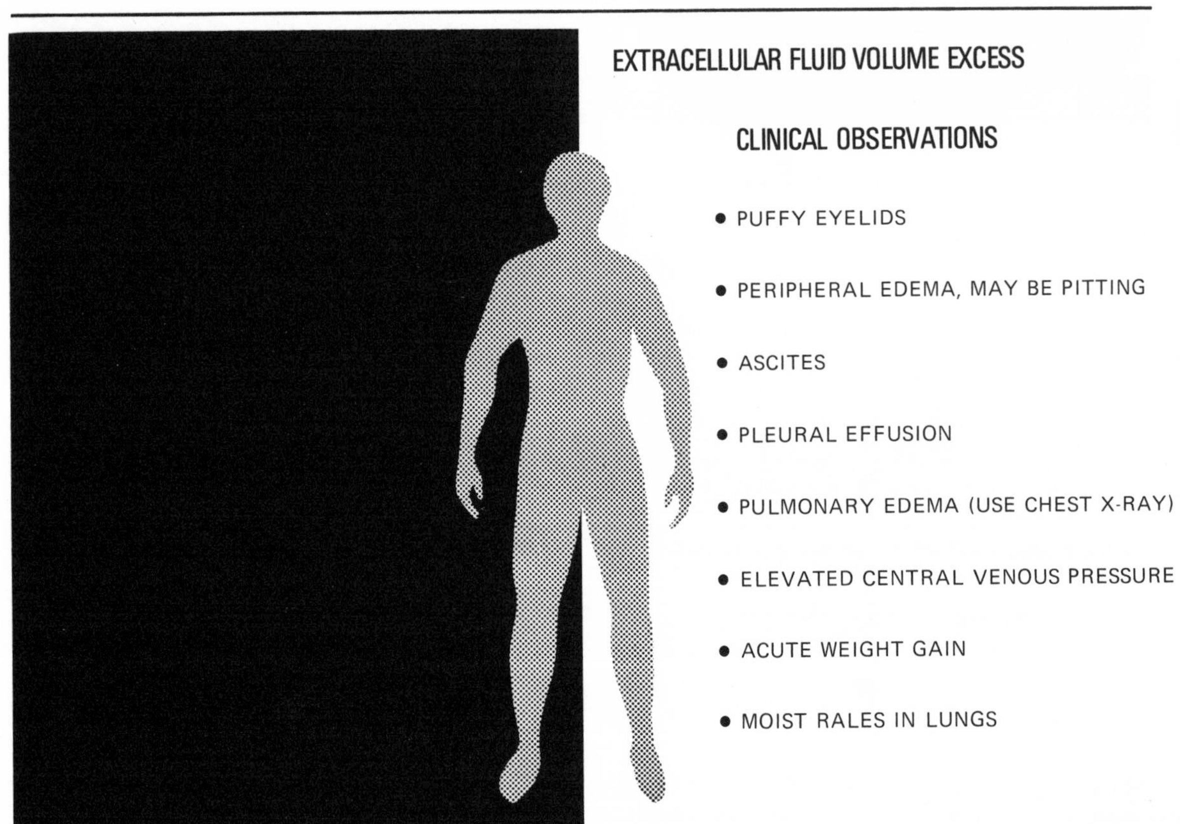

Fig. 8-2. Extracellular fluid volume excess.

Diagnosis of Extracellular Fluid Volume Excess

Expanding volume of extracellular fluid produces numerous clinical symptoms which contribute far more in diagnosing this imbalance than they do in the case of extracellular fluid volume deficit. Symptoms are as follows: puffy eyelids; peripheral edema, which may actually be pitting; ascites; pleural effusion; pulmonary edema—often visible by x-ray when undetectable by stethoscope; elevated venous pressure—either central or peripheral; acute weight gain, sometimes as much as 10 per cent of the normal body weight. In many patients, this imbalance occurs without frank edema because of the mysterious third factor, which causes diuresis before frank edema supervenes; in a severe excess, the patient may succumb from the pulmonary edema.

The laboratory gives little help in diagnosing extracellular fluid volume excess, except that the formed elements of the blood may be decreased because of plasma dilution. If renal impairment has occurred, both the blood urea nitrogen (BUN) and the plasma potassium may be elevated.

The goal of therapy in extracellular fluid volume excess is to rid the body of excess water and electrolytes without altering the electrolyte composition of the fluid. Primary treatment is directed toward the causative factors. Diuretics are often helpful in providing symptomatic relief, and in addition, it may be necessary to withhold all liquids for a time.

Clinical Example. An 8-year-old boy was unable to retain liquids following appendectomy, and he was therefore maintained on parenteral fluids. For 2 days he was given an intravenous infusion of 5 per cent dextrose in isotonic solution of sodium chloride in the amount of 4 L. On the morning of the third day, he complained of shortness of breath. His eyelids were puffy, his cheeks appeared full, and moist rales were heard in the lungs. He was weighed and was found to have gained approximately 6 per cent over his admission weight. His red blood cell count was found to be 4,000,000, and his hemoglobin was 10.5 Gm.

9 Composition Changes of Major Extracellular Electrolytes

Each electrolyte has special bodily functions, and although some play larger roles than others, all are necessary for the maintenance of life. Their normal concentrations are precisely geared to the body's needs, so they must be maintained at proper levels if the body is to remain healthy. Also vitally important are the concentrations of carbonic acid and base bicarbonate.

Discussed in this chapter are disturbances involving alterations in the normal concentration of the extracellular fluid's electrolytes, as expressed in mEq./L. of extracellular fluid. A change in the concentration of an electrolyte can be produced either by a change in total quantity of the electrolyte or in the total volume of water in extracellular fluid. For example, one could develop a sodium deficit either because of decreased intake or increased loss of sodium, or because of excessive intake or decreased loss of water. Similarly, one could develop an excess of sodium in extracellular fluid either because of increased intake or decreased loss of sodium, or because of decreased intake or increased loss of water. These mechanisms apply not only to changes in sodium concentration, but to all the other extracellular electrolytes as well.

SODIUM

Sodium is the most abundant cation of extracellular fluid and the second most important cation of cellular fluid. Chemically, sodium is a metallic element, and its chemical symbol, *Na*, stems from the Latin word *natrium*, meaning sodium. In pure form, the element is extremely unstable since it readily combines with oxygen either in air or in water. In nature and in body fluids, it exists only in combination with various anions, usually chloride; the compound sodium chloride is more commonly called table salt.

Sodium affects many vital functions of the human body. It is largely responsible for the osmotic pressure of extracellular fluid, and inside cells, sodium is a factor in numerous vital chemical reactions. The kidneys regulate body water and electrolytes, based in part on sodium concentration in the extracellular fluid. Therefore, when sodium concentration rises, the kidneys retain water in an effort to maintain the normal composition of the extracellular fluid. When the amount of water increases, the kidneys retain sodium. Other functions of the element are as follows: probably through some type of chemical-electrical action, sodium stimulates reactions within nerve and muscle tissues; as a component of sodium bicarbonate, it is highly important in maintaining the delicate balance between the acids and alkalies of the body fluid.

Since sodium plays such a vital role, it is not surprising that the body possesses a highly efficient mechanism for regulating the electrolyte so that its normal concentration of 142 mEq./L. of extracellular fluid can be maintained. During periods of decreased intake or increased loss, the mechanism acts to conserve sodium. Important in sodium conservation is the hormone aldosterone, secreted by the adrenal cortex, which promotes potassium loss and sodium retention via a complex and little understood feedback mechanism involving the afferent arterioles, the juxtaglomerular apparatus, and the macula densa of the distal tubule. When fluid volume deficit occurs, a resultant decrease in glomerular filtration aids in sodium conservation simply because there is less sodium in the tubular urine to be exchanged for potassium and hydrogen in the peritubular capillaries of the distal tubules. Body sodium conservation is usually so effective that patients being maintained on a low sodium diet for control of certain diseases, such as essential hypertension, are seldom in danger of developing sodium deficit as a result of the decreased intake.

When sodium intake increases, the regulating mechanism acts to rid the body of excesses, and there is a prompt increase both in sodium excretion and in the glomerular filtration rate. For many years, it was believed that the increased filtration of sodium through the glomeruli was responsible for the increased urinary excretion of the ion. Recent studies, however, indicate that the increase in sodium excretion is related to decreased reabsorption of sodium from the proximal tubules of the kidneys. A similar sodium loss occurs when salt-retaining hormones, such as aldosterone, are administered over a prolonged period to normal human subjects. It is believed that tubular excretion of sodium is controlled by a third factor, perhaps a hormone, whose chemical structure and site of origin are unknown. This mysterious third factor may explain why patients with primary hyperaldosteronism do not develop marked edema.

Although the sodium regulating mechanism is quite effective, an *acute* decrease or increase in the sodium level of extracellular fluid produces severe reactions.

Sodium Deficit of Extracellular Fluid

Sodium deficit of extracellular fluid occurs when the concentration of sodium in extracellular fluid falls below normal. Other names for this imbalance are *electrolyte concentration deficit, low sodium syndrome, hypotonic dehydration,* and *hyponatremia.*

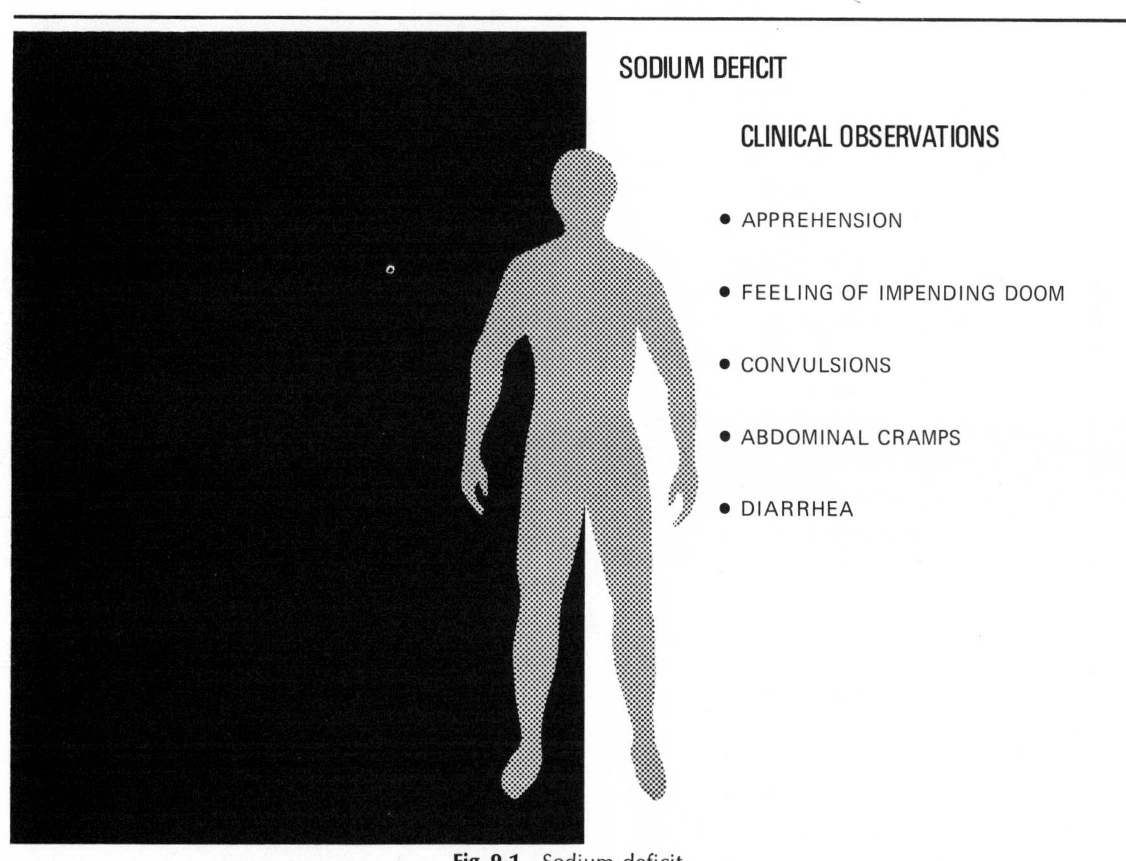

Fig. 9-1. Sodium deficit.

Sodium deficit can result either from losses of sodium without corresponding water loss—as with overzealous administration of diuretics, especially thiazide diuretics or furosemide—or from gains of water in excess of sodium—as when one perspires profusely and replaces the fluid lost with plain water. In the hospital, sodium deficit may develop when a severely burned patient—or one who is undergoing gastric or intestinal suction—is permitted to drink plain water in large amounts. In addition, the use of repeated tap water enemas causes sodium deficit, as does parenteral administration of electrolyte-free solutions; inhalation of fresh water, as occurs in fresh water drowning, also produces this imbalance.

The clinical findings in sodium deficit are virtually identical with those of so-called heat prostration, often the result of sodium deficit in unacclimatized persons. (Because of the body's sodium conservation mechanism, the properly acclimatized individual is remarkably resistant to heat stress disease caused by sodium loss.) The patient first suffers apprehension or anxiety, followed by a bizarre, undefinable feeling of impending doom. He is weak, confused, and perhaps even stuporous, and may suffer abdominal cramps or muscle twitching, and, in severe deficit, convulsions. In an effort to counterbalance the deficit, the adrenal glands secrete increased amounts of aldosterone, which stimulates the kidneys to conserve water, sodium, and chloride. This action results in depressed urinary output (oliguria) or complete absence of urinary output (anuria). If the deficit is severe, there is vasomotor collapse, with the following symptoms: hypotension; rapid, thready pulse; cold, clammy skin; and cyanosis. An interesting finding that may be observed is fingerprinting over the sternum, consisting of a visible fingerprint apparent after pressure is applied with a finger or thumb on the skin overlying the sternum. Fingerprinting is due to increased plasticity of the tissues, which results from the transfer of water from the abnormally dilute extracellular fluid into the cells. As a result of this osmotic transfer of water, an abnormally large portion of the body fluid lies within the confines of the cells, and the fluid volume of the extracellular fluid—both plasma and interstitial fluid—is decreased. Consequently, tissues become more plastic than normal and tend to retain any shape attained by pressure deformation.

Laboratory findings are helpful in diagnosis of sodium deficit, as the plasma sodium is below 137 mEq./L.—it may be as low as 110, 100, or even 90—and plasma chloride is below 98 mEq./L. The specific gravity of the urine is below 1.010.

The goal of therapy in sodium deficit of the extracellular fluid is to restore the sodium concentration to normal as quickly as possible without producing a fluid volume excess. If the fluid volume is normal or excessive, a 3 per cent or 5 per cent solution of sodium chloride is administered. This type of solution is hypertonic, so it will provide the needed sodium in a minimal amount of water. If the extracellular fluid volume is below normal, an isotonic solution of sodium chloride may be administered.

Clinical Example. Following the removal of her gallbladder, a 35-year-old woman complained of considerable gas and general abdominal discomfort. A gastric tube was inserted, suction drainage instituted, and the woman was given water to sip. Over a period of two days, approximately 2 L. of fluid were removed from the stomach by means of the gastric tube. During this period, the patient had nothing by mouth except sips of plain water, and on the morning of the third day, she complained of abdominal cramps. Nursing records showed that she had passed only 400 ml. of urine during the previous 24 hours, and physical examination revealed the finding of fingerprinting over the sternum. The plasma sodium was found to be 132 mEq./L., and the plasma chloride was 90 mEq./L. Urine was not available for a specific gravity determination.

Sodium Excess of Extracellular Fluid

Sodium excess of extracellular fluid, sometimes called *hypernatremia, salt excess, oversalting*, or *hypertonic dehydration*, is one of the most dangerous of all body fluid disturbances. It occurs when the sodium concentration of extracellular fluid rises above the normal level. The imbalance, which may be acute or chronic, results from

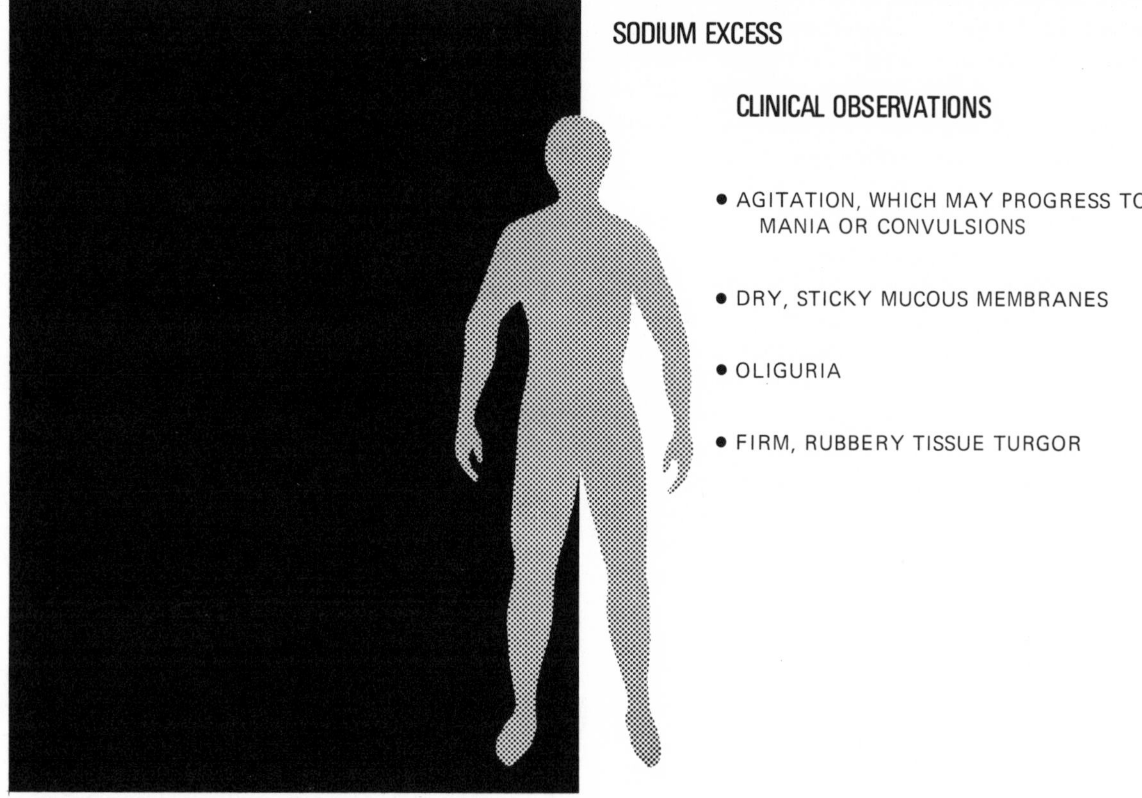

Fig. 9-2. Sodium excess.

decreased intake or increased output of water or from increased intake or decreased output of sodium.

Acute sodium excess may follow excessive administration of concentrated oral electrolyte mixtures; or it may occur in any condition in which more water is lost than electrolytes, as in tracheobronchitis—in which excessive water losses occur through the lungs due to fever and deep, rapid breathing—or in profuse watery diarrhea when treatment has been inadequate. Unconscious patients may develop sodium excess simply because they cannot drink water. The individual who has inhaled ocean water frequently develops a sodium excess, which must be corrected if the patient is to recover; indeed, sodium excess is often the actual cause of death in salt water drowning. Infants are particularly prone to develop acute sodium excess, and the mortality rate is quite high—about 50 per cent in hospital-treated infants with diarrhea and sodium excess.

Clinical findings in sodium excess include dry, sticky mucous membranes, flushed skin, intense thirst, and rough, dry tongue. Body tissues are firm since water from the cellular fluid, following the law of osmosis, flows into the more concentrated extracellular fluid. Oliguria or anuria is present, and the patient may have fever. He appears agitated and restless, may develop mania or convulsions, and his reflexes are decreased.

Laboratory findings are helpful in diagnosis, since the plasma sodium is usually above 147 mEq./L.—but may range far higher—plasma chloride is above 106 mEq./L., and the specific gravity of urine is above 1.030.

Long-term or chronic ingestion of large amounts of sodium, as when one salts his food excessively or eats extremely salty foods, also can cause sodium excess and may lead to hypertension. Although the daily requirement for sodium is probably below 100 mg. in acclimatized persons, most individuals ingest from 3,000 to 5,000 mg. daily, and inhabitants in certain areas of Japan have an average daily intake in excess of 20,000 mg. Hereditary factors largely determine whether this type of sodium excess will cause hypertension in a given individual, but researchers have induced uninherited but life-long hypertension in experimental animals by feeding them highly salted foods. Fairly recently, researchers questioned a group of Americans about normal use of salt and learned that only 1 per cent of those who never salted their food at the table suffered from hypertension, as compared to 8 per cent of those who salted to taste, and 10 per cent of those who salted before tasting. Another study revealed that a large segment of the population in areas of Japan where the usual diet is extremely salty suffers from hypertension.

The goal of therapy in sodium excess is to reduce the sodium concentration of the extracellular fluid before it reaches a critical level. Treatment involves administration of a Butler-type solution, which is only one-third to one-half as concentrated as plasma and which provides free water for formation of urine. Hypertension can often be controlled by use of a low sodium diet.

Clinical Example. A 6-year-old girl was admitted to the hospital because of extreme agitation and inability to sleep. The history revealed that for the past 4 days, she had suffered a mild diarrhea, which her mother treated by administering a solution of salt and soda in water. Apparently, the mother had added a tablespoon full of salt and a tablespoon full of baking soda to each pint of water and had forced the child to drink about a pint of this mixture a day. On physical examination, the child was found to have dry, sticky mucous membranes and a rough, dry tongue. Her skin was flushed, and she complained of thirst. The mother stated the child had not urinated for the past 24 hours. The plasma chloride was found to be 112 mEq./L., and the plasma sodium, 160 mEq./L.

POTASSIUM

Potassium, a soft, silver-white metal that exists outside the test tube only in combination with other elements, is the chief cation of cellular fluid. Its chemical symbol, K, is derived from the German word *kalium.* Potassium is indispensable in the human body, as it is necessary for the intricate chemical reactions needed for transformation of carbohydrate into energy and for reassembling amino acids into proteins. The ion helps maintain the normal water and electrolyte content of cellular fluid, and it is also needed for transmission of nervous impulses within the heart. Skeletal muscles and the muscles of the heart, intestines, and lungs could not function normally without potassium.

Ironically, although one cannot live without potassium, the human body contains enough of the electrolyte to kill dozens of people were it injected quickly into them. The extracellular fluid normally contains 5 mEq./L., or about 70 mEq.; the cellular fluid contains a total of 4,000 mEq. Secretions and excretions, especially sweat, saliva, gastric juice, and feces, are rich in potassium. The potassium content of urine varies with the intake, but it amounts to at least 40 to 50 mEq. daily. In the kidneys, along with water and other electrolytes and small molecules, potassium is completely filtered at the glomerulus and is then completely reabsorbed in the proximal convoluted tubules. Excretion occurs only in the distal convoluted tubules, and then in exchange for sodium.

Potassium Deficit of Extracellular Fluid

While the human body has an efficient mechanism for conserving sodium, it has no such mechanism for conserving potassium. Even in times of great need, the kidneys continue to pour out 40 to 50 mEq. of potassium daily in the urine; and with such continuing losses, potassium deficit, or *hypokalemia,* can develop quickly when the patient's intake is inadequate. This imbalance occurs frequently, not only as a result of prolonged inadequate intake of potassium, but also as a result of excessive losses of potassium-rich secretions or excretions, as occurs in diarrhea, for example.

Probably the leading cause of potassium deficit is administration of powerful diuretics, particularly the thiazides or furosemide, without adequate potassium supplementation. Surgical operations often cause losses of potassium-rich fluids, especially if the procedure involves the digestive tract. The imbalance is also often associated with gastrointestinal suction, diseases involving the intestinal tract, familial periodic paralysis, pyelonephritis, thyroid storm, aldosterone-secreting tumor of the adrenal cortex, crushing injuries, broken bones, extensive bruising, and wound healing. Even emotional or physical stress can cause the imbalance. Excessive sweating, fever, and high environmental temperatures are further causes. Indeed, potassium loss plays a major role in the development of heat stress disease, which affects people of all ages who are subjected to high environmental temperatures, especially if they are exercising. Factory workers, athletes, and others who are exposed to high environmental temperatures often use salt tablets to replace the sodium lost in sweat, but, since the body conserves sodium and continues to lose potassium, potassium supplementation, at least as important as sodium supplementation, is often neglected.

Potassium deficit is frequently associated with metabolic alkalosis, as discussed later in this chapter.

The clinical findings in potassium deficit can be remembered easily if one recalls that potassium is essential for the normal functioning of muscle cells; thus symptoms of potassium deficit are caused largely by muscle weakness. Early, symptoms are nonspecific, as the patient has malaise, or is simply not feeling well. In some patients, potassium deficit damages renal tubules,

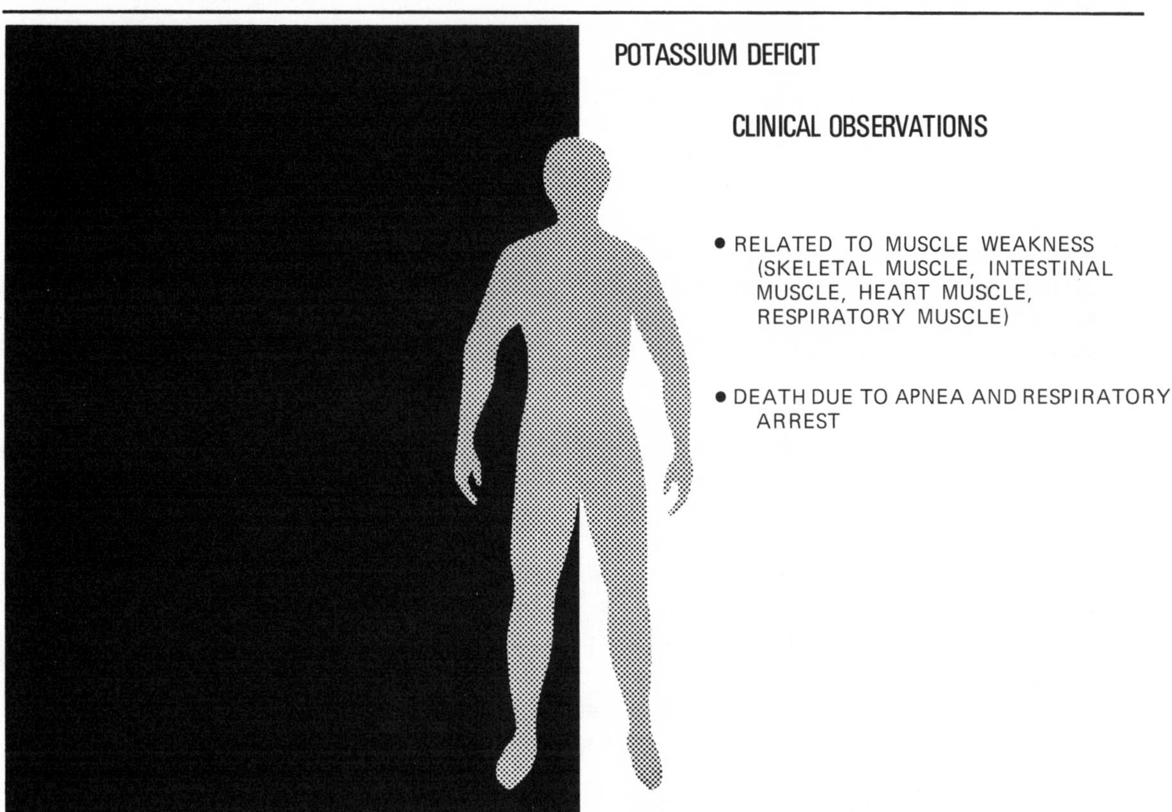

Fig. 9-3. Potassium deficit.

and thus impairs the concentrating ability of the kidney, the result of which is polyuria and thirst. Later, the skeletal muscles become weak, and the reflexes are decreased or absent, and eventually muscle weakness leads to flabbiness, with the patient lying flat, like a cadaver. Cardiac disturbances accompanying potassium deficit may include atrial and ventricular arrhythmia, diminution of the intensity of heart sounds, weak pulse, falling blood pressure, and heart block. Degeneration of the myocardium with loss of cellular striations may follow prolonged potassium deficit, and the intestinal muscles, too, are affected. The patient suffers anorexia, vomiting, gaseous intestinal distention, and paralytic ileus. Weakness of the respiratory muscles produces shallow respiration, and death in potassium deficit apparently results from apnea and respiratory arrest rather than from cardiac standstill.

Laboratory findings helpful in diagnosis include repeated serum potassium determinations of below 4 mEq./L. (a single determination can be seriously misleading). The plasma chloride is often below 98 mEq./L., and plasma bicarbonate is above 29 mEq./L. Potassium deficit also induces specific EKG findings, including low, flattened T wave, depressed S-T segment, and prominent U wave.

Fortunately, potassium deficit is not difficult to correct. Abnormal potassium losses may be counteracted by oral administration of a potassium salt or by providing a high potassium diet. A frank potassium deficit is best treated by oral administration of potassium chloride or other potassium salts or by parenteral infusion of a potassium-containing solution. A balanced, or Butler-type, solution is often used.

Clinical Example. A 60-year-old man was admitted to the hospital because of extreme weakness and a complete loss of appetite. The history revealed that he had been taking a thiazide-type diuretic for his hypertension for the past 6 months. Weakness and anorexia had been gradual in onset. The man had eaten an average diet with no particular emphasis on potassium-containing foods, nor did he receive a potassium supplement. Physical examination revealed a patient with soft, flabby muscles, which felt much like half-filled water bottles. Intestinal sounds impressed the physician as less than normal. There was minimal gaseous distention of the intestines, and the plasma potassium was found to be 3 mEq./L. An electrocardiogram presented findings consonant with potassium deficit.

Potassium Excess of Extracellular Fluid

Because the kidneys so efficiently rid the body of potassium, potassium excess, or *hyperkalemia*, does not develop as often as potassium deficit. However, this does not mean that excesses are any less dangerous than deficits; indeed, they can be extremely hazardous. In most cases, potassium excess is caused by leakage of the electrolyte from the body cells, and so following a severe burn or crushing injury, the extracellular fluid may be flooded with potassium from the damaged cells. If the kidneys are not functioning properly, the imbalance can result from excessive oral ingestion of potassium. It can also be caused by overzealous parenteral administration of potassium-containing solutions. Mercuric bichloride poisoning, which damages the kidneys, can lead to potassium excess, since the imbalance is inevitable following renal failure and may be the cause of death. Severe excesses also result from cellular hypoxia, uremia, adrenal insufficiency—as in Addison's disease, in which aldosterone is lacking—and administration of spironolactone, which opposes aldosterone. Metabolic acidosis may be associated with potassium excess, as discussed later in this chapter.

The clinical findings in potassium excess include irritability, nausea, diarrhea—a result, not a cause, of the imbalance—and intestinal colic. If the condition becomes severe, there is weakness and flaccid paralysis, perhaps difficulty in phonation and respiration, and there is oliguria, which may progress to anuria. Because transmission of stimuli through the heart muscle is slowed or prevented, intraventricular conduction disturbance occurs, with or without atrioventricular dissociation, and finally, ventricular fibrillation and cardiac arrest develop. Death in potassium excess results from poisoning of the heart muscle.

A repeated plasma potassium above 5.6

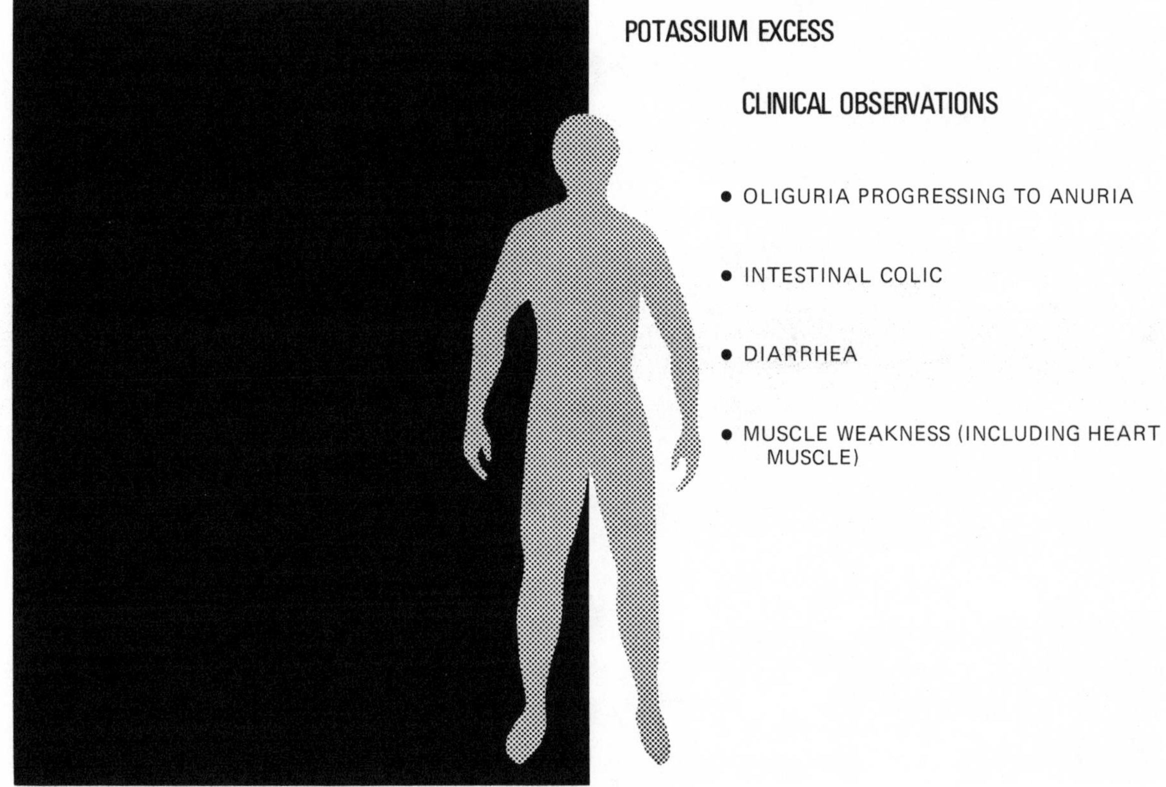

Fig. 9-4. Potassium excess.

mEq./L. indicates potassium excess, and a test for renal function usually will show renal impairment. The imbalance also presents specific EKG findings: early, T waves are peaked and elevated; later, P waves disappear; finally, there are biphasic deflections resulting from fusion of the QRS complex, RS-T segment, and the T wave.

When the kidneys are functional, an uncomplicated potassium excess can be corrected simply by avoiding additional intake of the electrolyte, either orally or parenterally. Should kidney function be drastically impaired, as in anuria, a diet that supplies fat and carbohydrates but not protein or potassium should be administered, or carbonic anhydrase inhibitors, insulin and dextrose, or ion exchange resins can be used. In some cases, hemodialysis or peritoneal dialysis may be necessary.

Clinical Example. A 40-year-old man was admitted to the hospital because of extreme irritability, abdominal cramps, and nausea. His urination had been scanty for the past month, and during the previous 24 hours had ceased altogether. He gave a history of chronic kidney disease, which began in childhood. The plasma potassium was found to be 7 mEq./L., and the electrocardiogram showed a high T wave and a depressed ST segment.

CALCIUM

The cation calcium (*Ca*) is the most abundant electrolyte in the body, and about 99 per cent is concentrated in bones and teeth, the remainder throughout the plasma and body cells. The normal concentration of calcium in the extracellular fluid is 5 mEq./L. Calcium is closely associated with phosphorus; together, they make bones and teeth rigid, strong, and durable. The plasma

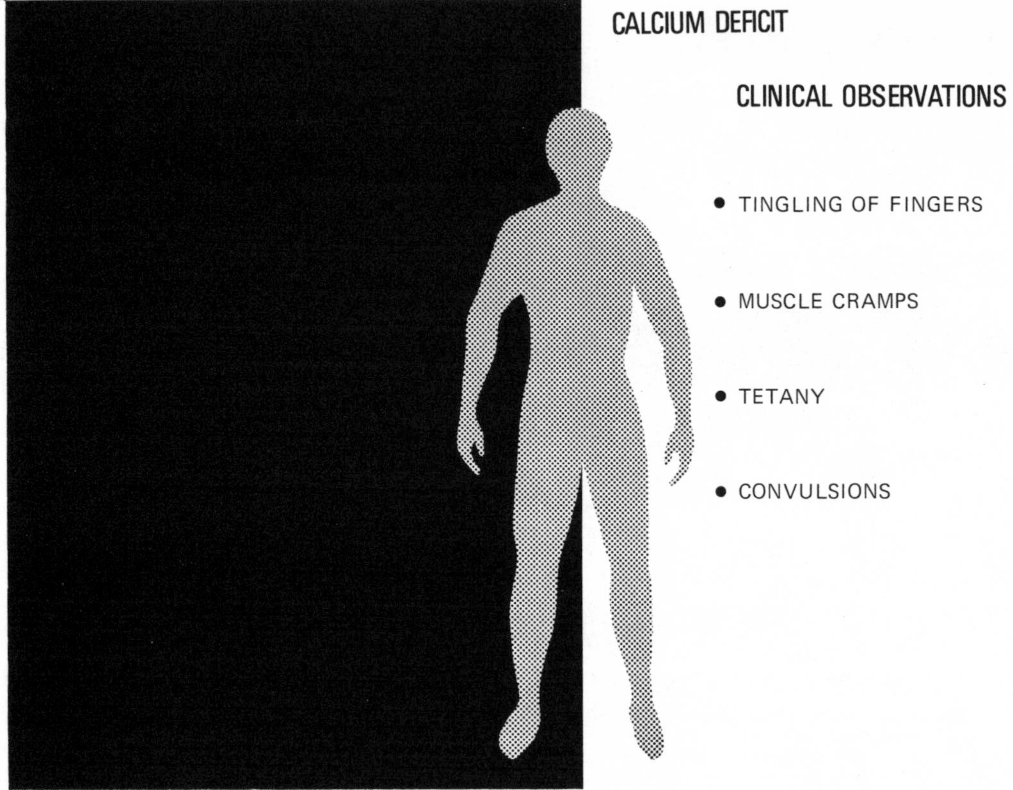

Fig. 9-5. Calcium deficit.

levels of calcium and phosphorus are regulated by the parathyroid glands, and normally, an increase or decrease in the serum phosphate concentration is associated with the opposite decrease or increase in the plasma calcium level, and vice versa. Vitamin D promotes intestinal absorption of calcium and increases kidney excretion of phosphate.

The element is also a necessary ingredient of cell cement, which holds the body cells together, and, in addition, it determines the strength and thickness of cell membranes. Calcium exerts a sedative effect on nerve cells, thus is important in maintaining normal transmission of nerve impulses. The electrolyte also aids in the transfer of energy and in the absorption and utilization of vitamin B_{12}. It activates enzymes that stimulate many essential chemical reactions in the body and plays a role in blood coagulation. Since only the ionized calcium is physiologically active, calcium bound to protein, which depends on the concentration of the plasma protein, is inactive. Usually from 50 to 75% of the serum calcium is ionized, and most of the rest is bound to serum albumin; when the total protein of the blood falls, more of the calcium becomes bound.

The normal adult needs about 1 gm. of calcium daily, and pregnant or lactating women require additional amounts. Vitamin D and protein are required for absorption and utilization of calcium.

Calcium Deficit of Extracellular Fluid

Calcium deficit of extracellular fluid, also called *hypocalcemia*, can result from abnormalities in body metabolism, from inadequate dietary intake of calcium, or from excessive losses of calcium in diarrheal stools or wound exudate. The imbalance is often associated with sprue, acute pancreatitis, hypoparathyroidism, surgical removal of the parathyroids, massive subcutaneous infections, burns, and generalized peritonitis. Excessive infusion of citrated blood, as in an exchange transfusion in an infant, may bring about calcium deficit, and the imbalance can also result from rapid correction or overcorrection of acidosis, wherein calcium ionization is increased. When the plasma pH returns to normal, or above normal, calcium ionization decreases, and unless adequate calcium is provided, the decreased ionization may cause hypocalcemia. Magnesium excess also tends to cause calcium deficit, possibly because magnesium plays a role in parathyroid function.

The clinical findings in calcium deficit are as follows: tingling of the ends of the fingers and of the circumoral region; muscle cramps, affecting both abdominal and skeletal muscles; carpopedal spasms; tetany; and convulsions. If calcium deficit is prolonged, calcium will be drawn from the bones to replenish the extracellular fluid, after which the bones become porous and break at the slightest provocation.

Laboratory findings helpful in diagnosis include a plasma calcium determination below 4.5 mEq./L. However, plasma calcium determinations can be misleading since only the ionized calcium is physiologically active. The ionized calcium can be measured by determining calcium levels before and after treatment with dextran gel or by ultrafiltration. In the simple and sometimes useful urinary Sulkowitch test, Sulkowitch reagent is added to urine and urinary calcium is precipitated as calcium oxalate. If no precipitate forms, hypocalcemia is present, whereas a fine white precipitate indicates normal plasma calcium, and a dense precipitate indicates calcium excess. The Sulkowitch test results do not correlate well with urinary calcium excretion, but the test is valuable in tetany, in hyperparathyroidism, and for regulation of vitamin D intake in a patient with hypoparathyroidism. And finally, a specific abnormal EKG finding in calcium deficit is a prolonged Q-T interval.

An interesting manifestation of prolonged calcium deficit is a condition called osteomalacia. In this condition, bones lose their calcium, phosphorus, and other electrolytes, becoming soft and pliable, and the patient actually shrinks in height. In the first recorded case of osteomalacia, the physician reported that his patient had shrunk some 17 inches. Fortunately, osteomalacia is rare, yet it is seen during famines and among pregnant and lactating women in countries where calcium intake is grossly inadequate.

A not so rare manifestation of calcium deficit is osteoporosis, which has a high incidence among women over 45 and men over 55; 25 per cent of women and 20 per cent of men over the age of 70 have osteoporosis. In this condition, the bones maintain their chemical composition but become thinner, lighter, and more porous. The ailment reveals itself in back pains, decreased height, and frequent and painful fractures of the vertebrae, ribs, and the bones of the arms, legs, hands, and feet.

Acute calcium deficit is treated by intravenous administration of a 10 per cent solution of calcium gluconate—of crucial importance if tetany or convulsions have occurred. Milder deficits may be corrected by a high calcium diet plus oral supplements of calcium lactate. In osteoporosis, no treatment has proved entirely successful, but physical therapy is useful to keep the bones active, and a high protein diet, plus generous supplements of vitamin D and calcium, is essential. Administration of parathormone is often helpful.

Clinical Example. A 70-year-old male was admitted to the hospital because of sprue of some two months' duration. During his first two weeks in the hospital, the patient had numerous large, foul-smelling stools daily. Because of the frequent bowel movements, he was given a potassium supplement in addition to a regular diet. During his third week in the hospital, he complained of tingling of the ends of his fingers and of abdominal cramps. Physical examination revealed hyperactive deep reflexes and bilateral carpopedal spasms. A Sulkowitch test on the urine revealed no precipitation, and the plasma calcium level was found to be 3.8 mEq./L.

Calcium Excess of Extracellular Fluid

Calcium excess of extracellular fluid, or *hypercalcemia,* can develop from drinking too much milk—as an ulcer patient might do to soothe his pain—or too much hard water with a high calcium content. The imbalance may be caused by tumor or overactivity of the parathyroid glands, multiple myeloma, or excessive administration of vitamin D (over 50,000 units daily) in the treatment of arthritis. Multiple fractures, bone tumors, and prolonged immobilization also produce symptoms of calcium excess when calcium stores released from bone flood the extracellular fluid. Osteomalacia and osteoporosis, although manifestations of calcium deficit, cause symptoms of hypercalcemia during the early stages when calcium is moving out of bones and into the extracellular fluid. Thus, while the bones may be dangerously deficient in calcium, there still exists calcium excess of the extracellular fluid.

The clinical observations in calcium excess include relaxed skeletal muscles, deep bony pain —due to honeycombing of bones—pathologic fractures, and flank pain—due to kidney stones, which form from the excess calcium presented to the kidneys for excretion.

The plasma calcium concentration is above 5.8 mEq./L., the urinary Sulkowitch test shows dense precipitation, and calcium excess is indicated by x-ray examination revealing generalized osteoporosis, widespread bone cavitation, or radiopaque urinary stones. An elevated blood urea nitrogen (BUN) indicates that the urinary stones have damaged the kidneys.

Hypercalcemic crisis is the most important syndrome of calcium excess, for it represents an emergency situation requiring immediate atten-

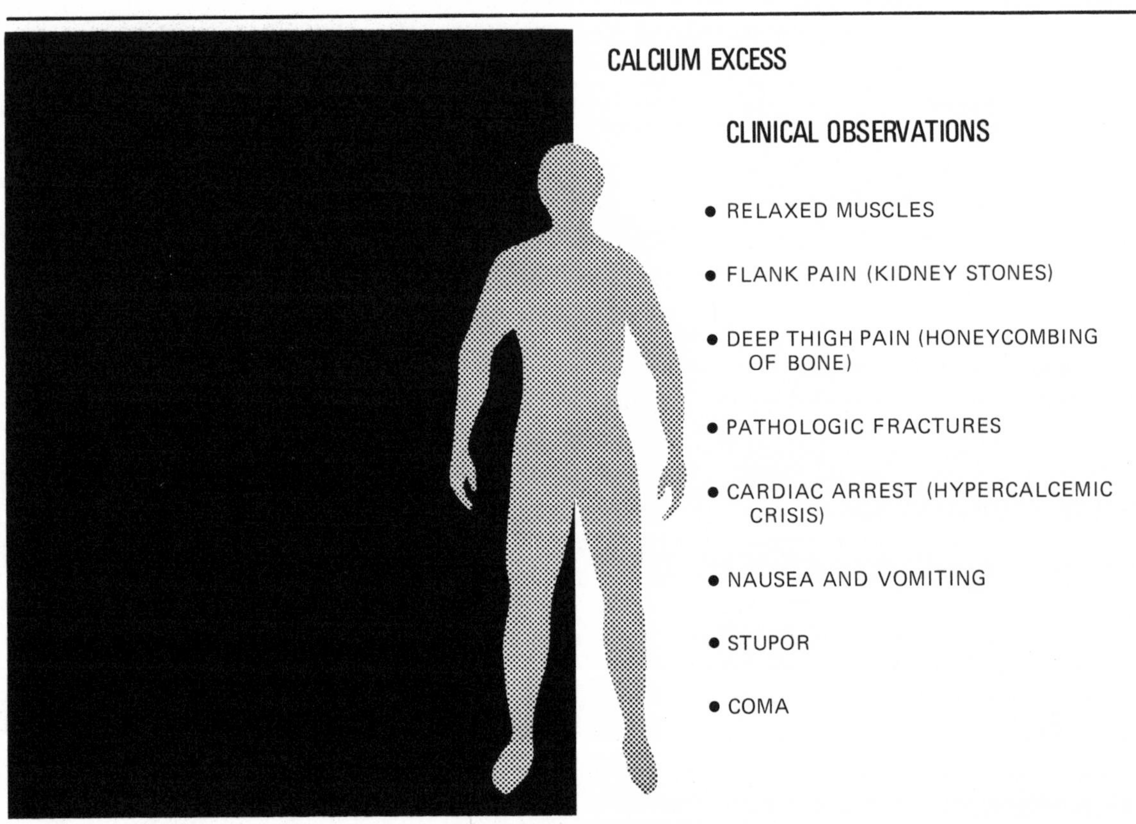

Fig. 9-6. Calcium excess.

tion to prevent cardiac arrest. The symptoms include intractable nausea and vomiting, dehydration, stupor, coma, and azotemia.

Medical management of hypercalcemic crisis has generally been unsatisfactory, since due to slow action or inherent toxicity, none of the many regimens tried has been consistently successful. Sulfate solutions and inorganic phosphate solutions are among the most frequently used, and in less critical situations, therapy is directed toward correcting the underlying cause. If the patient is also being treated for other fluid imbalances, only calcium-free solutions should be used.

Clinical Example. A 55-year-old female was admitted to the hospital because of pain in the right femur. She stated that she had suffered a slight fall, but hardly enough, in her opinion, to bruise her. X-ray examination revealed a fracture of the right femur, as well as numerous areas of decalcification. Physical examination revealed that her muscles were hypotonic, and the Sulkowitch test on urine produced heavy precipitation. The plasma calcium level was found to be 6.4 mEq./L., and a preliminary diagnosis of parathyroid tumor was confirmed at operation.

MAGNESIUM

Magnesium, known chemically as *Mg*, is the fourth most abundant cation in the human body. The average adult contains about 20 gm., about half of which is stored in bone cells; 49 per cent is distributed throughout the specialized cells of the liver, heart, and skeletal muscles. The extracellular fluid contains only 1 per cent, most of which is in the cerebrospinal fluid, and the normal serum level is 1.67 mEq./L.

The minimum daily requirement for magnesium is a matter of controversy, but most medical authorities agree on 250 mg. for the average adult, 150 mg. for the infant, and 400 mg. for the pregnant or lactating woman. The usual American diet provides from 180 to 300 mg. daily.

Calcium and magnesium, both of which are regulated by the parathyroid glands, share a common route of absorption in the intestinal tract and appear to have a mutually suppressive effect on one another. If calcium intake is unusually high, calcium will be absorbed in preference to magnesium, and conversely, if magnesium intake is high, more of it will be absorbed and calcium will be excluded. A normal intake of both allows for adequate absorption of both.

The body's magnesium content also directly affects the potassium concentration, because if magnesium is deficient, the kidneys tend to excrete more potassium. Consequently, potassium deficit may also develop.

Magnesium's importance was not understood until its recent recognition as the activator of numerous vital reactions related to enzyme systems. Among the systems that magnesium activates are those that enable the B vitamins to function and those associated with utilization of potassium, calcium, and protein. Magnesium is particularly important in nervous tissue, in skeletal muscle, and in the heart, having considerable therapeutic value in correcting arrhythmias and in counteracting the toxic side effects of certain powerful drugs used in the treatment of heart disease. When used in conjunction with hypotensive agents, magnesium is a useful therapeutic agent in treatment of hypertension. And lastly, toxemia of pregnancy, which formerly had a high mortality rate, responds to magnesium therapy.

Magnesium Deficit of Extracellular Fluid

Magnesium deficit of extracellular fluid, also referred to as *hypomagnesemia*, develops when the magnesium concentration of that fluid decreases.

Alcoholism looms high on the list of factors causing magnesium deficit, and indeed, ingestion of alcohol appears to promote the imbalance, even in the face of what normally would be an adequate intake. The combination of liver disease and sustained losses of gastrointestinal secretions is almost certain to produce magnesium deficit. Diabetes mellitus appears to predispose to magnesium deficit, and so does a high intake of calcium since absorption of magnesium from the intestinal tract varies inversely with calcium ab-

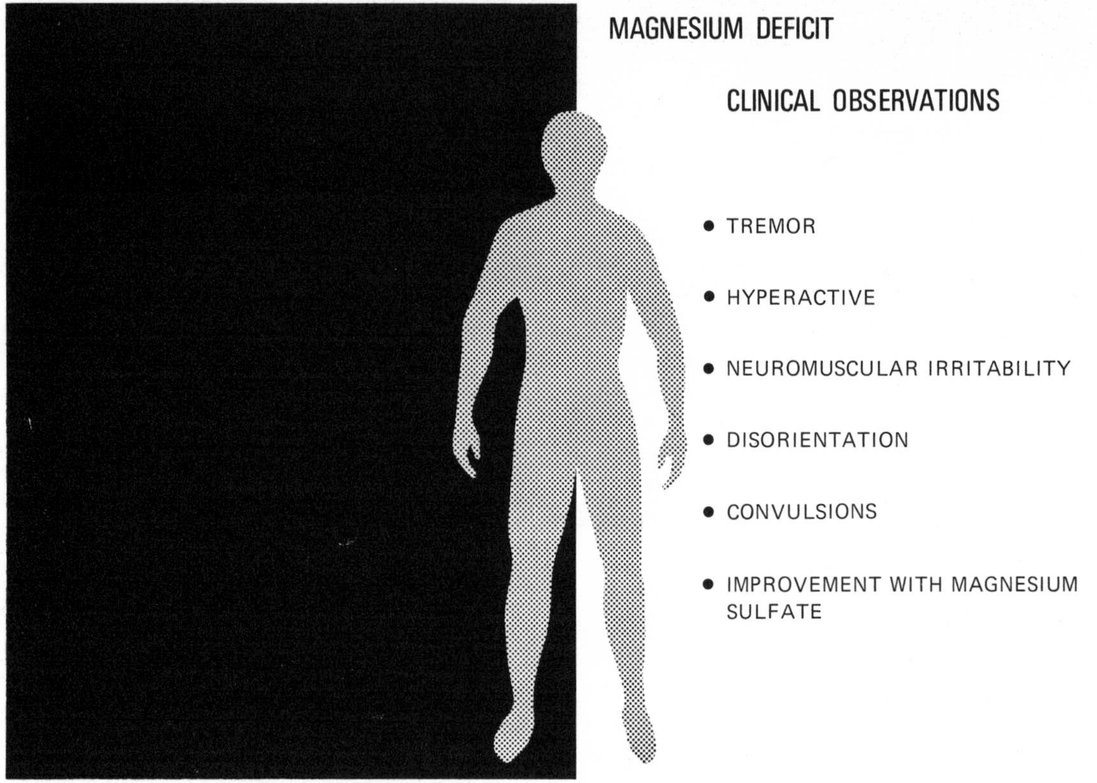

Fig. 9-7. Magnesium deficit.

sorption. Other causes are primary hyperaldosteronism, severe renal disease, toxemia of pregnancy, diseases of the small intestine that impair gastrointestinal absorption, vigorous drug-induced diuresis, or prolonged administration of magnesium-free solutions.

Although magnesium deficit is relatively simple to diagnose, a review of the literature suggests that many persons die of undiagnosed magnesium deficit. Perhaps the reason the imbalance is so frequently overlooked is that it is easily mistaken for potassium deficit, with which it is often associated. Magnesium deficit should always be considered a possible imbalance when a patient being treated for potassium deficit does not respond to appropriate therapy, or in the alcoholic with a body fluid disturbance.

While the clinical picture of magnesium deficit varies from patient to patient, certain symptoms are frequently seen. These include tremor, athetoid or choreiform movements, tetany, a positive Chvostek or Trousseau sign, excessive neuromuscular irritability, painful paresthesia, and—an ominous symptom—convulsions. The patient usually is confused and may hallucinate. Another symptom is tachycardia; when it occurs, the blood pressure rises. A therapeutic test consisting of administration of a 1 per cent solution of magnesium sulfate or magnesium citrate by mouth may prove of great value in diagnosing magnesium deficit. If the imbalance is present, there will be an immediate therapeutic response; all symptoms, however, may not disappear for some 60 to 80 hours.

The most useful laboratory test in magnesium deficit is the plasma magnesium determination, since if it is below 1.4 mEq./L., magnesium deficit is probably present.

Magnesium deficit is treated by administration of magnesium as magnesium sulfate or other salt, and when excessive amounts of magnesium-rich secretions or excretions are being lost, appropriate replacement solutions should be administered to prevent a deficit.

Clinical Example. A 27-year-old male was admitted to the hospital with regional enteritis accompanied by considerable diarrhea. He was given the usual hospital diet plus a potassium supplement. After a month in the hospital, the patient began to have periods of disorientation. Physical examination revealed a tremor of the fingers, hyperactive deep reflexes, and a positive Chvostek sign, and on one occasion, the patient had a convulsion of brief duration. Plasma potassium was normal, and plasma magnesium was found to be 1 mEq./L. Magnesium sulfate was administered as a therapeutic test, and immediate improvement was noted.

Magnesium Excess of Extracellular Fluid

Magnesium excess, or *hypermagnesemia,* represents a rare imbalance, hence we have not included it in our diagnostic classification. It can occur when magnesium is not being excreted normally, as in chronic renal disease or untreated diabetic acidosis. Administration of excessive quantities of magnesium, as in a child with congenital megacolon who is given magnesium sulfate rectally, can cause an excess, and the imbalance has also been reported when perfusion fluid used in hemodialysis contained excessive magnesium. Deficiency of aldosterone, as in Addison's disease, can cause it, as can hyperparathyroidism.

Symptoms of magnesium excess, including lethargy, coma, and impaired respiration, can terminate in death and appear when the plasma magnesium exceeds 6 mEq./L.

Clinical Example. A 26-year-old male was admitted to the hospital with hopelessly infected kidneys, and following bilateral nephrectomy, he was put on hemodialysis pending availability of a transplant. Following the third hemodialyzing session, he became extremely lethargic and appeared to have some difficulty in breathing. Complete serum electrolyte studies revealed a magnesium concentration of 3 mEq./L. The source of the excess was sought without success until one of the nurses recalled that water from a new supplier had been used for the last perfusion bath. When analyzed, the water was found to be unduly high in several electrolytes, including magnesium. The supplier of water for the perfusing equipment was immediately changed, and the patient's next hemodialyzing session was uneventful.

PROTEIN

Protein has been called the *keystone* of the nutritional arch. Because all living matter is composed largely of proteins, without protein, there would be no life. Through its drawing power for liquids—oncotic pressure—protein helps prevent leaking of plasma from the blood vessels. In addition, the amino acids of which proteins are composed are the building blocks for the growth of new tissue. Protein is also required for the elaboration of enzymes, for the fabrication of those blood-borne messengers we call hormones, for the manufacture of some vitamins, and in the immune mechanism since many antibodies are proteins. Since it is practically impossible to develop protein excess, this imbalance is not included in our diagnostic classification and will not be discussed.

Protein Deficit of Extracellular Fluid

Since protein is an anion (e.g., Ca + caseinate−), we have included protein deficit of extracellular fluid in our diagnostic classification. The imbalance is also known as *hypoproteinemia* and *protein malnutrition;* Kwashiorkor, or the pluricarencial syndrome, as it is called in Latin America, and hypoproteinosis are closely related clinical states.

Protein deficit, which develops slowly, frequently does not attract the attention of the attending physician, and can be deadly. The imbalance can result from decreased intake, increased loss, or impaired utilization of protein. Naturally, the individual on an inadequate diet—for whatever reason—will develop protein deficit, most extreme in starvation, which causes wasting and internal cannibalization of the body tissues. Bleeding, whether severe, repeated, or of long duration, drains the body's protein stores, sooner or later causing a deficit, as does infection. Burns, fractures, and surgical operations help deplete protein stores through the destruction and apparently purposeless wastage of tissues; this is called *toxic destruction of protein.* Diseases that affect the digestive tract interfere with protein intake and cause protein poverty. Protein deficit is often associated with potassium deficit since adequate potassium is essential for protein synthesis. Indeed, every patient with any disturbance of the body fluids is a candidate for protein deficit, particularly if he has been ill for a long time, since the sort of conditions that cause body fluid disturbances can also cause protein deficit.

The clinical findings of protein deficit include weight loss and wasting of the muscles; body tissues become flabby and soft. The patient complains that he is always tired, and becomes chronically depressed. His poor appetite becomes still poorer, and he may vomit repeatedly; and if he is injured, his wounds will not heal. His recuperative powers are greatly decreased; he may experience one infection after another. Lastly, the protein deficient patient frequently suffers from anemia, which may be either microcytic or macrocytic.

Laboratory aids in diagnosis of hypoproteinemia include depressed hemoglobin, depressed hematocrit, and low red blood cell count—these findings are significant only when iron intake is adequate. In severe imbalances, the plasma albumin may drop below 4 gm./100 ml.

The most desirable method of treating protein deficit is via a mixed diet providing high-quality protein, adequate calories, and sufficient amounts of vitamins and minerals. If the deficit

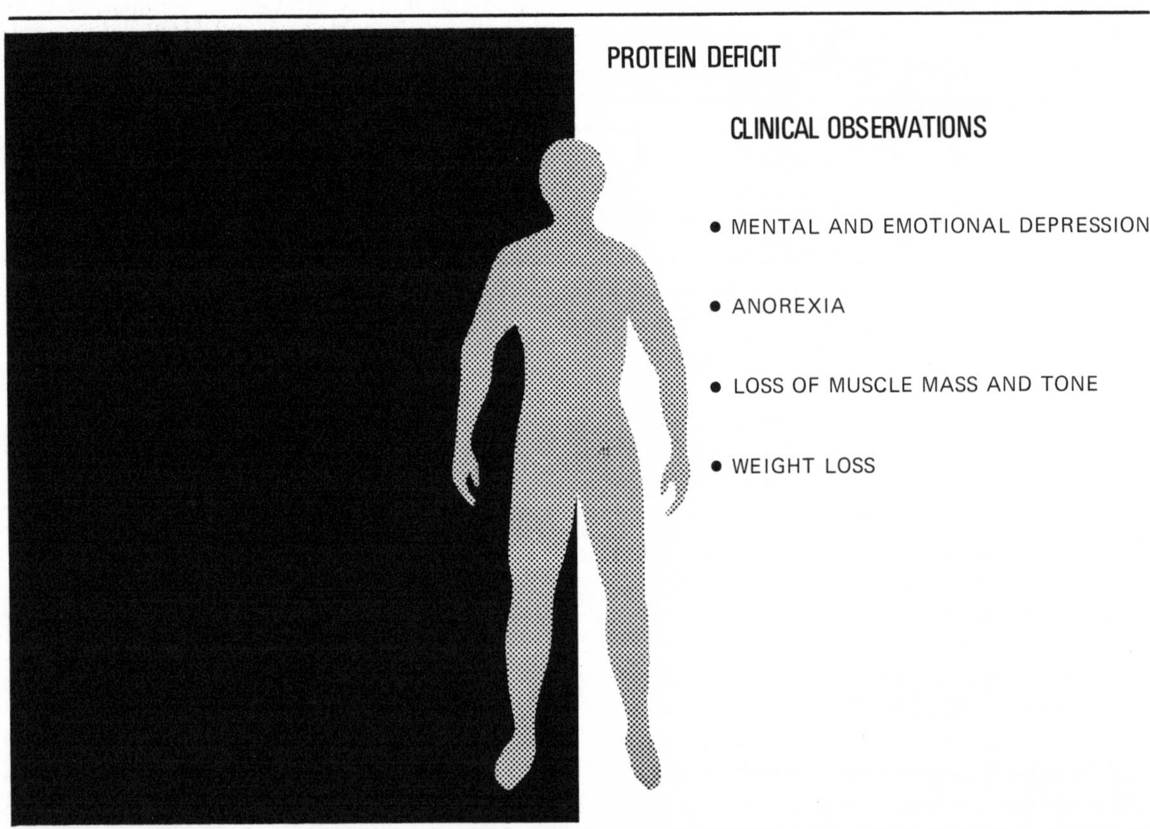

Fig. 9-8. Protein deficit.

must be corrected rapidly, either a high protein diet alone or one supplemented with high protein oral electrolyte mixtures can be used. If the patient cannot take nourishment by mouth, partial or complete feeding via nasogastric tube may be necessary. When oral or nasogastric feedings are impossible, difficult, or contraindicated, then protein may be administered parenterally.

Clinical Example. A 28-year-old female was admitted to the hospital following an automobile accident, in which she was severely injured. She had lost considerable blood and had sustained multiple fractures, one of which was compound. She received several blood transfusions during the first few days in the hospital, but after this period her only source of nutrients was the usual hospital diet, at which she only nibbled. Her fractures were slow in knitting, and her flesh wounds healed slowly. She was emotionally depressed and pale, her muscles were soft and flabby, and she lost 20 lbs. during the period of her stay in the hospital. Her plasma albumin was determined and found to be 3.8 Gm./100 ml. Her hemoglobin was found to be 9 Gm., and her red blood cell count, 3,000,000. (Recall that a depression of the hemoglobin or red blood cell count is indicative of protein deficit only if the patient has been receiving adequate iron.)

ACID-BASE BALANCE

The normal composition of the body fluid depends not only upon the concentration of the various electrolytes, but also upon the concentration of acids and alkalies. Acids are substances that contain hydrogen ions that they can release to other substances, whereas alkalies possess no hydrogen ions of their own, but are able to accept them from acids. The strength of an acid is determined by the number of hydrogen ions it contains per unit of weight, and the power of an alkali is measured by the number of hydrogen ions it can accept per unit of weight.

Together, the acids and alkalies of the body fluids produce the chemical reactions necessary for life, and in order for such reactions to proceed normally, the body must maintain a precarious balance between the burning acids on the one side and the corrosive alkalies on the other. This is called *acid-base balance.* When acid-base balance is maintained, the reaction of the body fluid is neutral, or normal, and if the balance becomes upset, the body fluid becomes either acid or alkaline in its reaction. It is the number of hydrogen ions present in the body fluid that determines whether its reaction is acid, neutral, or alkaline.

Recall that we use the term pH to express the reaction of the body fluid (see Chapter 6, Units of Measure). A pH scale ranges from 1 to 14; 7 is neutral, below 7 is acid, and above 7 is alkaline. The normal pH of extracellular fluid ranges from 7.35 to 7.45 (slightly alkaline). If the plasma pH drops below 7.35, acidosis, or acidemia, is said to be present—even though in the technical sense, a true acid reaction must be below 7. Rarely does plasma pH drop below 7, although it may be as low as 6.8 in extremely ill acidotic patients. If plasma pH rises above 7.45, alkalosis, or alkalemia, is said to be present. Death occurs when the plasma pH is below 6.8 or above 7.8.

What is it that determines the hydrogen ion concentration of the extracellular fluid? Basically, it is the *ratio* of carbonic acid to base bicarbonate. Carbon dioxide (CO_2) unites with water in the extracellular fluid to form carbonic acid, whereas the cations sodium, potassium, calcium, and magnesium unite with the anion bicarbonate to form base bicarbonate. Other body buffers enter into acid-base balance, but carbonic acid and base bicarbonate are far and away the most important ones. The normal ratio of carbonic acid to base bicarbonate is 1:20, and so, as long as there is 1 mEq. of carbonic acid for every 20 mEq. of base bicarbonate in the extracellular fluid, the hydrogen ion concentration lies within normal limits. Normally, there are 1.35 mEq. of carbonic acid to every 27 mEq. of base bicarbonate.

It is important to note that *absolute* quantities of carbonic acid and base bicarbonate are not important in maintaining the balance; it is the *relative* quantities that are important. For example, acid-base balance will not be disturbed if base bicarbonate is increased, perhaps doubled, as long as the carbonic acid is also increased by the same factor; or, both can be decreased by the same factor without upsetting the balance. Imbalances result only when the normal 1:20 ratio is upset.

Think of acid-base balance as a teeter-totter, with carbonic acid on one end and base bicarbonate on the other. In health, the teeter-totter is level, but any condition that increases carbonic acid or decreases base bicarbonate tilts the teeter-totter toward the carbonic acid side and causes acidosis, or acidemia, and any condition that increases base bicarbonate or decreases carbonic acid tilts the teeter-totter toward the base bicarbonate side and produces alkalosis, or alkalemia.

The balance can be tilted by two general types of body disturbances: one type adds or subtracts base bicarbonate; and the other type adds or subtracts carbonic acid. Body metabolism affects the base bicarbonate side of the balance, and for this reason, imbalances caused by alterations in base bicarbonate concentration are called *metabolic disturbances* of acid-base balance. The kidneys largely regulate base bicarbonate concentration.

The amount of carbon dioxide blown off by the lungs affects the carbonic acid side of the balance, since by speeding up or slowing down respiration, the lungs increase or decrease the level of carbonic acid in the extracellular fluid. When lung function is abnormal, acid-base balance is disturbed, causing the resultant imbalances referred to as *respiratory disturbances* of acid-base balance.

The pH of the plasma, of course, tells us whether we have acidosis or alkalosis, although it does not indicate the nature of the imbalance—i.e., whether it is metabolic or respiratory. pH can be measured directly by a pH meter or with a colorimeter, using either heparinized arterial blood or "arterialized" blood from a warmed ear lobe or fingertip. Blood from a vein can be used if it is promptly drawn and kept stoppered under oil.

Carbonic acid—really CO_2+HOH—can be measured by a pCO_2 meter, and from this, the amount of carbonic acid can be determined by use of a nomogram. Normal pCO_2 values range from 35-38 mm. Hg if arterial blood is used, and from 40-41 mm. Hg if venous blood is used.

Various laboratory tests can be used to measure the bicarbonate level of the plasma, including the carbon dioxide (CO_2) content, CO_2 capacity, and CO_2 combining power. The names of these tests can be misleading unless one recalls that what is being measured is not the carbon dioxide of plasma, but rather the bicarbonate. In all these tests, bicarbonate is treated with sulfuric acid, which causes it to release carbon dioxide. The carbon dioxide is then measured, and after an adjustment has been made to allow for the amount of carbon dioxide dissolved in the plasma, the bicarbonate concentration is calculated on the basis of the carbon dioxide released from the bicarbonate as a result of the chemical treatment.

The test for CO_2 content measures the total carbon dioxide freed when plasma is acidified, representing not only the carbon dioxide derived from bicarbonate—which is a measure of plasma alkali—but also carbon dioxide in the form of dissolved CO_2 or carbonic acid—which measures the acid portion of the plasma. The normal CO_2 content ranges from 24-33 mEq./L. If there is a respiratory acid-base disturbance, the CO_2 content will not represent an accurate measure of the bicarbonate. In carbonic acid excess (respiratory acidosis), because of the CO_2 retention by the lungs, the carbonic acid is elevated; in carbonic acid deficit (respiratory alkalosis), because of the blowing off of CO_2, it is depressed. But there are tests that give one a more accurate estimate of the plasma bicarbonate, even in the presence of a respiratory disturbance, and these include the CO_2 capacity test and the CO_2 combining power test.

In these tests, the actual carbonic acid and carbon dioxide concentration of the plasma is adjusted to normal either by bubbling a 5.5 per cent carbon dioxide gas mixture through the plasma (CO_2 capacity test) or by having the laboratory technician blow his breath through it (CO_2 combining power test). Thus, if the test plasma's CO_2 is elevated because of respiratory acidosis, bubbling the normal concentration of CO_2 through it will reduce it to normal, a process known as *equilibration.* If the plasma's CO_2 is depressed because of respiratory alkalosis, then equilibration will raise it to normal. In essence, equilibrating plasma amounts to recirculating the plasma through the lungs of a normal person so that it will achieve its normal CO_2-carbonic acid level. The result is that either the CO_2 capacity test or the CO_2 combining power test gives a fairly close approximation of the test specimen's bicarbonate. Normally, CO_2 capacity varies from 24-33 mEq./L., and CO_2 combining power varies from 24-35 mEq./L. (depending on reference source).

The CO_2 content, bicarbonate, pH, pCO_2, and carbonic acid content can all be calculated by use of a nomogram if two of the values are known. A straight line is drawn between the two known points and the desired value read from the other three scales.

Considerably more complex and somewhat more accurate methods of measuring acid-base disturbances have been introduced by Astrup, by Siggard-Andersen, and by Kintner, all involving logarithmic relationships, neither easy for the non-mathematician to visualize nor necessary for the usual clinical purposes.

Primary Base Bicarbonate Deficit of Extracellular Fluid

A primary deficit in the concentration of base bicarbonate in the extracellular fluid is usually called *metabolic acidosis* or *acidemia,* and is caused by any clinical event that decreases the concentration of base bicarbonate in the extracellular fluid. Thus, any condition that floods the extracellular fluid with acid metabolites, such as diabetic acidosis, infection, renal insufficiency, or salicylate intoxication, can cause this imbalance. When one or more other etiologic factors is present, metabolic acidosis can be caused by the parenteral infusion of an isotonic solution of sodium

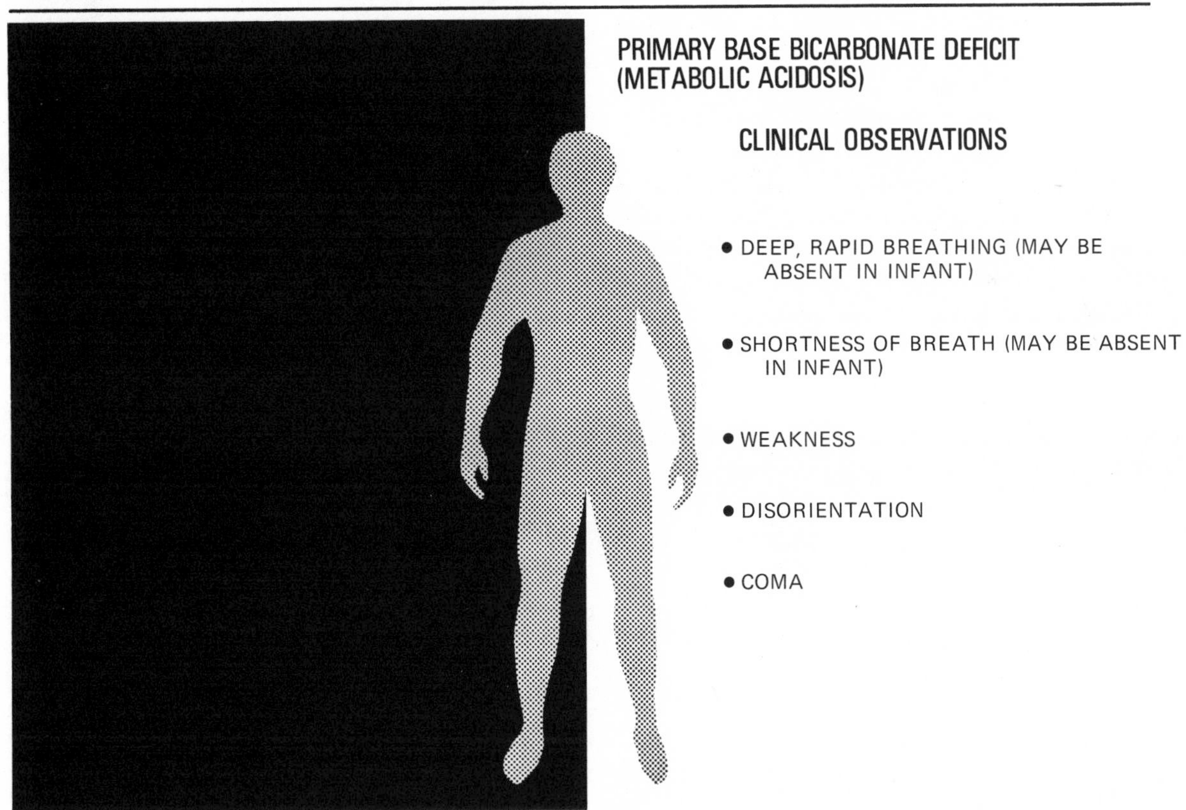

Fig. 9-9. Primary base bicarbonate deficit.

chloride (normal saline) since this imposes an excessive chloride load on the kidneys. A ketogenic diet can produce the imbalance. Metabolic acidosis is frequently associated with potassium excess, whereby the kidneys attempt to reduce the potassium concentration of the extracellular fluid by excreting the excess potassium in the urine. Therefore, potassium rather than hydrogen is exchanged for sodium in the distal convoluted tubules, and the hydrogen ion concentration of the extracellular fluid is thus elevated. To make matters still worse, treatment of potassium excess is directed toward forcing the excess potassium from the extracellular fluid back into the cells. When potassium enters the cells, hydrogen leaves them, further contributing to acidosis; conversely, metabolic acidosis promotes potassium excess. In metabolic acidosis, the kidneys exchange hydrogen rather than potassium for sodium in the distal convoluted tubules, and hydrogen replaces potassium in the cells, causing an excess of potassium in the extracellular fluid.

Among the clinical findings in metabolic acidosis are deep, rapid breathing (Kussmaul) and shortness of breath on exertion, each caused by the body's effort to rid itself of carbon dioxide—and, hence, of carbonic acid—and thus restore the acid-base balance to normal. However, these findings may be absent in a young infant or in extremely severe acidosis. Other symptoms include weakness, disorientation, and coma. Ultimately, metabolic acidosis, as well as the other acid-base disturbances, can lead to death if not corrected.

What help does the lab give us? In *uncompensated* metabolic acidosis, the urine pH is usually below 6 and plasma pH is below 7.35. Plasma bicarbonate is below 25 mEq./L. in adults, below 20 mEq./L. in children. The CO_2 combining power is roughly equivalent to the plasma bicarbonate. In *compensated* metabolic acidosis, whereby the carbonic acid concentration may be decreased by the lungs blowing off of CO_2, the plasma pH is about 7.35. The kidneys aid in compensation by retaining bicarbonate, but renal compensation is slower than pulmonary compensation.

If the compensatory efforts of the lungs and kidneys do not restore balance, metabolic acidosis may be treated by administration of bicarbonate or lactate parenterally or an alkaline solution by mouth.

Clinical Example. A 3½-year-old girl was admitted to the hospital approximately 2 hours after having ingested 10 5-grain tablets of sodium salicylate. At the time of admission, the child was stuporous, and breathing was both deep and rapid, of the typical Kussmaul variety. A pH determination on the urine revealed a reading of 5. The plasma bicarbonate was found to be 10 mEq./L., and plasma pH was 7.25.

Primary Base Bicarbonate Excess of Extracellular Fluid

A primary excess of base bicarbonate, usually referred to as *metabolic alkalosis* or *alkalemia*, can result from any clinical event that increases the amount of base bicarbonate in the extracellular fluid. This imbalance is frequently preceded by a loss of chloride-rich secretions, such as the gastric juice lost in vomiting or in gastrointestinal suction. Bear in mind that the total anions in the extracellular fluid must always equal the total cations, and so if one anion decreases, another anion must increase to maintain the balance. Hence, with excessive losses of chloride, bicarbonate rises precipitously and produces alkalosis. Excessive intake of alkalies, such as baking soda, can also cause this imbalance, as can administration of adrenocortical hormones. Infusion of potassium-free solutions, administration of a potent diuretic, or any other condition that leads to potassium deficit can also produce metabolic alkalosis. Indeed, there is a close association between metabolic alkalosis and potassium deficit, since although potassium deficit does not cause alkalemia, it leaves the body peculiarly vulnerable to the imbalance should chloride loss occur. In potassium deficit, hydrogen rather than potassium is exchanged for sodium in the distal convoluted tubules, and in addition, hydrogen moves into cells so that cellular potassium can enter the extracellular fluid to raise its potassium concentration. If chloride has already been lost, with a resultant increase in base bicarbonate, the decrease in hydrogen concentration that occurs

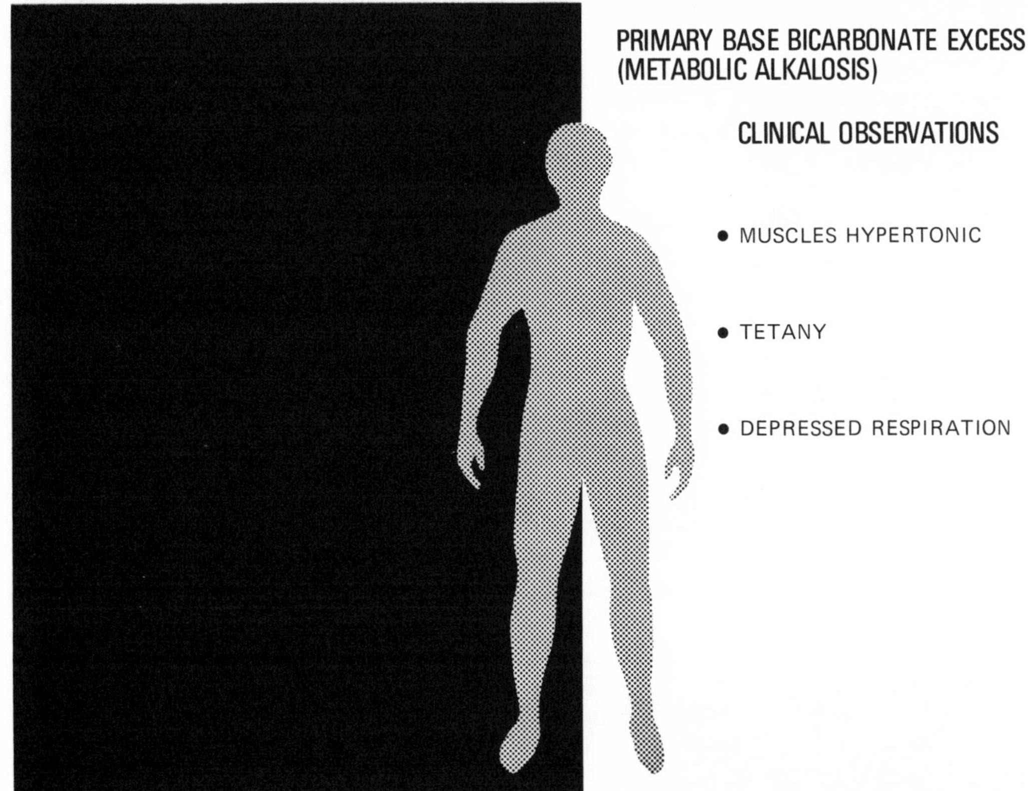

Fig. 9-10. Primary base bicarbonate excess.

in potassium deficit only exaggerates the alkalosis; conversely, metabolic alkalosis promotes development of potassium deficit. In alkalosis, potassium enters the cells in exchange for hydrogen, which leaves the cells, lowering the pH of the extracellular fluid. In addition, potassium rather than hydrogen is exchanged for sodium in the distal convoluted tubules.

Among the clinical observations in metabolic alkalosis are hypertonicity of the muscles, tetany, and depressed respiration, the latter of which retains carbon dioxide, thus causing an increase in the carbonic acid concentration of extracellular fluid and helping to restore the acid-base balance to normal. Correction of metabolic acidosis to normal or to metabolic alkalosis may precipitate tetany or convulsions for the following reason: a latent calcium deficit of the extracellular fluid becomes active and causes hyperirritability, manifesting itself in tetany and convulsions if the deficit is severe. The effective calcium of the extracellular fluid is the ionized portion, with the degree of ionization directly proportional to the acidity of the fluid. In the acid body fluid of acidosis, calcium ionization is high, even if the total calcium concentration is decreased, and for this reason, tetany and convulsions from calcium deficit do not occur in acidosis, even though muscle twitching may. In the alkaline fluid of alkalosis, ionization is greatly decreased, and so with the correction of the acidosis to normal, or with its overcorrection to alkalosis, the latent calcium deficit becomes manifest and symptoms of hyperirritability occur.

Laboratory findings are helpful in diagnosis of metabolic alkalosis. The urine pH is often above 7, but it may actually be 6 or below if the imbalance is associated with potassium deficit—because hydrogen rather than potassium is being exchanged for sodium in the distal convoluted tubules, causing the urine to be acid. The plasma pH is above 7.45, plasma bicarbonate is above 29 mEq./L. in adults and above 25 mEq./L. in children, and the plasma potassium is below 4 mEq./L. If the alkalosis is hypochloremic, the plasma chloride will be below 98 mEq./L. The above findings obtain in uncompensated metabolic alkalosis. Should there be sufficient retention of carbonic acid (compensated metabolic alkalosis), the plasma pH may be within the limits of normal.

Body correction is both renal and pulmonary, with the kidneys excreting the excessive bicarbonate as rapidly as they can. If these efforts fail, chloride should be administered.

Clinical Example. A 22-year-old woman was admitted to the hospital with the diagnosis of anorexia nervosa. During the first three days of her hospital stay, she ate very little and vomited what she did eat. She was given no supplements or parenteral fluid therapy. On the fourth day, she exhibited tetanic movements of the fingers. Physical examination revealed that her muscles were hypertonic, and the physician thought that breathing was depressed. The urine pH was found to be 7.5, plasma bicarbonate level determined as 38 mEq./L., and plasma potassium was 3.5 mEq./L.

COMMENT While the acid side of the acid-base balance goes up and down in the two imbalances just described, it is important to remember that base bicarbonate is the cause, and changes in the carbonic acid side occur only secondarily to alterations in the concentration of base bicarbonate. In the next two imbalances, the carbonic acid side becomes the cause, whereby changes in

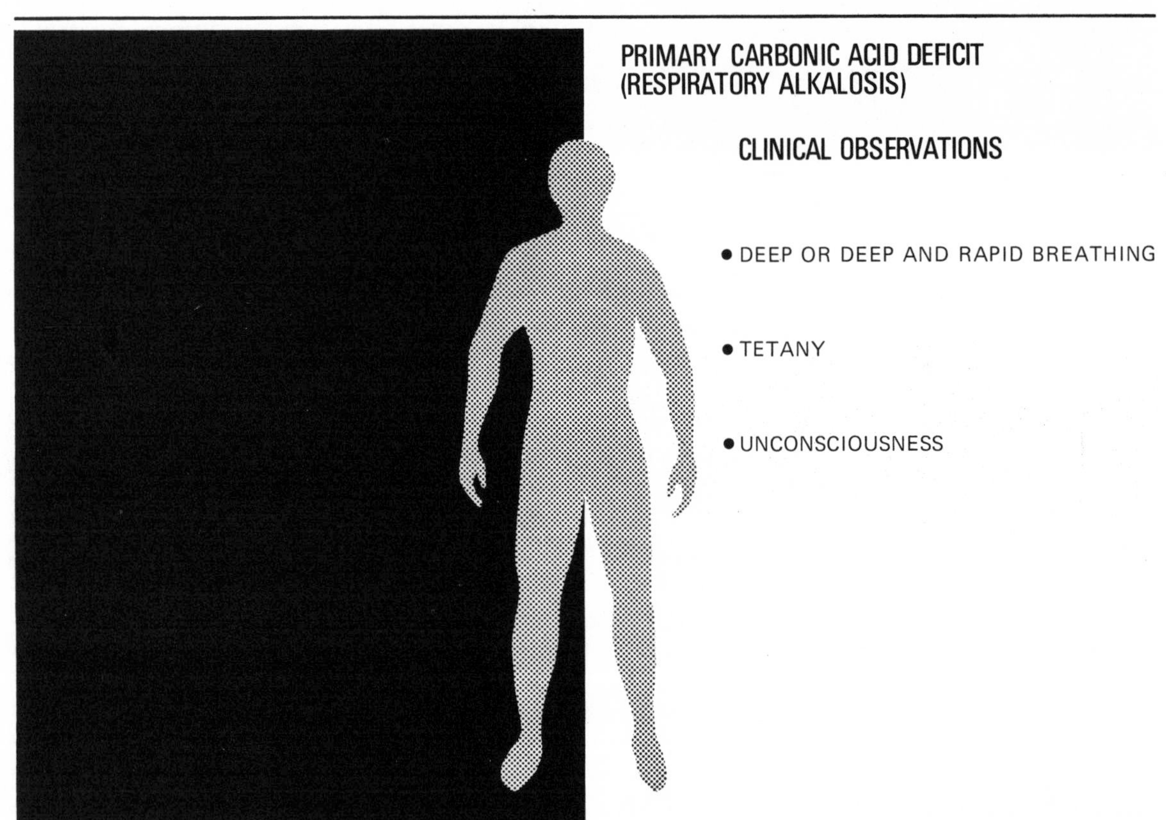

Fig. 9-11. Primary carbonic acid deficit.

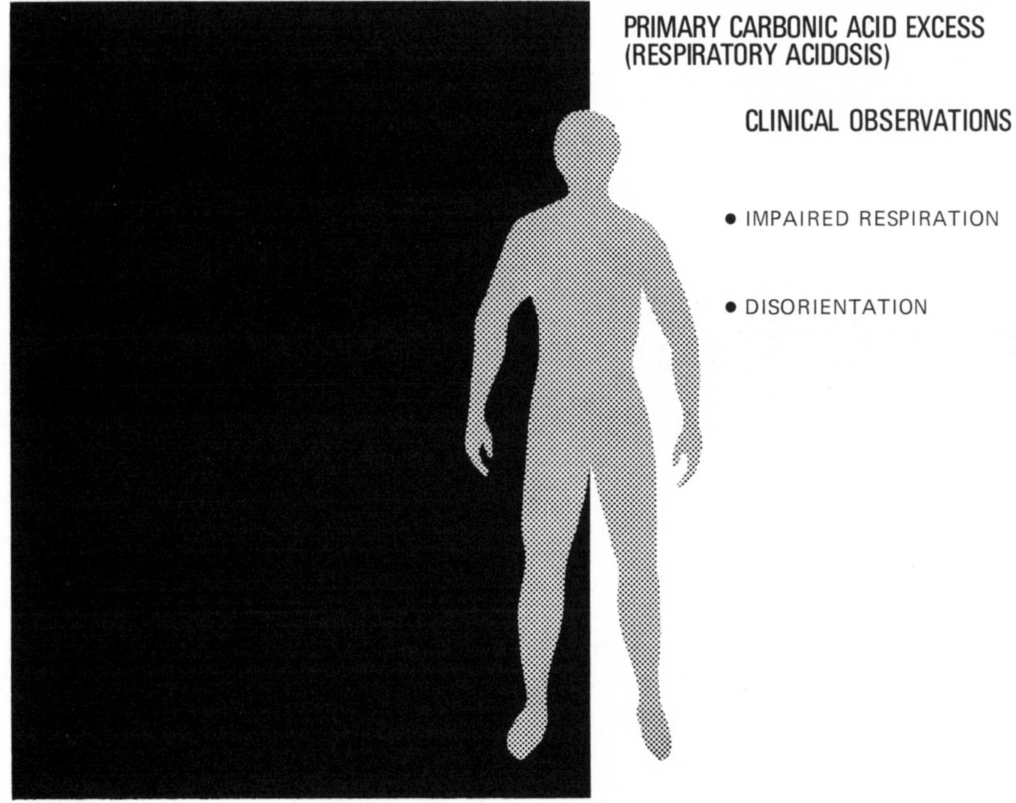

Fig. 9-12. Primary carbonic acid excess.

the base bicarbonate side become secondary to alterations in the concentration of carbonic acid.

Primary Carbonic Acid Deficit of Extracellular Fluid

Any condition that produces an increased rate and depth of respiration, thereby accelerating carbon dioxide loss, can cause a primary deficit of carbonic acid in the extracellular fluid. This imbalance is usually called *respiratory alkalosis* or *alkalemia.* Its principal cause, *hyperventilation,* may be voluntary, as is the case with the individual who overbreathes so that he can swim a long distance underwater; or it may be caused by oxygen lack, as in high altitudes, or by fever, anxiety, or hysteria. It is also seen in the early stages of salicylate intoxication and in encephalitis.

The clinical observations of respiratory alkalosis include deep breathing or deep and rapid breathing, light-headedness, circumoral paresthesia, tetany, convulsions, and, finally, unconsciousness. (The clinical picture of this imbalance, with the exception of the hyperventilation, can be experimentally induced in normal subjects by an intravenous infusion of sodium lactate.) Following hyperventilation, a period of apnea frequently occurs. One can anticipate that the patient will start breathing again as the CO_2 builds up in the blood and stimulates the respiratory center in the medulla, but, cases have been reported where the individual did not resume breathing.

As for laboratory findings, the urine pH is characteristically above 7, and the plasma pH above 7.45. Plasma bicarbonate is depressed; it will usually be below 25 mEq./L. in adults, below 20 mEq./L. in children, representing a body compensatory measure designed to maintain level the acid-base balance. pCO_2 is below normal.

For obvious reasons, the lungs are unable to participate in correction of respiratory alkalosis, and so compensation must depend upon the kidneys alone, which excrete bicarbonate and retain acid. Therapy is directed toward correcting the condition that initially caused the overbreathing. Parenteral infusion of a solution containing chloride ions to neutralize bicarbonate may be helpful in restoring balance while the pulmonary problem is being corrected.

Clinical Example. An 18-year-old girl was admitted to the hospital for study because of tetanic spasms of the fingers and occasional convulsions. The history revealed that she had been extremely apprehensive because of her fear of failing in school. Her mother noticed that she had been breathing deeply and rapidly for several weeks. Physical examination revealed hyperactive reflexes. The urine pH was 7.5, and the plasma bicarbonate, 20 mEq./L.

Primary Carbonic Acid Excess of Extracellular Fluid

Primary carbonic acid excess of extracellular fluid, commonly called *respiratory acidosis* or *acidemia,* is caused by any condition that obstructs respiratory exchange. Such conditions as emphysema, asthma, pneumonia, occlusion of the respiratory passages, barbiturate poisoning, and morphine poisoning cause respiratory depression, with impaired expiration of carbon dioxide. Inspiration of excessive carbon dioxide, as in spaces with poor ventilation, can also cause respiratory acidosis. Other causes include acute pulmonary edema, atelectasis, pneumothorax, poliomyelitis, and even hypoventilation (as can occur in the extremely obese patient).

The clinical observations in this imbalance include weakness, respiratory embarrassment, giddiness, disorientation, and coma.

Laboratory findings include a urine pH below 6, and a plasma pH below 7.35. As a body compensatory measure, plasma bicarbonate rises to above 29 mEq./L. in adults, above 25 mEq./L. in children. pCO_2 is elevated to above normal.

The lungs, of course, are unable to participate in compensation, but the kidneys help by retaining bicarbonate and excreting hydrogen, although with the kidneys working alone, compensation is slow. Therapy is directed primarily toward correcting the condition that is responsible for the impaired lung function, and administration of bicarbonate or lactate may also be necessary to restore balance while the lung ailment is being corrected.

Clinical Example. A 50-year-old male was admitted to the hospital in a state of coma. The history revealed that he had suffered from emphysema for the past six years, and that during the past two weeks, he had become increasingly weak and disoriented. His urine pH was 5.5, the plasma bicarbonate 40 mEq./L., the plasma pH, 6.8.

Trends in uncompensated and compensated acid-base disturbances are shown in Tables 9-1 and 9-2.

Many clinicians regard the term acidosis as any clinical situation tending to produce acidemia, even though it has not produced it. Similarly, they regard the term alkalosis as any clinical situation tending to produce alkalemia, whether or not it has succeeded in so doing.

Using this terminology, one might encounter such a paradoxical situation as alkalemia (caused by carbonic acid deficit, or respiratory alkalosis) coexisting with base bicarbonate deficit (metabolic acidosis). In this instance, the respiratory alkalosis would, in effect, overpower the effects of the metabolic acidosis. Similarly, one might conceivably find acidemia (caused by carbonic acid excess, or respiratory acidosis) coexisting with base bicarbonate excess (metabolic alkalosis). In this instance, the respiratory acidosis would overpower the metabolic alkalosis.

Some would refer to the former situation as a compensated metabolic acidosis coexisting with a respiratory alkalosis, and to the latter as a compensated metabolic alkalosis coexisting with a respiratory acidosis. Obviously, mixed metabolic and respiratory acid-base disturbances can be enormously complex.

Table 9-1. Early Uncompensated pH Disturbances

Imbalance	*HCO_3*	*Arterial pCO_2*	*H_2CO_3*	*Plasma pH*
Metabolic Alkalosis	Above 29 mEq./L.	Normal	Normal	Above 7.45
Metabolic Acidosis	Below 25 mEq./L.	Normal	Normal	Below 7.35
Respiratory Alkalosis	Normal	Below 35 mm. Hg	Below 1.33 mEq./L.	Above 7.45
Respiratory Acidosis	Normal	Above 38 mm. Hg	Above 1.33 mEq./L.	Below 7.35

Table 9-2. Partially Compensated pH Disturbances

Imbalance	*HCO_3*	*Arterial pCO_2*	*H_2CO_3*	*Plasma pH*	*Urine pH*
Metabolic Alkalosis	Above 29 mEq./L.	Above 38 mm. Hg	Above 1.33 mEq./L.	Still above 7.45, but closer to normal	Above 7
Metabolic Acidosis	Below 25 mEq./L.	Below 35 mm. Hg	Below 1.33 mEq./L.	Still below 7.35, but closer to normal	Below 6
Respiratory Alkalosis	Below 25 mEq./L.	Below 35 mm. Hg	Below 1.33 mEq./L.	Still above 7.45, but closer to normal	Above 7
Respiratory Acidosis	Above 29 mEq./L.	Above 38 mm. Hg	Above 1.33 mEq./L.	Still below 7.35, but closer to normal	Below 6

10 Position Changes of Water and Electrolytes of Extracellular Fluid

Normally, about one-fourth of the extracellular fluid exists as plasma, and about three-fourths as interstitial fluid. These two fluids are quite similar in composition, except for the amount of protein they contain: plasma has about 18 mEq./L., and interstitial fluid only 1 mEq./L. It is the oncotic pressure exerted by the plasma protein that prevents large amounts of the plasma's water and electrolytes from being forced into the interstitial fluid by the hydrostatic pressure produced by the pumping action of the heart. However, under certain circumstances, water and electrolytes do shift into the interstitial fluid, and in other cases, water and electrolytes of interstitial fluid shift into the plasma.

We can readily understand why such shifts occur when the plasma protein content is altered. However, shifts also take place when plasma protein is normal, although the mechanisms for these shifts are obscure and appear to be of little value.

PLASMA-TO-INTERSTITIAL FLUID SHIFT

In plasma-to-interstitial fluid shift, sometimes called *hypovolemia*, abnormal quantities of water and electrolytes move from plasma into the interstitial fluid. This decreases the volume of plasma and increases the volume of interstitial fluid; the normal three to one ratio is upset. The imbalance is closely related to shock and to edema and is almost invariably seen on the first or second day following a severe burn. The shift is also often seen following a massive crushing injury, severe trauma, or perforation of a peptic ulcer and may be observed with intestinal obstruction or following the acute occlusion of a major artery. Plasma-to-interstitial fluid shift may occur in the patient undergoing surgery, producing the condition known as *surgical shock*.

The clinical symptoms of plasma-to-interstitial fluid shift include pallor, tachycardia, low blood pressure, weak pulse—perhaps undetectable—cold extremities, disorientation, and, finally, coma. The clinical picture usually suffices for diagnosis of this imbalance, but laboratory tests are helpful, as the red blood cell count, hemoglobin, and packed cell volume will be elevated because of the decrease in plasma volume.

Hypovolemia appears similar, if not often identical, to the condition known as *shock*. The exact mechanism of shock is not known, but certainly a shift of water and electrolytes from plasma to interstitial fluid can cause it. Pooling of blood in dilated blood vessels of the abdomen may play a role. Shock is a frequent aftermath of injury, and even patients with minor injuries, such as a sprain, broken finger, or a small cut, sometimes suffer severe shock and die from it, before reaching the hospital.

When plasma-to-interstitial fluid shift develops slowly over a long period of time, as in starvation, the patient displays a huge belly, as well as swollen ankles, legs, wrists, and arms—a condition known as *starvation edema*.

In general, treatment of plasma-to-interstitial fluid shift is directed toward the underlying cause of the shift and toward replacing the shifted fluid with solutions given by mouth or vein. Localized shifts may be relieved by application of a binder, and mild or moderate shifts caused by depletion of plasma protein can be corrected via a high protein diet plus commercially prepared protein supplements. In severe protein deficiency, plasma volume is restored by parenteral administration of plasma, dextran, or an electrolyte solution that

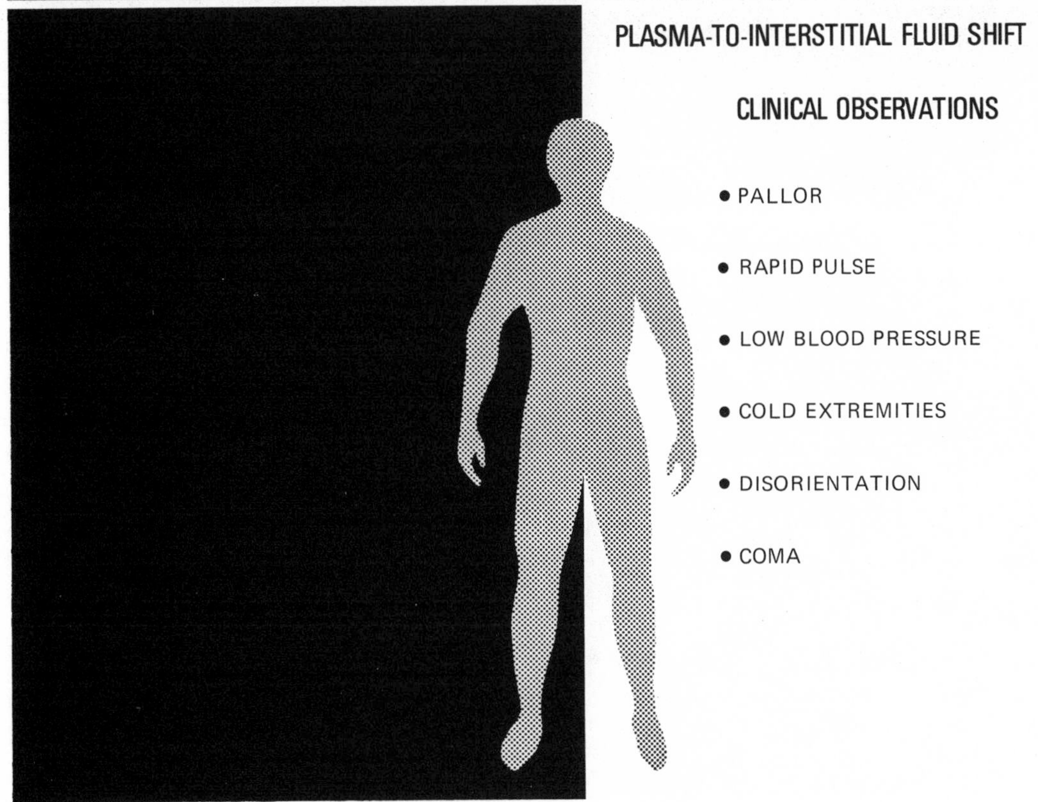

Fig. 10-1. Plasma-to-interstitial fluid shift.

has approximately the same composition as plasma. Injured persons should be given emergency treatment for shock *at the scene of the accident,* not after they reach the hospital.

Clinical Example. An 11-year-old girl was admitted to the hospital with two-thirds of her body covered by second- and third-degree burns, suffered when an inflammable party dress caught fire. The burn team of the hospital immediately took charge and carried out the usual excellent burn program of that hospital. Nevertheless, during her second 24 hours in the hospital, her hemoglobin and red blood cell count rose rapidly. Her blood pressure dropped to 90/70, her pulse increased to 125, and she complained of cold hands and feet. The burned area appeared boggy, as if filled with fluid. (This is an example of the plasma-to-interstitial shift that almost invariably occurs early following a severe burn. On the third to fifth day, the opposite shift occurs—interstitial space-to-plasma shift, the so-called remobilization of edema fluid.)

INTERSTITIAL FLUID-TO-PLASMA SHIFT

In interstitial fluid-to-plasma shift, or *hypervolemia,* water and electrolytes from interstitial fluid flow into the plasma. This imbalance always occurs during the recovery phase of a condition that previously caused a plasma-to-interstitial fluid shift, such as burn or fracture. In this case, the shift is called *remobilization of edema fluid.* If too much fluid is administered during the initial shift, the secondary shift may endanger life. Following hemorrhage, water and electrolytes move from interstitial space to plasma in an effort to replace those that were lost in blood. The shift also can occur when the

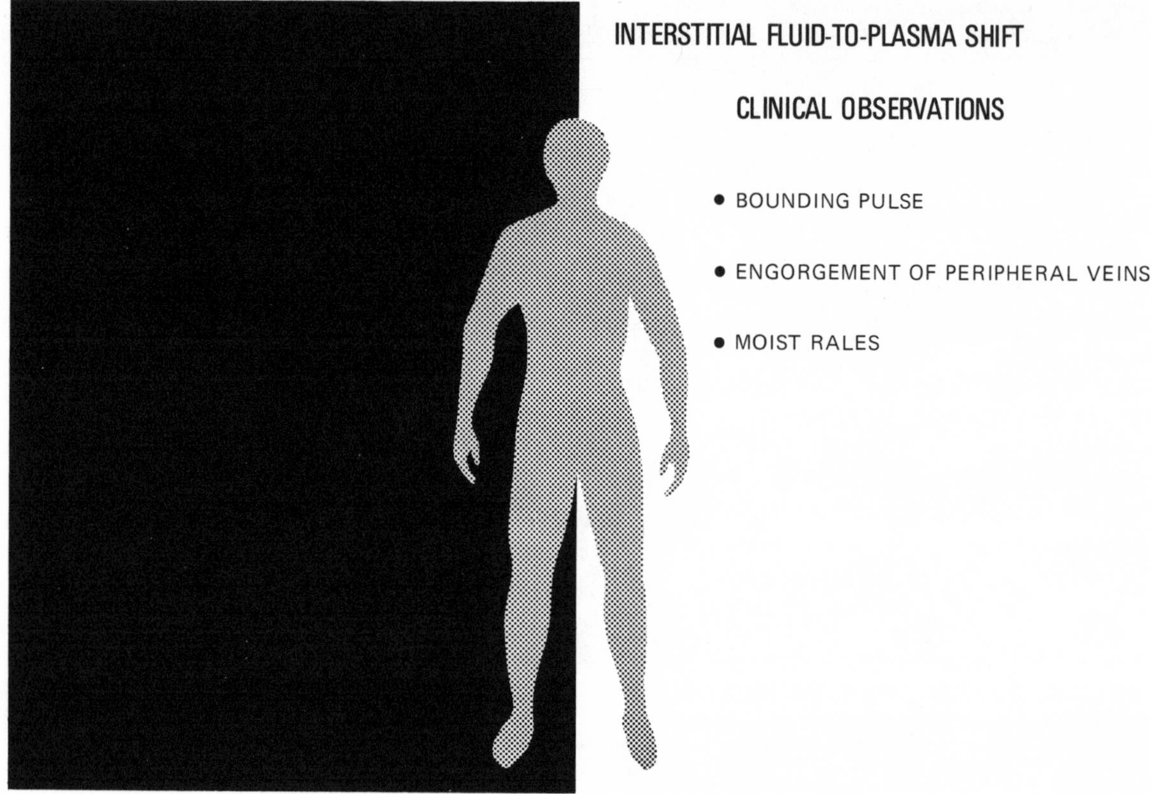

Fig. 10-2. Interstitial fluid-to-plasma shift.

oncotic pressure of the plasma has been increased by administration of excessive amounts of blood, plasma, dextran, or hypertonic solutions.

In many respects, the clinical observations of interstitial fluid-to-plasma shift are just the opposite of those seen in plasma-to-interstitial fluid shift. They include a bounding pulse, engorgement of the peripheral veins, moist rales in the lungs, pallor, weakness, and air hunger. Cardiac dilatation and ventricular failure may occur as well. Laboratory findings helpful in diagnosis include a decrease in the red blood cell count, hemoglobin, and packed cell volume.

Treatment of interstitial fluid-to-plasma shift varies according to the cause and, of course, is directed toward lowering plasma volume. If the shift is severe, phlebotomy may be necessary, and application of tourniquets is helpful in other cases. If the shift develops as a compensatory effort to replace water and electrolytes lost in blood, then transfusion of whole blood is the proper treatment. If the shift is not large enough to require urgent therapy, a balanced diet supplemented by iron tablets will correct it.

Clinical Example. A 14-year-old boy was admitted to the hospital with second- and third-degree burns over 60 per cent of his body. His initial water and electrolyte therapy was, perhaps, over-zealous. On the third day, he complained of being unable to get his breath, and physical examination at that time revealed a bounding pulse, with engorgement of the peripheral veins. Moist rales were heard in both lungs, and the red blood cell count was found to be 3,500,000, and the hemoglobin, 10 Gm. (This patient was suffering from the well-known remobilization of edema fluid that occurs during the third to fifth day following a severe burn. This shift will be more severe if the patient has received excessive quantities of water and electrolytes during the first one or two days of his treatment.)

COMMENT The clinical examples of body fluid disturbances were chosen so as to represent relatively pure examples of single disturbances. Actually, these examples are not uncommon. Sometimes, one sees combined imbalances, and in some patients a considerable number of imbalances can be present simultaneously. Usually, however, one or two imbalances dominate the clinical picture. The infant with an acute onset of vomiting and diarrhea, for example, early has volume deficit of extracellular fluid, and shortly thereafter, if not properly treated, will develop primary base bicarbonate deficit. If potassium is not given and the diarrhea continues, he will, after 3 or 4 days, develop potassium deficit. If he continues to have loose, watery stools and, particularly, if he is also given salt mixtures by mouth, he may well develop a sodium excess.

The addition of each one of these fluid balance disturbances has the effect of increasing, perhaps doubling, the mortality. Various disease states are characterized by a wide variety of body fluid disturbances, depending upon the severity of the disease. Among these conditions might be mentioned burns, severe trauma, diabetes mellitus, gastrointestinal disease and intestinal obstruction. As an example, obstruction of the large intestine can manifest the following disturbances:

Extracellular fluid volume deficit, caused by decreased intake of water and electrolytes, and by losses through vomiting and through secretion of intestinal juices into the dilated obstructed bowel;

Extracellular fluid volume excess, caused by

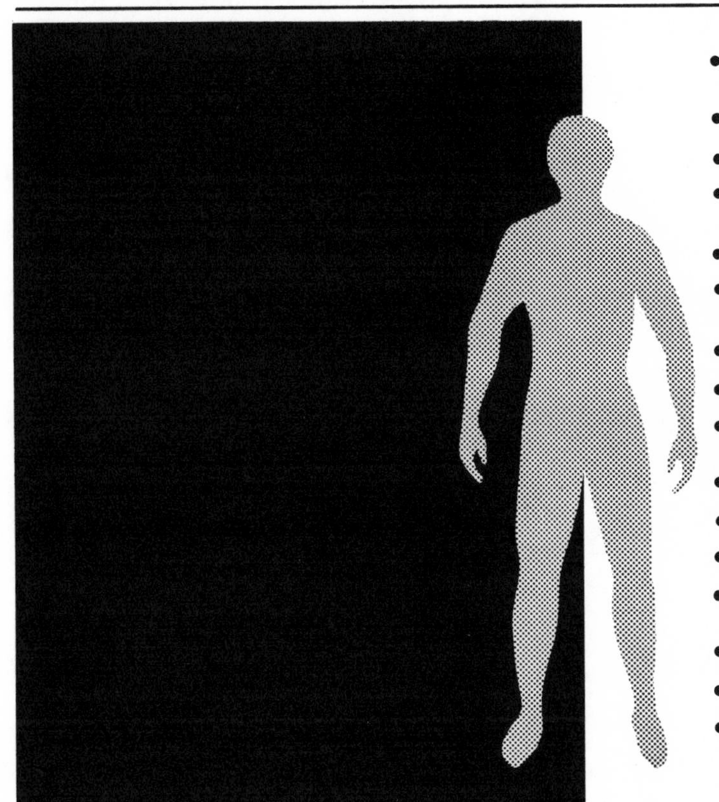

Fig. 10-3. The systematic approach to understanding body fluid disturbances brings order out of confusion.

administering excessive quantities of isotonic saline following surgical intervention;

Sodium deficit, resulting from failure to supply water and electrolytes when gastric or intestinal suction tubes are functioning;

Sodium excess, caused by cessation of eating and drinking and the resultant loss of water in excess of electrolytes—may also occur when isotonic saline is given without adequate quantities of electrolyte-free solutions;

Potassium deficit, an imbalance which results when potassium is not supplied to the patient with intestinal obstruction;

Potassium excess, resulting from extensive tissue damage caused by gangrenous bowel, as in volvulus, by the administration of excessive potassium, or by impaired renal function;

Calcium deficit, seen with strangulating obstruction of the small intestine, much less frequently in large bowel obstruction, but massive repeated transfusions of blood can precipitate it;

Primary base bicarbonate excess, seen when gastric juice has been lost in considerable amounts through vomiting; there is a compensatory rise in bicarbonate since the body's anions must always equal the cations. In some instances, loss of gastric juice is counterbalanced by loss of alkaline intestinal secretions.

It cannot be overemphasized that if one is to understand either combined or complex body fluid disturbances, she must understand the single imbalances, the mechanism of their development, plus their relationships to each other and to disease.

TERMINOLOGY PROBLEMS

Understanding body fluid disturbances is made considerably more difficult by the fact that so many terms frequently apply to the same condition. In an attempt to resolve this problem, we are including in this chapter a table showing in parallel columns each chemical imbalance, then the conventional term applied to the imbalance, and finally, the related clinical term, if any. A careful study of Table 10-1 will help to resolve apparent conflicts in terms.

Table 10-1. Terminology Chart For Physico-Chemical Imbalances and Related Clinical States

Physico-Chemical Imbalance	*Conventional Terminology*	*Closely-Related Clinical States*
Extracellular Fluid Volume Deficit	Fluid deficit Dehydration (incorrect term, since ECF volume deficit means loss of water *and* electrolytes) Hypovolemia	
Extracellular Fluid Volume Excess	Fluid volume excess Overhydration (incorrect term, since this imbalance means an excess of both water *and* electrolytes)	
Sodium Deficit	Electrolyte concentration deficit Hyponatremia Low sodium syndrome Hypotonic dehydration	Heat exhaustion Sodium-losing kidney
Sodium Excess	Hypernatremia Hypertonic dehydration Salt excess Oversalting	
Potassium Deficit	Hypokalemia Potassium deficiency	Potassium-losing kidney

Table 10-1. (Continued)

Physico-Chemical Imbalance	*Conventional Terminology*	*Closely-Related Clinical States*
Potassium Excess	Hyperkalemia	
Calcium Deficit	Hypocalcemia	Calicum deficiency leg cramps
Calcium Excess	Hypercalcemia	Pathologic fractures
Primary Base Bicarbonate Deficit	Metabolic acidosis Acidemia	Diabetic ketosis Renal acidosis
Primary Base Bicarbonate Excess	Metabolic alkalosis Alkalemia	
Primary Carbonic Acid Deficit	Respiratory alkalosis Alkalemia	Hyperventilation
Primary Carbonic Acid Excess	Respiratory acidosis Acidemia	
Protein Deficit	Hypoproteinemia Protein malnutrition	Kwashiorkor Pluri-carencial syndrome Hypoproteinosis
Magnesium Deficit	Hypomagnesemia	
Shift of Water and Electrolytes from Plasma to Interstitial Space	Hypovolemia	Shock Edema
Shift of Water and Electrolytes from Interstitial Space to Plasma	Hypervolemia	Remobilization of edema fluid

11 Help from the Lab

For some years there hung on the office wall of a friend, Dr. Alex Steigman (then Professor of Pediatrics at the University of Louisville School of Medicine), an editorial that told of a pilot who was attempting to land his airplane at a coastal airport during a heavy fog. Unknown to the pilot, the airplane's instruments, by which he was attempting to land the plane, were out of kilter. The instrument readings, therefore, conflicted with what his senses told him. He was faced with an awesome choice: believe the instruments, or believe his own God-given faculties. He chose to place his faith in the instruments; the plane plunged into the sea, and all aboard were killed. The moral that the editor drew from the tragedy was this: modern mechanistic aids are wonderful, and they frequently help us invaluably; but now and then we must choose between believing the robot and believing our own impressions.

Certainly this lesson applies to the use of laboratory findings in body fluid disturbances. We must always direct our attention to the recovery of the patient, rather than to the manipulation of his biochemical findings. The famous pediatrician, Dr. Edward Park, used to tell of the nurse whose grief over the death of an infant with diarrhea was considerably eased by the fact that, before the baby died, he had had a "beautiful stool." The "beautiful stool" was no more satisfaction to the baby than the correction of an abnormal biochemical finding would be to the patient who does not live to enjoy it. We must view the clinical picture as being of primary importance; we must regard the laboratory findings as confirmatory rather than diagnostic; we must always treat *patients* rather than *biochemical findings*. In short, we must place the clinical Dobbin before the biochemical cart, which is, of course, where he belongs. Dr. Robert E. Cook stated the matter well when he said: "Regardless of the multiplicity of laboratory determinations, proper interpretation and therapy depend nonetheless upon frequent and accurate clinical evaluation."

LIMITATIONS OF THE LABORATORY

What are some of the limitations of the laboratory? First of all, many of the usual test procedures have difficulties inherent in them that make consistently accurate results difficult to attain, even though the tests are performed by highly-skilled technicians. Moreover, physicians do not always know the "normal" laboratory values for ill persons, since our tables of values are based on those found in healthy persons. It may sometimes be undesirable—even dangerous—to attempt to restore the "abnormal" value of a patient to "normal," since what we regard as an abnormal value may be the result of a defensive action on the part of the body. For example, in primary carbonic acid deficit (respiratory alkalosis), the body lowers the level of base bicarbonate in order to maintain the carbonic acid-base bicarbonate balance. The plasma level of base bicarbonate is, therefore, lower than normal; but the normal referred to is the normal for health, not for this particular imbalance. The normal level of base bicarbonate for carbonic acid deficit is much lower than the level for health, and so to bring this properly low base bicarbonate level up to the normal level for health by the injection of base bicarbonate into the blood would make the disturbance worse and might well kill the patient.

We can cite many other examples showing

why we must take the laboratory reading with the proverbial grain of salt. For example, the level of potassium in plasma is only one indication of the cellular stores. These, of course, are far more important than the plasma level, which may be elevated in the face of a cellular deficit or depressed in the face of a cellular excess. It may, of course, be normal in either case, since the cellular stores of potassium are only one of the several factors that determine the plasma level. All that the plasma level actually shows is potassium in transport.

Another example is the state of urine, ordinarily acid in acidosis, but sometimes alkaline even though acidosis is present. This fact is demonstrated in several clinical conditions, such as chronic renal disease, in which the infecting organism converts urea in newly-formed urine to ammonia. And, although the urine is usually alkaline in alkalosis, we may find an acid urine when alkalosis is accompanied by a severe potassium deficit. Nevertheless, the physician can almost always improve diagnosis and treatment of body fluid disturbances when he has laboratory aids available. The essence of the problem is how to use the aids intelligently.

LABORATORY AIDS AVAILABLE

In addition to the chemical methods for determining the plasma levels of calcium, chloride, phosphorus, proteinate, albumin, bicarbonate, nonprotein nitrogen and urea, the *flame photometer* has been immensely useful in determining the level of sodium and potassium in body fluids. The flame photometer reading depends upon the color of the flame given out when the electrolyte in question is burned.

The *electrocardiograph* is useful in diagnosing potassium deficit, potassium excess, calcium deficit and calcium excess, although, like other laboratory tests, it is confirmatory rather than primarily diagnostic. The *x-ray*, too, is a useful diagnostic aid, helping to diagnose certain imbalances in the calcium level. An important development in laboratory techniques is the number of tests that can be performed on a small quantity—for example, a few drops of blood. These *microchemical determinations* are particularly useful in the case of the small baby, who does not have much blood to spare for laboratory tests. The use of *radioisotopes* is becoming more and more important in medicine and may soon be of value to the practicing physician as he diagnoses abnormalities of the body fluid. In addition to laboratory tests that require complex equipment, there are many tests that physicians can do in their offices, including tests to determine the acidity or specific gravity of the urine, the hemoglobin level of the blood, the red blood cell count, and the packed cell volume.

There are other measurements which are not strictly laboratory tests but which are extremely valuable, including the determination of body weight and measurements of fluid intake and fluid output. Indeed, a careful measurement of both the kind and quantity of fluids going into and passing from the patient is of utmost importance for the proper treatment of body fluid disturbances. Since the nursing staff has responsibility for the 24-hour supervision of the patient, the important duty of measuring intake and output falls to them. Basic knowledge of body fluid disturbances and their treatment makes it apparent to nurses that accurate intake-output records are often worth their weight in gold to the patient. There is usually no substitute for them, as they are often the chief basis for accurate diagnosis and effective treatment. Knowledge of intake-output figures is vital to the physician treating a patient with an imbalance of the body fluids.

EVALUATION OF TEST RESULTS

Variations in laboratory values for individuals of different ages are important considerations when evaluating the results of laboratory tests. Normal values for the red cell count, hemoglobin, packed cell volume and plasma bicarbonate differ in infants, children and adults. This is true not only for *average values*, but *normal ranges* as well; both are presented in Table 11-1. Plasma levels are best reported as milliequivalents per liter (mEq./L.), but when they are reported as milligrams (mg.), they can be quickly converted by reference to the conversion table.

A reasonable minimal daily program for laboratory surveillance of the patient should include, if facilities are available, plasma sodium, plasma

Table 11-1. Laboratory Values

I. Normal Ranges

*A. Blood Formed Elements**

	Birth	*3 mo.*	*1 yr.*	*5 yr.*	*12 yr.*	*Women*	*Men*
RBC—million/cu. mm.	4.1-5.7	3.1-4.7	3.9-4.7	4.0-4.8	4.3-5.1	4.2-5.0	4.8-6.0
Hemoglobin—Gm./100 ml.	14-20	9-13	11-12.5	12-14.7	13.4-15.8	13-16	15-18
Hematocrit—% Vol. of packed RBC/100 ml.	43-63	28-40	32-40	36-44	39-47	39-47	44-52

B. Plasma Chemical Constituents

Plasma Na^+	137-147 mEq./L.
Plasma K^+	4.0-5.6 mEq./L.
Plasma Ca^{++}	4.5-5.8 mEq./L.
Plasma Cl^-	98-106 mEq./L.
Plasma Magnesium	1.4-2.3 mEq./L.
Plasma Protein	6-8 Gm./100 ml.
Plasma HCO_3^-	Adults: 25-29 mEq./L. Children: 20-25 mEq./L.
Plasma Cl^- plus Plasma HCO_3^-	123-135 mEq./L.
Plasma pH	7.35-7.45
Plasma HPO_4^-	1.7-2.6 mEq./L.

C. Urine Values

Urine pH	4.5-8.2
Urine specific gravity	1.010-1.030

* Covers 94% of normal population.

II. Average Values in Health

A. Blood Formed Elements

	Birth	*3 mo.*	*1 yr.*	*5 yr.*	*12 yr.*	*Women*	*Men*
RBC—million/cu. mm.	4.9	3.9	4.3	4.4	4.7	4.6	5.4
Hemoglobin—Gm./100 ml.	17.1	11.1	11.7	13.3	14.5	14.5	16.5
Hematocrit—% Vol. of packed RBC/100 ml.	53	43	36	40	43	43	48

B. Plasma Chemical Constituents

Plasma Na^+	142 mEq./L.
Plasma K^+	5 mEq./L.
Plasma Ca^{++}	5 mEq./L.
Plasma Cl^-	103 mEq./L.
Plasma Magnesium	1.67 mEq./L.
Plasma Protein	7.0 Gm./100 ml. (16 mEq./L.)
Plasma HCO_3^-	Adults: 27 mEq./L. Children: 23 mEq./L.
Plasma pH	7.4
Plasma HPO_4^-	2 mEq./L.

C. Urine Values

Urine pH	6.0
Urine specific gravity	1.015

potassium, plasma bicarbonate, and plasma chloride. Initially, the hemoglobin, urinary pH and urinary specific gravity should be tested, and measurement of the plasma pH is always helpful if facilities are available for its determination. When tests are abnormal, they should be repeated daily until they return to normal. Although body weight and fluid intake-output measurements are not strictly laboratory procedures, they do provide important objective information, which helps to guard against gross over-provision of water and electrolytes. If possible, these measurements should be performed daily until fluid balance is achieved.

The ancient Hebrews must have been interested in something akin to modern laboratory diagnosis, since they had a proverb that states: "The causes of all diseases are to be found in the blood." Today, the examination of blood, particularly of plasma, and of other body fluids is invaluable in the management of the patient with body fluid disturbances.

12 The Role of Nursing Observations in the Diagnosis of Body Fluid Disturbances

FORMULATION OF NURSING DIAGNOSIS

Although her role is not diagnostic in a medical sense, the nurse must possess enough knowledge of body fluid disturbances to make an intelligent nursing diagnosis, in order to locate pertinent nursing problems. Once the problems (or potential problems) are identified, the nurse can plan for meaningful observations, measures to prevent imbalances, intelligent execution of medical directives, and other effective nursing care measures. The emphasis of this chapter is observations.

The nurse must be a careful observer in all areas of nursing—fluid balance is no exception. Changes in the patient developing a fluid imbalance are often subtle and perceptible only to those familiar with him and his condition. Thus, observations made by the nurse are particularly valuable, because she spends more time with the patient than does the physician. The observations must be planned and based on an understanding of basic physiologic processes; otherwise, they are of little or no value.

To assist in nursing diagnosis formulation, the nurse should answer the following:

1. Is there present any disease state that can disrupt body fluid balance? (For example: diabetes mellitus, emphysema, or fever) What type of imbalance does this condition usually result in? (See Table 12-1.)
2. Is the patient receiving any medication or treatment that can disrupt body fluid balance? (For example: steroids or thiazide diuretics) If so, how might this therapy upset fluid balance? (See Table 12-2.)

Table 12-1. Imbalances Likely to Occur in Various Clinical Conditions

Condition	*Imbalances Likely to Occur*	*Condition*	*Imbalances Likely to Occur*
	Acute Illnesses:		
Uncontrolled severe diabetes mellitus	Metabolic acidosis Potassium deficit	Oxygen lack with hyperpnea	Respiratory alkalosis
Adrenal insufficiency	Potassium excess	High external temperature with physiologic hyperpnea	Respiratory alkalosis
Acute pancreatitis	Calcium deficit	Fever	Respiratory alkalosis Fluid volume deficit
Perforated peptic ulcer	Plasma-to-interstitial fluid shift	Systemic infection	Metabolic acidosis Fluid volume deficit
Pneumonia (exudate blocks exchange of CO_2)	Respiratory acidosis	Acute occlusion of major artery	Plasma-to-interstitial fluid shift
Occlusion of breathing passages (inability to exchange CO_2)	Respiratory acidosis	Massive infection of subcutaneous tissues	Calcium deficit
Tracheobronchitis	Sodium excess		
	Chronic Illnesses:		
Emphysema	Respiratory acidosis	Renal disease	Metabolic acidosis Potassium excess Fluid volume excess
Asthma	Respiratory acidosis		
Congestive heart failure	Fluid volume excess	Hyperaldosteronism	Fluid volume excess Potassium deficit
Pulmonary edema	Respiratory acidosis		

Table 12-1. *(Continued)*

Condition	*Imbalances Likely to Occur*	*Condition*	*Imbalances Likely to Occur*
		Chronic Illnesses:	
Hyperparathyroidism	Calcium excess	Multiple myeloma	Calcium excess
Primary hypoparathyroidism	Calcium deficit	Gastric disease with repeated vomiting	Metabolic alkalosis Potassium deficit
Meningitis	Respiratory alkalosis		
Encephalitis	Respiratory alkalosis	Chronic alcoholism	Magnesium deficit
		Burns or Injuries:	
Burn, early	Potassium excess Plasma-to-interstitial fluid shift	Severe trauma	Protein deficit Plasma-to-interstitial fluid shift
Burn after third day	Potassium deficit Protein deficit Interstitial fluid-to-plasma shift	Fractures	Protein deficit Plasma-to-interstitial fluid shift
		Inhalation of fresh water (drowning)	Sodium deficit
Massive crushing injury	Potassium excess Plasma-to-interstitial fluid shift	Inhalation of salt water (drowning)	Sodium excess

Table 12-2. Imbalances Caused by Medical Therapy

Condition	*Imbalances Likely to Occur*	*Condition*	*Imbalances Likely to Occur*
Administration of adrenal cortical hormones	Fluid volume excess Potassium deficit Metabolic alkalosis	Excessive infusion of large molecular solution	Interstitial fluid-to-plasma shift
		Excessive administration of citrated blood	Calcium deficit
Administration of potent diuretics	Potassium deficit Sodium deficit Metabolic alkalosis	Excessive ingestion of sodium chloride	Sodium excess (if water intake is inadequate) Fluid volume excess (if water intake is adequate)
Morphine or meperidine in excessive doses	Respiratory acidosis		
Barbiturate poisoning	Respiratory acidosis	Excessive ingestion of sodium bicarbonate	Metabolic alkalosis
Oral intake of potassium exceeding renal tolerance	Potassium excess		
Early salicylate intoxication	Respiratory alkalosis	Gastric suction plus drinking water	Sodium deficit Metabolic alkalosis Potassium deficit
Salicylate intoxication (not early)	Metabolic acidosis		
Mercuric bichloride poisoning	Potassium excess	Water enemas	Sodium deficit Potassium deficit Metabolic acidosis
Excessive administration of vitamin D	Calcium excess	Recent correction of acidosis	Calcium deficit
Excessive parenteral infusion of isotonic solution of sodium chloride	Fluid volume excess Metabolic acidosis	Mechanical respirator inaccurately regulated (causing too deep or too fast breathing)	Respiratory alkalosis
Excessive parenteral administration of calcium-free solutions	Calcium deficit	Mechanical respirator inaccurately regulated (causing too shallow or too slow breathing)	Respiratory acidosis
Excessive parenteral administration of magnesium-free solutions	Magnesium deficit	Prolonged immobilization	Calcium excess
		Inhalation anesthesia	Respiratory acidosis
Excessive or too rapid parenteral administration of potassium	Potassium excess	Tight abdominal binders or dressings	Respiratory acidosis

3. Is there an abnormal loss of body fluids and, if so, from what source? What type of imbalance is usually associated with the loss of the particular body fluid or fluids? (See Table 12-3 and Table 12-4.)

4. Have any dietary restrictions been imposed? (For example: low sodium diet) If so, how might fluid balance be affected or altered in this case?

5. Has the patient taken adequate amounts of water and other nutrients orally or by some other route? If not, how long?

6. How does the total intake of fluids compare with the total fluid output?

Table 12-3. Imbalances Likely to Result from Loss of Specific Body Fluid

	Gastric Juice	*Intestinal Juice*	*Sensible Perspiration*	*Insensible Water Loss*	*Ascites*	*Wound Exudate*	*Bile*	*Pancreatic Juice*
ECF Volume Deficit	X	X	X		X	X		X
ECF Volume Excess								
Sodium Deficit	X	X	X		X	X	X	X
Sodium Excess				X				
Potassium Deficit	X	X						
Potassium Excess								
Calcium Deficit						X		X
Calcium Excess								
Magnesium Deficit	X							
Protein Deficit					X	X		
Metabolic Acidosis		X					X	X
Metabolic Alkalosis	X							
Respiratory Alkalosis								
Respiratory Acidosis								
Plasma-to-Interstitial Fluid Shift					X			
Interstitial Fluid-to-Plasma Shift								

Table 12-4. Electrolyte Content of Body Fluids Expressed in Milliequivalents per Liter

Body Fluid	*Na+*	*K+*	*Cl−*	*HCO_3−*
Saliva	9	25.8	10	10–15
(fasting) Gastric juice	60.4	9.2	84	0–14
(suction) Small bowel	111.3	4.6	104.2	31
(recent) Ileostomy	129.4	11.2	116.2	..
(adapted) Ileostomy	46	3.0	21.4	..
(fistula) Bile	148.9	4.98	100.6	40
(fistula) Pancreatic juice	141.1	4.6	76.6	121
Cecostomy	79.6	20.6	48.2	..
Urine: normal	40–90	20–60	40–120	..
abnormal	0.5–312	5–166	5–210	..
(normal) Perspiration	45	4.5	57.5	..
Plasma*	137–147	4–5.6	98–106	..
Transudates**	130–145	2.5–5	90–110	..

* *Also contains protein, 6–8 Gm./100 ml.*
** *Protein content is similar to plasma.*
Weisberg, H.: Water, Electrolyte, and Acid-Base Balance, ed. 2, p. 143. Baltimore, Williams & Wilkins, 1962.

ANTICIPATION OF FLUID IMBALANCES ASSOCIATED WITH SPECIFIC BODY FLUID LOSSES

Because the anticipation of an imbalance makes its appearance easier to detect, the nurse should learn to anticipate imbalances. It is extremely difficult to recognize significant changes in the patient when one does not know what to look for, and prevention is easier to practice when one knows which imbalance is likely to occur.

The type of imbalance (or imbalances) that accompanies the loss of a specific body fluid varies with the content of the lost fluid. The nurse can learn to anticipate specific imbalances when she knows the chief constituents of the lost fluids and how they function.

Table 12-4 lists the sodium, chloride, potassium and bicarbonate concentration of many of the body fluids.

A brief discussion of some of the body fluids and types of imbalances associated with their loss may help to clarify how the nurse can learn to anticipate fluid disturbances.

Gastric Juice

The usual daily volume of gastric juice is 2,500 ml. and the pH is usually 1 to 3, but the amount of gastric fluid can vary from 100 to 6,000 ml. in abnormal states. Gastric juice contains hydrogen (H^+), chloride (Cl^-), sodium (Na^+) and potassium (K^+) ions. Imbalances that may result from severe vomiting or prolonged gastric suction include:

1. *Extracellular Fluid Volume Deficit:* This imbalance is due to the loss of both water and electrolytes.
2. *Metabolic Alkalosis (Primary Base Bicarbonate Excess):* Alkalosis develops because H^+ and Cl^- are lost from the body. Since pH is a measure of H^+ concentration, the more H^+ present, the more acid the solution; conversely, with the loss of H^+ from the body the pH becomes more alkaline. The carbonic acid—base bicarbonate buffer system compensates for Cl^- loss by increasing the amount of HCO_3^-; thus, base bicarbonate excess develops. Because both Cl^- and HCO_3^- are anions, as the amount of Cl^- decreases, the body releases more HCO_3^- to keep the total number of anions at an appropriate balancing level. Because HCO_3^- is basic, however, the pH becomes more alkaline.
3. *Sodium Deficit:* Note in Table 12-4 that sodium is rather plentiful in gastric juice.
4. *Potassium Deficit:* There is sufficient potassium in gastric juice to result in a potassium deficit if vomiting or gastric suction is prolonged.

   Sodium is more plentiful in gastric juice than is potassium (see Table 12-4). Recall that sodium is the chief extracellular ion and that potassium is the chief cellular ion. The loss of sodium occurs more rapidly because extracellular ions move easily out of the body.
5. *Tetany (if metabolic alkalosis is present):* Although there is no loss of calcium in gastric juice, the patient may develop tetany from a deficit of *ionized* calcium. Since calcium ionization is readily influenced by pH and calcium ionization is decreased in alkalosis, the tetany accompanying alkalosis is corrected when the pH is restored to normal.
6. *Ketosis of Starvation:* Patients with gastric suction or with prolonged vomiting are usually allowed nothing by mouth. The parenteral route may supply only a fraction of the caloric need; hence the patient undergoes starvation. Ketosis results from the excessive catabolism of body fat during starvation. The accumulation of ketone bodies in the blood stream may tend to counteract metabolic alkalosis caused by loss of gastric juice, but, since ketosis is a form of acidosis, the accumulation of sufficient ketones can convert the alkalosis into acidosis.
7. *Magnesium Deficit:* Although this imbalance is rare, it can occur with the loss of gastric juice, particularly when prolonged nasogastric suction is used and magnesium-free parenteral fluids are given. There is 1 mEq./L. of magnesium in gastric juice.

Intestinal Juice

The daily volume of intestinal juice is usually about 3,000 ml. and its pH is usually alkaline. Diarrhea, intestinal suction and fistulas can result in the loss of Na^+ and HCO_3^- in excess of Cl^-. Losses from these sources can lead to:

1. *Extracellular Fluid Volume Deficit:* This imbalance is due to the loss of both water and electrolytes.
2. *Metabolic Acidosis (Primary Base Bicarbonate Deficit):* The loss of HCO_3^- is compensated for by an increase in the number of Cl^-. (As mentioned earlier, this change occurs to keep the total number of anions equal to the total number of cations in the body.) The loss of HCO_3^-, which is basic, results in acidosis.
3. *Sodium Deficit:* The amount of sodium lost from the intestines in diarrhea or intestinal suction can be great.
4. *Potassium Deficit:* This imbalance develops because relatively large amounts of potassium are lost in the secretions.

Bile

The normal daily secretion of bile is 500 ml. and the pH is alkaline. Abnormal losses of bile can occur from fistulas or from T-tube drainage following gallbladder surgery. Imbalances that can result from excessive loss of bile include:

1. *Sodium Deficit:* Note in Table 12-4 that the sodium content of bile is quite high.
2. *Metabolic Acidosis:* This imbalance develops because of the loss of HCO_3^- and the relative increase of Cl^-.

Pancreatic Juice

The normal daily secretion of pancreatic juice is 700 ml. and the pH is 8 (alkaline). Losses of pancreatic juice result in depletion of Na^+, HCO_3^- and Cl^-. The loss of HCO_3^- exceeds the loss of Cl^- because it is more plentiful in pancreatic juice (see Table 12-4), which is an integral part of intestinal secretions; thus, loss of pancreatic juice is accompanied by losses of other intestinal secretions. Imbalances that can result from pancreatic fistulas include:

1. *Metabolic Acidosis:* This imbalance occurs because the basic ion, HCO_3^-, is lost in excess of Cl^-.
2. *Sodium Deficit*
3. *Calcium Deficit*
4. *Decrease in Extracellular Fluid Volume*

Sensible Perspiration

Excessive sweating due to fever or to high environmental temperature can result in large losses of water, sodium and chloride. Normally, sweat is a hypotonic fluid containing sodium, chloride, potassium, ammonia and urea. Severe perspiration can lead to:

1. *Sodium Deficit:* This is especially apt to occur when plain water is ingested in large amounts after profuse sweating, replacing the lost water but not the electrolytes.
2. *Sodium Excess:* This imbalance can occur if the heavily perspiring individual has an inadequate water supply. The sodium concentration in sweat averages around 50-80 mEq./L. (considerably less than the sodium content of plasma). Thus, proportionately more water than sodium is lost in sweat and results in a relative plasma sodium increase. If water intake is deficient, plasma sodium elevates further.
3. *Extracellular Fluid Volume Deficit:* Both water and electrolytes are lost in sweat, and an imbalance may result if there is no provision for fluid intake.

Insensible Water Loss

The insensible loss of water without solute through the lungs and skin is normally about 600 to 1,000 ml. daily and is increased by anything that accelerates metabolism. For example, the increase in insensible water loss is roughly 50 to 75 ml. per degree of Fahrenheit temperature elevation for a 24-hour period.

Increased respiratory activity causes an increased loss of water vapor by way of the lungs.

Damage to the skin's surface also results in loss.

Increased insensible water loss can lead to:

1. *Water Deficit (Dehydration)*: Because only water is lost by means of the insensible route, water deficit results.
2. *Sodium Excess:* A loss of water alone results in an increased concentration of sodium in the extracellular fluid.

Large Open Wounds

Considerable quantities of water, electrolytes and protein are lost in the drainage from large open wounds. Such drainage has a composition similar to plasma. (Note the similarity between transudates and plasma in Table 12-4.) Severe losses from wound drainage can lead to:

1. *Protein Deficit*
2. *Sodium Deficit*
3. *Fluid Volume Deficit*

Ascites

Ascites is the accumulation of fluid within the abdominal cavity. The composition of ascitic fluid is similar to plasma; the amount varies, but occasionally as much as 20 L. can form in a week, creating an enormous loss of protein. The accumulation of large quantities of ascitic fluid requires periodic paracentesis, which can result in considerable losses of protein and electrolytes, sometimes leading to sodium deficit. Ascites can lead to:

1. *Protein Deficit*
2. *Sodium Deficit*
3. *Plasma-to-Interstitial Fluid Shift:* This imbalance may be serious if the formation of ascites is rapid.
4. *Fluid Volume Deficit*

PLANNED NURSING OBSERVATIONS RELATED TO BODY FLUID DISTURBANCES

The following summary of familiar nursing routines will show how meaningful observations can reveal a wealth of information concerning the patient's fluid balance status.

When the nurse detects significant symptoms, she can relay them to the physician, thus facilitating early diagnosis and treatment. The ability to sort out observations demanding urgent action comes with a working understanding of fluid balance and experience in applying this knowledge. The tables presented in this section refer to symptoms and the diagnoses that they may possibly indicate.

Body Temperature

Usually the body temperature is checked at least twice daily, and when indicated, every 4 hours or oftener. Fever causes an increase in metabolism and thus in formed metabolic wastes, which require fluid to make a solution for renal excretion; in this way, fluid loss is increased. Fever also causes hyperpnea, an increase in breathing resulting in extra water vapor loss via the lungs. Because fever increases loss of body fluids, it is important that temperature elevations be reported and appropriate orders be sought.

Changes in the temperature of the extremities may be noted by touch; external skin temperature gives some insight into the state of peripheral circulation.

Table 12-5. Significance of Body Temperature Variations

Symptom	*Imbalance Indicated by Symptom*
Depressed body temperature	Fluid volume deficit Sodium depletion
Elevated body temperature	Sodium excess (excessive water loss)
Extremities cold to touch	Plasma-to-interstitial fluid shift Profound sodium depletion Profound fluid volume deficit

Pulse

The pulse should be evaluated in terms of rate, volume, regularity and ease of obliteration. The average rate for the adult at rest is 70 to 80 beats per minute. When abnormalities are noted, the pulse should be checked for a full minute. It is wise to observe it for no less than 30 seconds even though the patient does not appear to be seriously ill; a shorter period might not reveal an irregularity. (Variables that may have influenced the pulse, such as activity and emotional upsets, should be considered.)

The pulse should be checked whenever the temperature is taken, more often if indicated, and the nurse should check the pulses of all seriously ill patients whenever she makes rounds.

Because the nurse often delegates TPRs to auxiliary personnel, it is important to teach them the importance of observing pulse volume and regularity as well as pulse rate. (See Table 12-6 for possible implications of pulse variations.)

Table 12-6. Significance of Pulse Variations

Symptom	*Imbalance Indicated by Symptom*
Weak, irregular, rapid pulse	Severe potassium deficit
Weak, irregular, slowing pulse	Severe potassium excess
Increased pulse rate	Sodium excess Magnesium deficit
Decreased pulse rate	Magnesium excess
Bounding pulse (not easily obliterated)	Fluid volume excess Interstitial fluid-to-plasma shift
Bounding, easily obliterated pulse	Impending circulatory collapse
Rapid, weak, thready pulse, easily obliterated	Circulatory collapse Sodium deficit Hemorrhage Plasma-to-interstitial fluid shift
Decrease in pulse volume on changing position	Impending circulatory collapse Sodium deficit

Respiration

The nurse should become skilled in observing respiration for indications of body pH changes, as the lungs play a major role in regulating body pH by varying the amount of carbon dioxide retention.

In order to detect variations from normal, the nurse must evaluate respiration in terms of rate, depth, and regularity and be familiar with the respiratory changes accompanying both metabolic alkalosis and metabolic acidosis.

Severe metabolic alkalosis affects all aspects of breathing: (1) the rate is decreased; (2) the depth is shallow; (3) the respiratory pattern is disrupted by periods of apnea lasting from 5 to 30 seconds. Note that the lungs attempt to compensate for the alkalosis by retaining carbon dioxide. (Slow, shallow respiration favors carbon dioxide retention.)

Severe metabolic acidosis affects primarily the rate and depth of breathing: (1) the breathing rate is increased and may be as fast as 50 per minute; (2) depth is greatly increased. The increased volume of lung ventilation is striking; all of the respiratory accessory muscles are used to increase the capacity of the thorax. Note that the lungs attempt to compensate for the acidosis by "blowing off" carbon dioxide. (Fast, deep respiration favors a loss of carbon dioxide from the lungs.)

Usually, respiration is observed for 30 seconds and multiplied by two for a full minute's count; when abnormalities are noted, respiration should be observed for two full minutes. More accurate results are obtained if the patient is unaware that his breathing is being observed. Variable factors, such as increased activity or emotional upsets, may influence respiration.

Respiration is checked routinely when temperatures are taken and more often if indicated. Again, because auxiliary personnel frequently take TPRs, the importance of observing depth and rhythm as well as rate should be impressed upon them. The nurse should make it a practice to observe the respiration of seriously ill patients when she makes rounds.

Other factors related to fluid balance may also influence respiration. (See Table 12-7.)

Blood Pressure

Blood pressure measurement is usually taken over the brachial artery. Normal adults have an average systolic pressure of 90 to 145 mm. Hg and an average diastolic pressure of 60 to 90 mm. Hg. The pulse pressure (difference between systolic

Table 12-7. Significance of Variations in Breathing

Symptom	*Imbalance Indicated by Symptom*
Shallow, slightly irregular, slow breathing	Metabolic alkalosis
Shortness of breath on mild exertion (in absence of cardiopulmonary disease)	Mild metabolic acidosis
Deep rapid breathing (close observation reveals an effort with expiration)	Metabolic acidosis
Shortness of breath (in absence of cardiopulmonary disease)	Fluid volume excess
Moist rales (at first, heard only with stethoscope)	Fluid volume excess Interstitial fluid-to-plasma shift Pulmonary edema
Shallow breathing (secondary to weakness or paralysis of respiratory muscles)	Potassium deficit (severe) Potassium excess (severe)
Respiratory stridor	Calcium deficit (severe)
Severe dyspnea	Acute pulmonary edema

and diastolic pressures) is usually between 30 to 50 mm. Hg. The systolic pressure indicates the pressure within the blood vessels when the heart is in systole, whereas the diastolic indicates the pressure when it is in diastole. Pulse pressure varies directly with cardiac output.

Blood pressure variations are immensely helpful in evaluating body fluid disturbances and should be used often as a means of evaluation when there is a real or potential water and electrolyte balance problem. When an abnormal reading is obtained, it is wise to check the pressure in both arms. Variables that may influence blood pressure, such as increased activity, position change and emotional upsets, should be considered.

The physician may order blood pressure checks at regular intervals, or he may request them when special situations arise, such as a surgical procedure or the development of new symptoms. Symptoms such as dizziness while standing, sudden apprehension, or a weak pulse are indications to check the blood pressure.

Infrequently the nurse may notice an unusual reaction while checking the blood pressure of a patient with calcium deficit, wherein tightening of the blood pressure cuff to systolic pressure for 3 minutes may elicit a spasmodic reaction in which the hand assumes a clawlike position. (See Table 12-8 for possible implications of blood pressure variations.)

Table 12-8. Significance of Blood Pressure Variations

Symptom	*Imbalance Indicated by Symptom*
Hypotension	Sodium deficit Plasma-to-interstitial fluid shift Contracted plasma volume due to hemorrhage Severe potassium deficit or excess Magnesium excess Late interstitial fluid-to-plasma shift
Hypertension	Early interstitial fluid-to-plasma shift Fluid volume excess Magnesium deficit
Normal blood pressure while patient is flat in bed—hypotension and syncope develops when head of bed elevated	Contracted plasma volume Impending circulatory collapse Sodium deficit

Peripheral Veins

Observation of peripheral veins can be helpful in evaluating the patient's plasma volume. Usually, elevation of the hands causes the hand veins to empty in 3 to 5 seconds; placing the hands in a dependent position causes the veins to fill in 3 to 5 seconds. (See Figures 12-1, 12-2.)

A decreased plasma volume causes the hand veins to take longer than 3 to 5 seconds to fill when the hands are in a dependent position. The decreased plasma volume may be secondary to an extracellular fluid volume deficit or to a shift of fluid from the plasma to the interstitial space. The veins are not readily apparent when plasma volume is reduced. The slow filling of hand veins often precedes hypotension when the patient is in the early stage of shock.

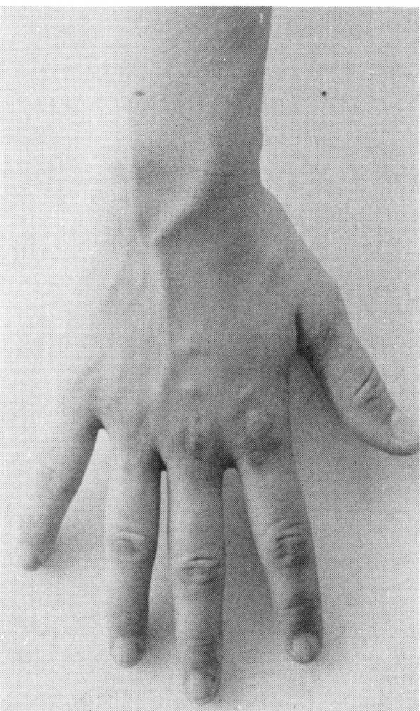

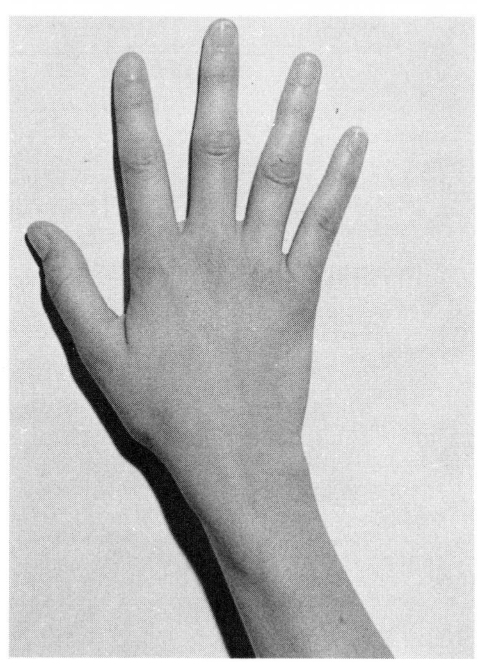

Fig. 12-1. (*Left*) Appearance of hand veins when the hand is held in a dependent position.

Fig. 12-2. (*Right*) Appearance of hand veins when the hand is held in an elevated position.

An increased plasma volume causes the hand veins to take longer than 3 to 5 seconds to empty when the hands are elevated. The increased plasma volume may be secondary to an increased extracellular fluid volume or to a shift of fluid from the interstitial space into the vascular compartment. When this is the case, the peripheral veins are engorged and clearly visible.

Skin and Mucous Membranes

Changes in skin elasticity and in mucous membrane moisture are important for evaluation of changes in fluid volume and electrolyte concentration, as pointed out in previous chapters.

A dry mouth may be due to a fluid volume deficit or may be due to mouth breathing. When in doubt, the nurse should run her finger along the oral cavity and feel the mucous membrane where the cheek and gum meet; dryness in this area indicates a true fluid volume deficit. (See Table 12-9 for possible implications of skin and mucous membrane variations.)

Table 12-9. Significance of Skin and Mucous Membrane Variations

Symptom	*Imbalance Indicated by Symptom*
Poor skin turgor	Fluid volume deficit
Dry mucous membranes with longitudinal wrinkles on tongue	Fluid volume deficit
Dry sticky mucous membranes with rough, red, dry tongue	Sodium excess
Flushed, dry skin	Sodium excess
Pallor of skin	Protein deficit Interstitial fluid-to-plasma shift Plasma-to-interstitial fluid shift
Cold, clammy skin	Sodium deficit Plasma-to-interstitial fluid shift
Pitting edema	Fluid volume excess
Fingerprinting on sternum	Sodium deficit

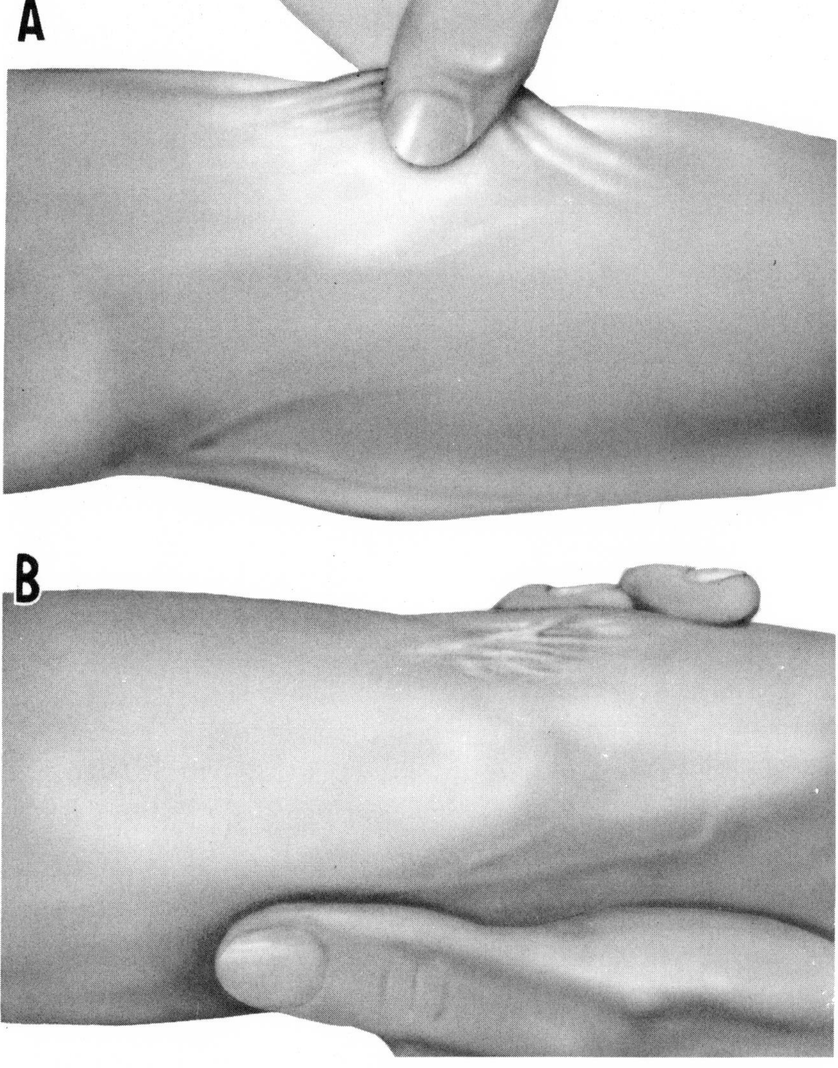

Fig. 12-3. (A & B). Poor skin turgor. (Moyer, C. A.: Fluid Balance, A Clinical Manual. p. 71. Chicago, Year Book Pub., 1952)

In a normal person, pinched skin will fall back to its normal position when released. In an individual with fluid volume deficit, the skin may remain slightly raised for many seconds. (See Figure 12-3, Parts A and B.) In part A, the skin of the forearm is picked up; in part B, 30 seconds later, the skin has not returned to its normal position. The patient in this instance is a young man with moderately severe extracellular fluid volume deficit.

Phonation

Speech variations can be significant in the evaluation of the patient's state of water and electrolyte balance, and so the nurse should observe for the presence of subtle changes in quality, content and formation of speech.

Hoarseness may indicate extracellular fluid volume excess, whereas irrelevant, hyperactive speech may be indicative of potassium deficit.

Difficulty in forming words can be secondary to dry mucous membranes, or it may be due to a generalized muscular weakness. (See Table 12-10 for possible implications of speech changes.)

Table 12-10. Significance of Speech Changes

Symptom	*Imbalance Indicated by Symptom*
Difficulty in forming words without first moistening mouth	Sodium excess Fluid volume deficit
Hoarseness	Fluid volume excess
Hyperactivity of speech with tendency to irrelevancy	Potassium deficit
Difficulty in speaking due to muscular weakness or paralysis	Severe potassium deficit Severe potassium excess
Voice change—progresses to a crowing noise associated with dyspnea (laryngospasm)	Severe calcium deficit

Fatigue Threshold

Many factors contribute to a low fatigue threshold, but those related to fluid balance may include deficits in extracellular fluid volume, potassium, sodium and protein. The nurse should compare the patient's activities and fatigue level with that of previous days to note significant changes. Episodes of muscular weakness, fatigability, and diminution of stamina and endurance should be noted—the latter symptoms are particularly descriptive of potassium deficit.

Facial Appearance

A patient with a severe extracellular fluid volume deficit has a drawn facial expression; the eyes are sunken and feel much less firm than normal.

A patient with an excess of extracellular fluid may have puffy eyelids and the cheeks may appear fuller than usual.

Behavior

Behavior changes may be indicative of water and electrolyte disturbances. (See Table 12-11 for possible implications of behavior changes.)

These changes are subtle at first and often the patient's family is the first to notice them. The attitude of the patient toward his illness is significant; a severely depleted patient is usually aware that he is seriously ill. Aged patients are particularly prone to develop personality changes and impaired mental function with fluid imbalances, because their homeostatic mechanisms do not normally function as efficiently as those of younger persons.

Table 12-11. Significance of Behavior Changes

Symptom	*Imbalance Indicated by Symptom*
Lassitude and indifference	Fluid volume deficit Sodium deficit
Apathy and weakness	Potassium deficit
Emotional depression	Protein deficit Magnesium deficit
Carphologia (picking at bedclothes)	Potassium deficit Magnesium deficit
Irritability, apprehension, and extreme restlessness	Potassium excess
Apprehension and giddiness	Sodium deficit
Apprehension	Plasma-to-interstitial fluid shift
Hallucinations (particularly visual)	Magnesium deficit
Hallucinations and delirium (may become maniacal)	Severe sodium excess
Hallucinations and delusions	Sodium deficit
Disorientation and confusion	Respiratory acidosis Severe potassium deficit Magnesium deficit
Stupor progressing to unconsciousness	Profound alkalosis Profound acidosis Profound shock

Skeletal Muscles

Usually the condition of skeletal muscles is readily observable by the nurse. Subjective complaints from the patient, such as weakness or cramping, should be noted. (See Table 12-12 for possible implications of symptoms related to skeletal muscles.)

Table 12-12. Significance of Skeletal Muscle Changes

Symptom	*Imbalance Indicated by Symptom*
Hypotonus	Potassium deficit Calcium excess
Flabbiness	Potassium deficit Protein deficit
Flaccid paralysis	Potassium deficit (severe) Potassium excess (severe)
Hypertonus: a. Chvostek's sign* may be positive b. Tremors in mild deficit c. Convulsions in severe deficit	 Calcium deficit Alkalosis (decreased calcium ionization) Magnesium deficit
Cramping of exercised muscles	Calcium deficit
Muscle rigidity (particularly in limbs and abdominal wall)	Calcium deficit
Carpopedal spasm	Calcium deficit

** Chvostek's sign is a local spasm following a tap on the side of the face.*

Table 12-13. Significance of Sensation Changes

Symptom	*Imbalance Indicated by Symptom*
Tingling of ends of fingers and toes; circumoral paresthesia	Calcium deficit Alkalosis (decreased calcium ionization)
Light-headedness	Respiratory alkalosis
Abdominal cramps	Sodium deficit Potassium excess
Painful muscle cramps	Calcium deficit Potassium deficit
Numb, dead feeling—particularly in extremities (precedes flaccid paralysis)	Potassium deficit Potassium excess
Numbness of extremities	Calcium deficit
Nausea	Calcium excess Potassium excess Potassium deficit
Deep bony pain	Calcium excess
Flank pain	Calcium excess
Tinnitus	Respiratory alkalosis
Abnormal sensitivity to sound	Magnesium deficit

Sensation

Patients with water and electrolyte imbalances frequently report changes in sensation. Some of the more common sensation changes are listed in Table 12-13.

Desire for Food and Water

ANOREXIA The patient's interest in food and water is useful in evaluating his body fluid status. Anorexia is common in potassium deficit and in protein deficit. Many fluid imbalances are accompanied by nausea, vomiting, and anorexia.

THIRST Thirst is a subjective sensory symptom and has been defined as an awareness of the desire to drink.

The desire to drink can be initiated by cellular dehydration, which may accompany (1) a decreased extracellular fluid volume or (2) a hypertonic extracellular fluid such as occurs with intravenous administration of excessive amounts of hypertonic salt solution, with or without extracellular fluid volume excess.

Cellular dehydration will occur when the body's water needs are not met. Gamble has estimated the daily water requirement of the adult at rest as 1,500 ml. Butler and his associates cite a somewhat higher figure, 1,500 ml. per square meter of body surface per day. These figures are minimal, since the average active adult, not ill, requires from 2,000 to 3,000 ml. of water per day, including 1,000 to 1,500 ml. for insensible perspiration and 1,000 to 1,500 ml. for urine excretion. Among the conditions that can increase the requirement for water are:

- Fever
- Excessive perspiration
- Abnormal loss of fluids from vomiting, diarrhea, intestinal suction, and fistulas
- Hyperthyroidism or any other cause of increased metabolic rate
- Diminished renal concentrating ability, such as occurs in old age

Of interest in this connection is the comparison of the water needs in patients with no complications with those of patients with increased water loss, as shown in Table 12-14.

Table 12-14. Calculation of Daily Water Requirements

	cc. Average Variation
Uncomplicated Cases:	
For vaporization	1,000 – 1,500
For urine	1,000 – 1,500
	2,000 – 3,000
Complicated Cases (sepsis, elevation of temperature, humid weather, renal disease):	
For vaporization	2,000 – 2,500
For urine	1,000 – 1,500
	3,000 – 4,000
Seriously Ill Patients With Drainage:	
For vaporization	2,000
For urine	1,000
For replacement of body fluid losses:	
1,000 ml. bile	1,000
3,000 ml. Wangensteen	3,000
	7,000

Wohl, M., and Goodhart, R.: Modern Nutrition in Health and Disease, ed. 3, p. 1055. Philadelphia, Lea and Febiger, 1964.

The nurse should constantly remember how important it is to meet the daily water requirement of the patient, by keeping accurate records of his intake and output, and by carefully observing the patient for signs of water deficit.

Thirst is often caused by dryness of the mouth resulting from decreased salivary flow, which can be caused by extracellular fluid volume deficit. In this case, true thirst exists. Decreased salivary flow can also be caused by administration of atropine, in which case, there is a desire to relieve the unpleasant dry sensation, but no true thirst.

Thirst is not always a reliable indicator of need and should not be the sole factor influencing fluid intake. The aged patient often does not recognize thirst and, even if he does, may be too weak to reach his water supply. Confusion or aphasia may stop him from making known his desire to drink. Patients with fluid volume excess due to cardiac and renal damage are sometimes quite thirsty; a problem in this situation is to meet their need without adding to their fluid overload, and the nurse must use caution in allowing patients to ingest as much water as they desire. Seriously burned patients experience great thirst; if allowed to drink all the water they desire, serious sodium deficit will develop. Thirst in the burned patient should be met with specially prepared oral electrolyte solutions. (See Table 12-15 for implications of changes in desire for food and water.)

Table 12-15. Significance of Changes in Desire for Food and Water

Symptom	*Imbalance Indicated by Symptom*
Anorexia	Potassium deficit Protein deficit Calcium excess
Thirst	Sodium excess (hypertonic extracellular fluid) Blood volume deficit due to hemorrhage Blood volume deficit due to acute heart failure Calcium excess (hypertonic extracellular fluid)
Absence of thirst	Sodium deficit (hypotonic extracellular fluid)

Character and Volume of Urine

SPECIFIC GRAVITY OF URINE To maintain fluid and osmolar balance, the kidneys must be able to dilute and concentrate urine. The specific gravity test is a convenient and simple method for evaluation of the kidneys' ability to perform this function.

The specific gravity of urine is its weight compared with the weight of an equal volume of distilled water; it indicates the amount of dissolved solids in the urine. The specific gravity of distilled water is 1.000; the specific gravity of urine, in health, ranges from 1.003 to 1.030. The higher the solute content of urine, the higher the specific gravity.

The chief urinary solutes are nitrogenous end-products (urea), sodium and chloride; others include potassium, phosphate, sulfate and ammonia. Urinary solutes are mainly derived from ingested foods and from metabolism of endogenous protein and other substances. Diet, then, influences specific gravity of the urine. The usual diet supplies approximately 50 Gm. of urinary solutes in 24 hours. Patients on low sodium or low protein diets cannot concentrate urine to high levels because they are ingesting an inadequate amount of solute. The inability of the patient eating a normal diet to concentrate urine is an indication of renal disease.

The patient's state of hydration can be assessed by measuring specific gravity, provided the kidneys are healthy. A highly concentrated urine implies water deficit; a dilute urine implies adequate hydration or possibly over-hydration.

Urine specific gravity measurement can help differentiate between the scanty urinary output of acute renal failure and that of water deficit. In acute renal failure, the specific gravity is fixed at a low level (1.010 to 1.012); in water deficit, the specific gravity is high.

The nurse may be asked to measure the urinary specific gravity of patients with burns, renal disease, cardiovascular disease, febrile conditions and general surgical conditions. She should keep the following points in mind:

1. The nurse should be familiar with the equipment used to test the specific gravity of urine:
   a. The apparatus used for the test consists of two parts—the cylinder to contain the urine, and the urinometer. (See Figure 12-4.)
   b. Note that the urinometer is calibrated in units of .001, beginning with 1.000 at the top and progressing downward to 1.060. A urinometer is read from top to bottom. (See Figure 12-5.)
   c. New urinometers should be checked for accuracy against distilled water before use, and rechecked from time to time thereafter—even a slight discrepancy can be significant.
2. The urine sample must be fresh.
3. The urine sample must be well mixed—remember, the specific gravity test measures solute concentration and a uniform solution must be used to yield an accurate reading.
4. The cylinder should be filled ¾ of the way with urine.
5. After the urinometer is placed in the cylinder, it is given a gentle spin with the thumb and forefinger to prevent it from adhering to the cylinder's sides. (See Figure 12-4.)
6. Should there be an insufficient amount of urine to float the urinometer, the reading cannot be made. In such an event, *q.n.s.* (quantity not sufficient) is charted.
7. To read specific gravity, it is necessary that the urinometer be at eye level. It is read by imagining a line where the lower portion of the meniscus crosses the scale on the urinometer. (See Figure 12-6.)

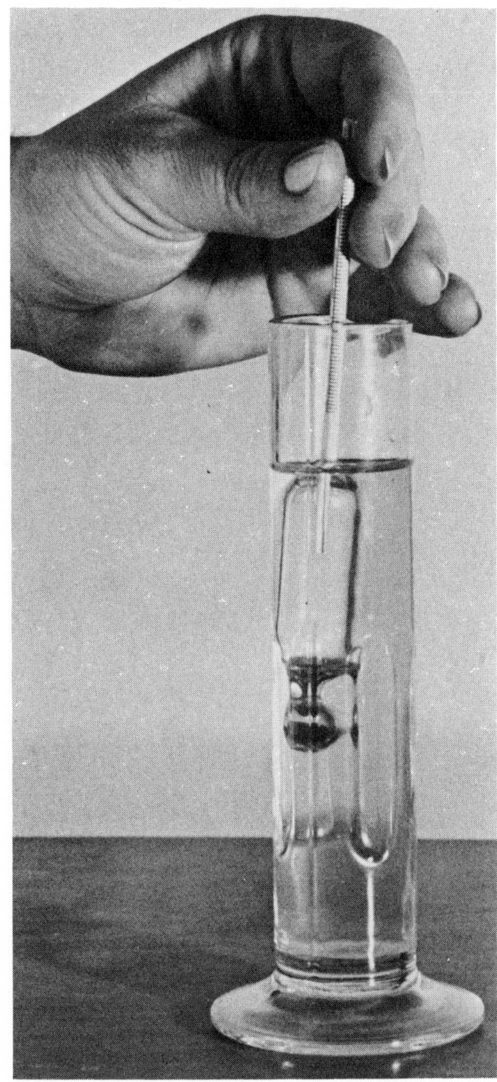

Fig. 12-4. Urinometer.

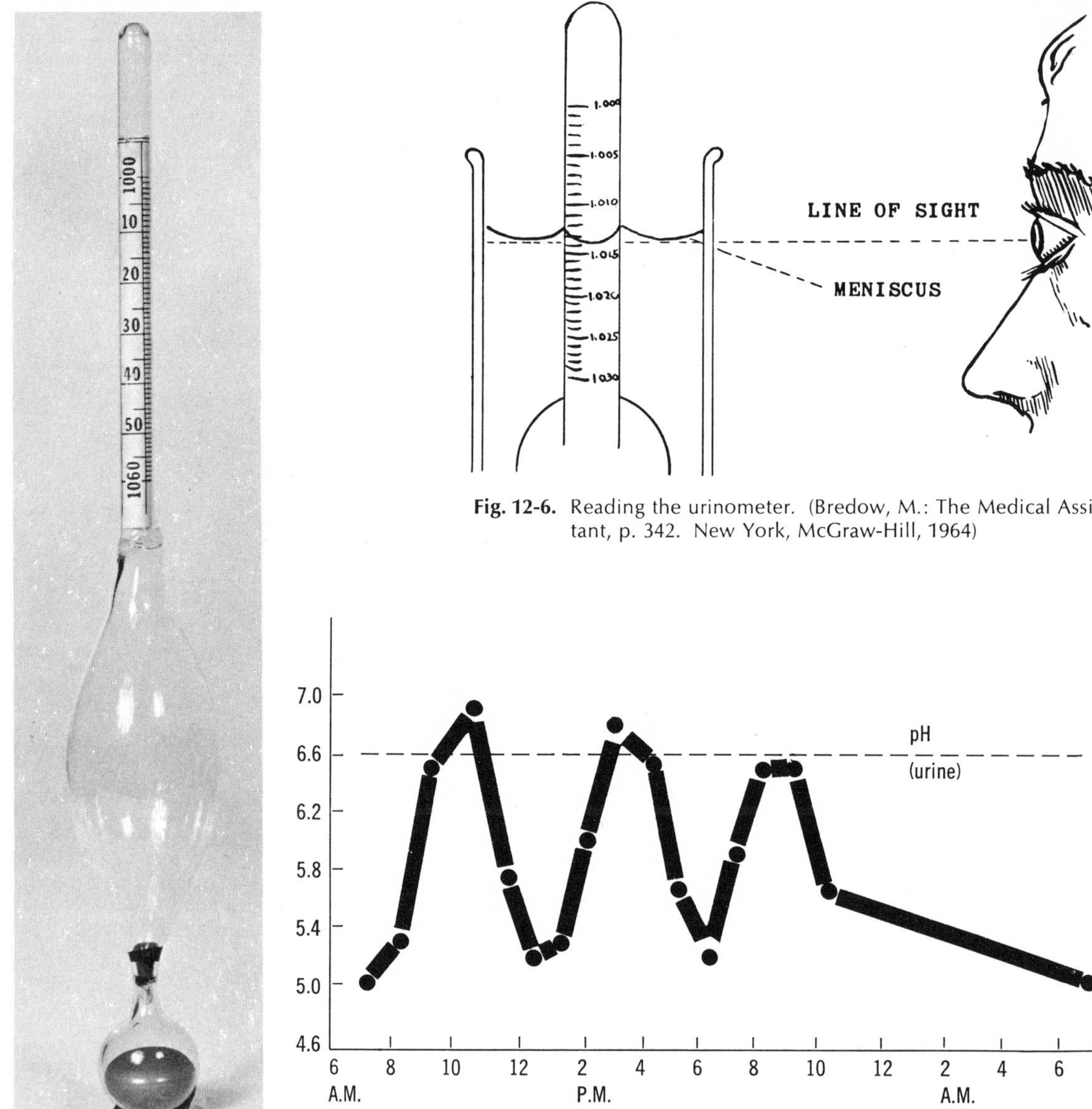

Fig. 12-5. Urinometer Scale.

Fig. 12-6. Reading the urinometer. (Bredow, M.: The Medical Assistant, p. 342. New York, McGraw-Hill, 1964)

Fig. 12-7. Daily fluctuations of urinary pH. (Pictoclinic, 9:6, No. 6, Ames Co., Elkhart, Indiana, 1962)

The results of specific gravity tests are evaluated in relation to other clinical signs shown by the patient. (See Table 12-16 for conditions that may cause low or high specific gravity of urine.)

pH OF URINE The kidneys play a major role in maintaining the acid-base balance in the body, by excreting electrolytes that are not required and by retaining those that are needed in the body. When an acid factor is in excess, the kidneys excrete hydrogen ions and conserve basic ions; when an alkaline factor is in excess, the kidneys excrete basic ions and retain hydrogen ions.

Urinary pH tests measure the hydrogen ion concentration in urine, and because the excreted electrolytes vary according to the body's need,

Table 12-16. Conditions Associated With Persistently Low or High Urinary Specific Gravity

Low Specific Gravity (1.010 or less)	Sodium deficit: Drinking large quantities of water Excessive parenteral administration of electrolyte-free solutions Severely restricted dietary intake of sodium chloride Diuresis from potent diuretics Diabetes insipidus (deficiency of antidiuretic hormone) Renal disease: Acute renal failure Pyelonephritis Hydronephrosis Severe potassium deficiency Calcium excess
High Specific Gravity (1.030 or higher)	Sodium excess: Decreased water intake Excessive loss of water Excessive ingestion of sodium chloride Glycosuria

the urinary pH can range widely (from 4.5 to 8.0) and still be within normal limits. However, the pooled daily urine output averages around 6. Several factors may cause normal fluctuations in urinary pH.

1. Sleep causes urine to become highly acid, as respiration is depressed during sleep and a mild state of respiratory acidosis is induced. (Shallow respiration favors retention of carbon dioxide, and an increase in the acid side of the carbonic acid:base bicarbonate ratio.) Note the low pH during the night hours in Figure 12-7. A rise in pH usually occurs upon awakening.
2. A rise in pH usually occurs following meals, since they stimulate the production of hydrochloric acid, a process causing hydrogen ions to be extracted from the blood. The type of food ingested affects pH. (See Table 14-5 for the acid-base reactions of various foods). Note the rise in pH following meals in Figure 12-7.
3. Certain drugs significantly alter urinary pH. Drugs that cause urine to become more acid include ammonium chloride, methenamine mandelate (Mandelamine), or sodium acid phosphate, and those that can cause urine to become alkaline include alkaline salts, such as sodium bicarbonate or potassium citrate.

In spite of the variables that influence urinary pH, most random urine samples show a pH of less than 6.6.

The nurse may be asked to perform urinary pH tests at the bedside for patients with a variety of metabolic disorders. Table 12-17 lists conditions in which urine is persistently acid or alkaline.

Several simple methods may be used by the nurse to measure urinary pH:

1. *Squibb Nitrazine Paper:* Nitrazine paper consists of a chemical (sodium dinitro-

Table 12-17. Clinical Conditions Associated With Persistently Acid or Alkaline Urine

Symptom	*Imbalance Indicated by Symptom*
Acid Urine	Metabolic acidosis: Diabetic acidosis Ketosis of starvation Severe diarrhea Respiratory acidosis: Emphysema Asthma Metabolic alkalosis accompanied by severe potassium deficit
Alkaline Urine	Metabolic alkalosis: Excessive ingestion of alkalis Severe vomiting Respiratory alkalosis: Oxygen lack Fever with its hyperpnea Primary hyperaldosteronism Acidosis accompanied by the following clinical conditions: *Chronic renal infection,* in which the infecting organism converts urea in newly-formed urine to ammonia *Milkman's syndrome,* a severe chronic acidosis apparently secondary to renal tubular dysfunction *Fanconi's syndrome,* a form of chronic acidosis secondary to renal tubular dysfunction *Sulfanilamide intoxication* secondary to renal tubular dysfunction *Pharmacologic alkalinuria* produced by a carbonic anhydrase inhibitor [such as acetazolamide (Diamox) or chlorothiazide (Diuril)] *Persistent acidosis* secondary to renal tubular dysfunction in infants

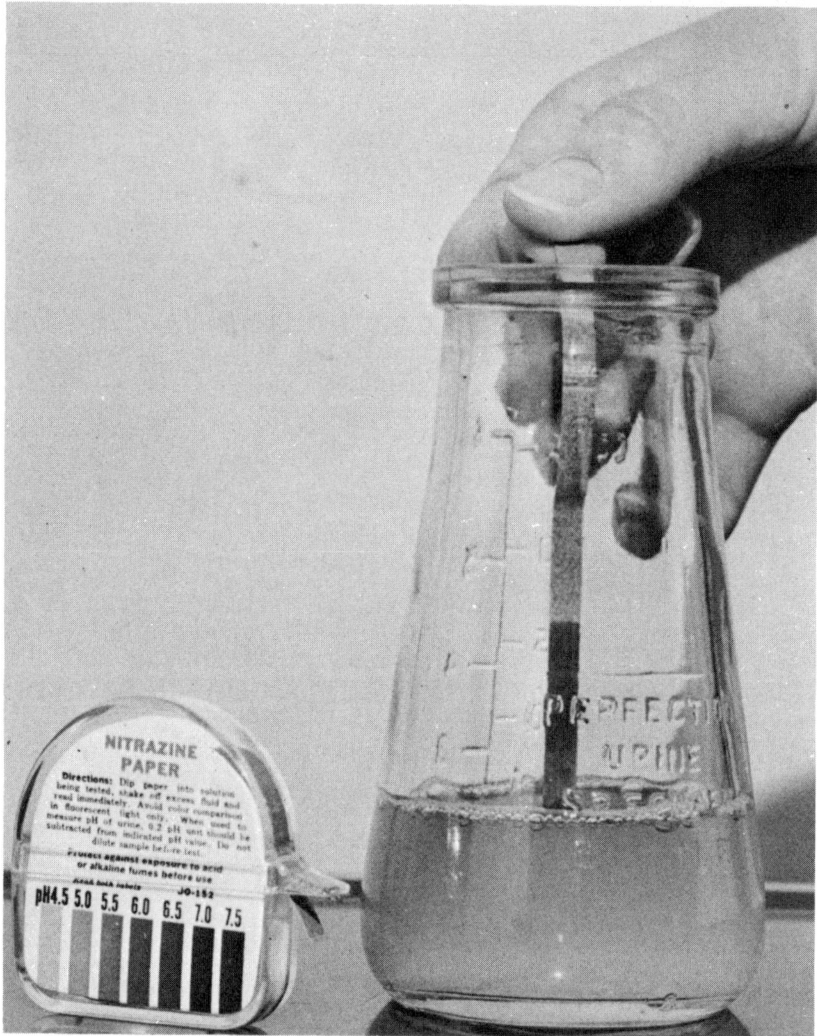

Fig. 12-8. Measuring urinary pH with Nitrazine paper.

phenolazonaphthol disulfonate) impregnated in cellulose. When Nitrazine paper is dipped into urine, a chemical change takes place that causes the paper to change color. The color can vary from yellow to blue and is matched against the scale on the paper dispenser. The color changes correspond to specific pH levels ranging from 4.5 to 7.5. (See Figure 12-8.) The nurse should keep the following points in mind while performing this test:

A. Only fresh urine should be used. (When urine is allowed to set for a time, urea breaks down into ammonia and the pH becomes more alkaline.)
B. The paper should be well moistened with urine but should not be left in the urine more than a few seconds—excessive fluid can wash away the chemicals from the paper.
C. After the paper has been dipped into the urine, the excess urine should be shaken off and the reading made immediately.

D. The color comparison between the Nitrazine paper and the color scale on the dispenser should be made in a good light—avoid color comparison in pure fluorescent light.

2. *Ames Combistix Dip Sticks:* Combistix is a dip-and-read combination test for urine protein, glucose and pH. Barriers are impregnated in the dipstick to separate the three areas; otherwise, the chemicals from each portion would run together when moistened. The pH portion of the reagent strip is impregnated with methyl red and bromthymol blue. When dipped into urine, a color change takes place. The color varies from orange to blue and represents a pH range of from 5 to 9. The nurse should keep the following points in mind while performing this test:
   A. Only fresh urine should be used.
   B. Care should be taken to prevent excessive urine from washing chemicals from the other portions of the reagent strip onto the pH portion.

Regardless of the type of test used, it is important that the nurse read the manufacturer's directions carefully. Accurate results can be expected only when instructions are followed as directed.

CHANGES IN URINARY VOLUME Generally speaking, urinary output can safely range from 25 to 500 ml. per hour. The nurse should report hourly output below 25 ml. or above 500 ml., also an output of less than 500 ml. in a 24-hour period.

The expected urinary volume varies with each patient and is influenced by many factors.

Urine volume is dependent on:

1. The amount of fluid intake
2. Water needs of the lungs, skin, and gastrointestinal tract
3. The amount of waste products to be excreted by the kidneys
4. The ability of the kidneys to concentrate urine
5. Blood volume
6. Hormonal influences
7. Age

Table 12-18. 24-Hour Average Intake and Output of Water in an Adult

Intake		*Output*	
Oral liquids	1,300 ml.	Urine	1,500 ml.
Water in food	1,000 ml.	Stool	200 ml.
Water of oxidation	300 ml.	Insensible:	
		Lungs	300 ml.
		Skin	600 ml.
Total	2,600 ml.	Total	2,600 ml.

Bland, J.: Clinical Metabolism of Body Water and Electrolytes, p. 48. Philadelphia, Saunders, 1963.

Fluid Intake

1. In health, urinary volume is approximately equal to the volume of liquids taken into the body—this rule does not hold true in illness. (See Table 12-18.)
2. A large intake of liquids causes a large urinary output; a small intake causes a small urinary output.
3. Adults usually pass between 1,000 to 1,500 ml. of urine in 24 hours. (Most persons void 5 to 10 times during the waking hours; each voiding is usually between 100 to 300 ml.)

Water Needs of the Lungs, the Skin, and the Gastrointestinal Tract

1. Water is available for urine formation only after the needs of the skin, the lungs and the gastrointestinal tract have been met.
2. Excessive sweating causes a decreased urinary volume—daily urinary volume is several hundred ml. less in the summer.
3. Increased water loss from the lungs occurs with hyperpnea—this loss can cause a reduction in the urinary volume.
4. Excessive losses of fluid in vomiting and diarrhea can also cause a decreased urinary volume.

Amount of Waste Products to Be Excreted

1. Under most circumstances, urine volume varies directly with the urinary solute load —a solute excess causes an increased need for water excretion.

2. Excessive fluid loss may occur as the result of the increased solute loads found in diabetes mellitus, thyrotoxicosis, fever and response to stress.
3. A decreased solute load causes a decreased urinary volume.

Ability of the Kidneys to Concentrate Urine

1. Kidneys able to concentrate urine normally have less need for water than damaged kidneys—a normal individual with a urinary specific gravity of 1.029 to 1.032 requires 15 ml. of water to excrete 1 Gm. of solute; an individual with nephritis, and a urinary specific gravity of 1.010 to 1.015, requires 40 ml. of water to excrete 1 Gm. of solute.
2. Low concentrating ability of the kidneys results in large urinary output.
3. Provided renal concentration is normal, the least amount of urine needed for excretion of daily metabolic wastes is 400 to 500 ml.
4. An acutely ill patient, or one with poor kidney function, may need to excrete as much as 3,000 ml. of urine daily to rid the body of waste products.

Blood Volume

1. A decreased blood volume causes decreased urinary output primarily due to changes in arterial pressure and pressure in the glomeruli. (This phenomenon explains the oliguria or anuria of profound shock.)
2. An increased blood volume causes increased urinary output, again primarily due to changes in arterial pressure and pressure in the glomeruli.

Hormonal Influences

1. An increased secretion of antidiuretic hormone occurs when the blood volume is decreased—the kidneys increase water reabsorption, and the urinary volume is decreased.
2. An increased secretion of aldosterone occurs when the blood volume is decreased—the kidneys increase sodium reabsorption, and the urine volume is decreased.
3. A decreased secretion of antidiuretic hormone occurs when the blood volume is increased—the kidneys decrease water reabsorption, and the urinary volume is increased.
4. A decreased secretion of aldosterone occurs when the blood volume is increased—the kidneys excrete more sodium and the urinary volume is increased.

Age

1. Data presented by Behnke indicate that the aged have a smaller urinary output (0.8 ml./minute) than do younger adults (1.0 ml./minute).
2. The decreased urinary volume in the aged is related to a decreased renal blood flow, secondary to vascular changes—the narrowed vessels decrease plasma filtration and cause less urine to be formed.
3. The decreased urinary volume in the aged may also be related to diet—most aged persons consume much more carbohydrate than protein. (Carbohydrate presents less of a solute load than the nitrogenous end-products of protein.)
4. The aged tend to drink less than younger adults.
5. The aged have a decreased concentrating power. It is important for the nurse to remember that when an increased solute load is presented to such patients, a large urinary volume will result. Such patients require a larger water intake when the renal solute load is high. (See Table 12-19 for conditions associated with urinary volume changes.)

Measuring and Recording Fluid Intake and Output

INTAKE-OUTPUT RECORDS A workable intake-output record has appropriate columns for all types of fluid gains and losses. The volumes

Table 12-19. Significance of Urinary Volume Changes

Symptom	*Imbalance Indicated by Symptom*
Oliguria	Fluid volume deficit Sodium deficit Potassium excess Severe sodium excess Renal calcification due to calcium excess Shock Renal insufficiency (late in disease)
Polyuria	Interstitial fluid-to-plasma shift Diabetes insipidus Increased renal solute load: Diabetes mellitus Infection Calcium excess Hyperthyroidism Renal insufficiency (early) "Salt-losing" nephritis

and types of fluid taken into the body are entered on the left side of the record, and the volumes and types of fluids lost from the body are entered on the right. The intake side of most records provides a column for oral intake and another column for parenteral fluids or other avenues of fluid gain. The output side usually provides a column for urine output and another column for gastrointestinal fluid losses or other routes of fluid loss. The record should be sufficiently simple so that the method of its use is self-evident, and necessary instructions should be incorporated in the record.

It is easy to become confused by intake-output records because they vary from hospital to hospital and even within the same hospital. For example, a burn unit requires a different intake-output record from that required in a general surgical unit.

The type of intake-output record used often depends on the patient's condition. A patient with a severe fluid balance problem may require an hourly summary of his fluid gains and losses, so that the physician can plan treatment according to immediate needs. Figure 12-9 depicts a bedside record suitable for an hourly fluid gain and loss summary. Many patients require only 8-hour summaries of their fluid gains and losses. Figure 12-10 depicts a bedside record suitable for this purpose. Both of these records provide for a 24-hour total. Some hospitals use a small intake-output slip at the bedside; at the end of each shift, the total is transferred to a summary sheet on the patient's chart. Completed intake-output records are attached to the patient's chart and kept as permanent records.

The use of the bedside intake-output record is facilitated when the chart is kept on a clipboard with an attached pen.

INDICATIONS FOR INTAKE-OUTPUT MEASUREMENT Physicians often indicate which patients are to have records kept of their daily fluid intake and output. However, the failure of the physician to request intake-output measurement is no reason to omit it when the patient has a real or potential water and electrolyte balance problem. Many physicians assume that the nurse will initiate intake-output measurement when necessary, without a written order. Patients with the following conditions should automatically be placed on the fluid intake-output measurement list:

Following major surgery
Thermal burns or other injuries
Suspected or known electrolyte imbalance
Acute renal failure
Oliguria
Congestive heart failure
Abnormal losses of body fluids
Lower nephron nephrosis
Diuretic therapy
Corticoid therapy
Inadequate food and fluid intake

NEED FOR ACCURATE INTAKE-OUTPUT RECORDS Most discrepancies between gains and losses of body fluids can be detected when an accurate record is kept of the total fluid intake-output. The content of the gained and lost fluids is as important as their volume, and because the electrolytic content of the individual body fluids varies widely, the amount of each fluid lost should be designated on the intake-output record. The amounts and kinds of fluids taken into the body should also be recorded.

LIQUID INTAKE AND OUTPUT RECORD	Patient's Last Name / First Name / History Number
	Location / Service / Date

Time A.M. or P.M.	INTAKE (in cc.)					OUTPUT (Measured or estimated in cc.)				
	Oral or tube		Parenteral		Running Total	Sweat	Urine	Other (feces, vomitus. etc.)		Running Total
	Type	Amount	Composition	Amount		+ to ++++		Type	Amount	

Fig. 12-9. Liquid intake and output record suitable for hourly measurement. (Bland, J.: Clinical Metabolism of Body Water and Electrolytes, p. 215. Philadelphia, Saunders, 1963)

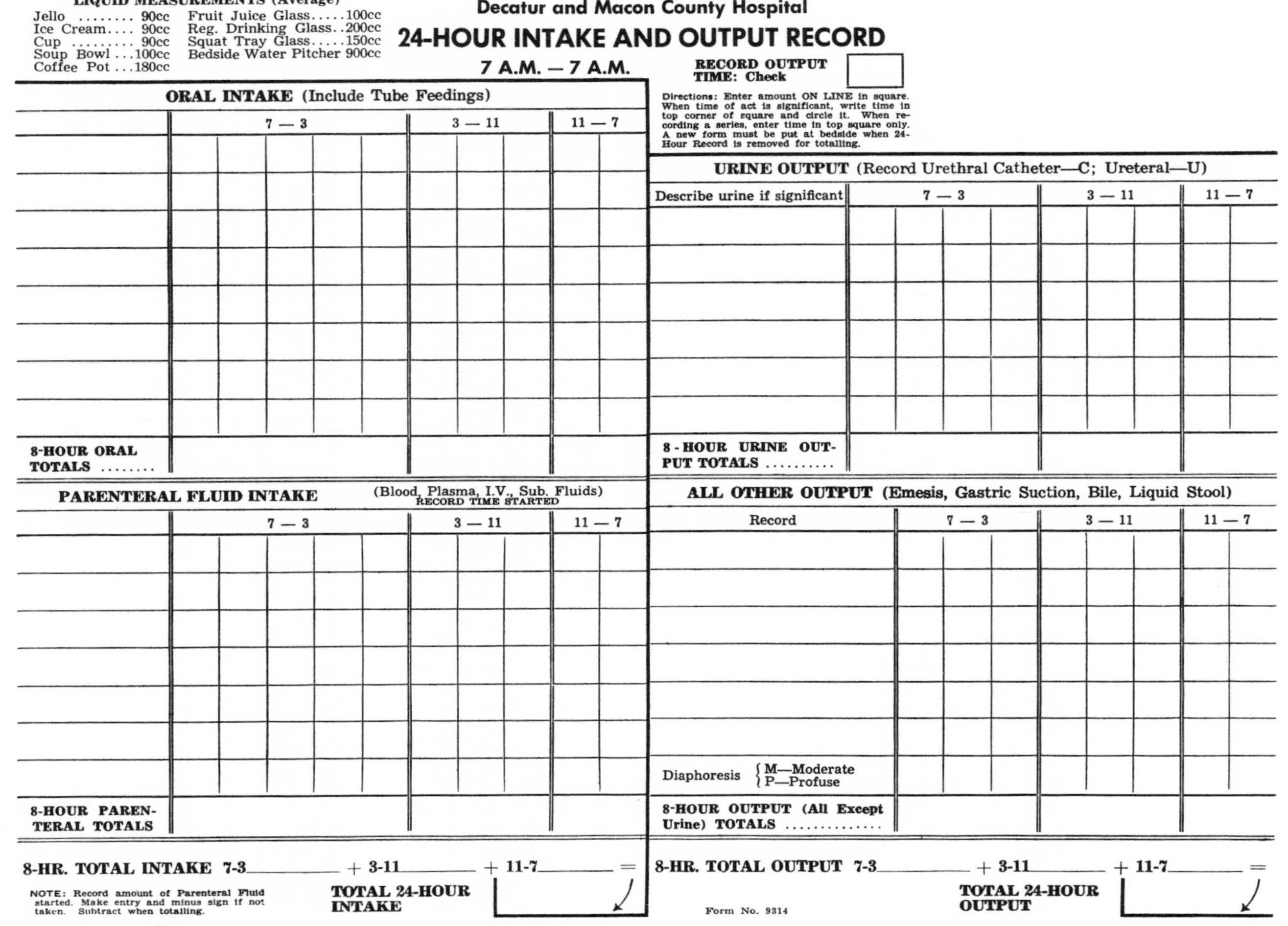

LIQUID MEASUREMENTS (Average)

Jello	90cc	Fruit Juice Glass	100cc
Ice Cream	90cc	Reg. Drinking Glass	200cc
Cup	90cc	Squat Tray Glass	150cc
Soup Bowl	100cc	Bedside Water Pitcher	900cc
Coffee Pot	180cc		

Decatur and Macon County Hospital

24-HOUR INTAKE AND OUTPUT RECORD

7 A.M. — 7 A.M.

RECORD OUTPUT TIME: Check ☐

Directions: Enter amount ON LINE in square. When time of act is significant, write time in top corner of square and circle it. When recording a series, enter time in top square only. A new form must be put at bedside when 24-Hour Record is removed for totalling.

ORAL INTAKE (Include Tube Feedings)

	7 — 3	3 — 11	11 — 7
8-HOUR ORAL TOTALS			

PARENTERAL FLUID INTAKE (Blood, Plasma, I.V., Sub. Fluids) RECORD TIME STARTED

	7 — 3	3 — 11	11 — 7
8-HOUR PARENTERAL TOTALS			

8-HR. TOTAL INTAKE 7-3 _____ + **3-11** _____ + **11-7** _____ =

NOTE: Record amount of Parenteral Fluid started. Make entry and minus sign if not taken. Subtract when totalling.

TOTAL 24-HOUR INTAKE ☐

URINE OUTPUT (Record Urethral Catheter—C; Ureteral—U)

Describe urine if significant	7 — 3	3 — 11	11 — 7
8-HOUR URINE OUTPUT TOTALS			

ALL OTHER OUTPUT (Emesis, Gastric Suction, Bile, Liquid Stool)

Record	7 — 3	3 — 11	11 — 7
Diaphoresis {M—Moderate, P—Profuse}			
8-HOUR OUTPUT (All Except Urine) TOTALS			

8-HR. TOTAL OUTPUT 7-3 _____ + **3-11** _____ + **11-7** _____ =

Form No. 9314

TOTAL 24-HOUR OUTPUT ☐

Fig. 12-10. Twenty-four hour intake-output record. (Decatur and Macon County Hospital, Decatur, Illinois)

Ideally, the physician should be able to use the nursing intake-output records as a major tool in diagnosis, as well as in the formulation of fluid replacement therapy. However, most physicians regard the usual intake-output record with the proverbial grain of salt. They are justified in complaining that an accurate account of a patient's intake-output is extremely difficult to obtain in the average hospital.

CAUSES OF INACCURATE INTAKE-OUTPUT RECORDS Neglect in keeping accurate nursing intake-output records is widespread and causative factors are extremely difficult to pinpoint. However, the difficulty seems to be related to a combination of the following factors:

- Failure to comprehend the value of accurate intake-output records
- Understaffed patient-care units
- Lethargic and improperly motivated personnel
- Lax supervision
- Unqualified personnel giving direct care to seriously ill patients
- Inadequate in-service education programs for all levels of personnel
- Failure to devise or implement a workable intake-output record

ACHIEVING ACCURATE INTAKE-OUTPUT RECORDS It is not technically difficult to measure fluid intake and output or to record the measurements. Yet, persistent effort is required if one is to achieve an accurate account of gains and losses of fluids.

There are innumerable possibilities for error in the measurement and recording of fluid gains and losses; however, some errors occur much more frequently than others.

Common errors and suggestions on how to overcome them are presented below:

Table 12-20. Overcoming Common Errors

Common Errors	*Suggestions*
Errors Involving Both Intake and Output:	
1. Failure to communicate to the entire staff about those patients requiring intake-output measurement (Body fluids are often discarded without being measured, and oral fluids are not recorded, merely because staff members are not aware of the patients on intake-output)	a. A "measure intake-output" sign should be attached to the patient's bed to serve as a reminder. b. A list of all patients requiring intake-output measurement should be posted in a convenient work area for quick reference. c. Also for quick reference, the cardex should contain a list of all patients requiring intake-output measurement. d. An adequate patient report should be given to all personnel.
2. Failure to explain intake-output to the patient and his family (Most patients will cooperate *if* they know what is expected of them)	a. Both the patient and his family should receive a simple explanation of why intake-output measurement is necessary. b. Careful instructions are necessary to acquaint the patient and his family with their role in helping to achieve an accurate intake-output record.
3. Well meaning intentions to record a drink of water or an emptied urinal at a later, more convenient time are often forgotten	Measurements should be recorded at the time they are obtained.
4. Failure to measure fluids that can be directly measured because it takes less time to guess at their amounts	Measure *all* fluids amenable to direct measurement—guesses should be reserved for fluids that cannot be measured directly.
Errors Related to Intake:	
5. Failure to designate the specific volume of glasses, cups, bowls and other fluid containers used in the hospital (Each person may ascribe a different volume to the same glass of water)	The bedside record should list the volumes of glasses, cups, bowls and other fluid containers used in the hospital (see Figure 12-10).

Table 12-20. *(Continued)*

Common Errors	*Suggestions*
6. Failure to obtain an adequate measuring device for small amounts of oral fluids (Patients frequently drink small quantities of fluids; the amounts must be estimated unless a calibrated cup is available—frequent estimates increase the margin of error)	Small calibrated paper cups should be kept at the bedside for such a purpose.
7. The amount of fluid taken as ice chips is frequently under-estimated	The nurse should consider that a full glass of ice chips is approximately one-half of a glass of water when melted; for example: a 200 ml. glass filled with ice chips will contain approximately 100 ml. of water after the ice is melted (see Figure 12-11).
8. Failure to consider the volume of fluid displaced by ice in iced drinks frequently causes an overstatement of ingested oral fluids	Only small amounts of ice should be used for iced drinks so that the accurate amount of fluid ingested can be recorded.
9. Assuming that the contents of empty containers were drunk by the patient (Patients sometimes give their coffee or juice to a visiting relative or to other patients in the room; they may forget to tell the person checking the tray)	The patient should be asked what fluids he drank.
10. Failure to detect that a patient has exaggerated his fluid intake, perhaps to avoid unwanted oral fluids or a parenteral infusion	Patients who frequently try to convey the idea that they will drink fluids after the nurse has left the room should be suspected.
11. Failure to accurately record the amount of parenteral fluid administered on each shift (Because it takes less time, there is a tendency to record the total infusion volume at the time it is started or when it is discontinued)	a. The actual amount of parenteral fluid run in on each shift should be recorded. b. The amount of solution left in the bottle at the end of a shift should be noted, in pencil, on the bedside record—this makes it easier for the next shift to determine the amount run in on their time.
12. Failure to note inadequate intake of solid foods (It is frequently forgotten that solid foods are mainly water, and failure to eat solids causes an increased need for liquids)	Notations concerning inadequate food intake should be made in the appropriate place on the patient's chart.
Errors Related to Output:	
13. Failure to estimate fluid lost as perspiration (Many nurses fail to recognize perspiration as a major source of fluid loss)	a. An attempt should be made to describe the amount of clothing and bed linen saturated with perspiration—it has been estimated that one necessary bed change represents at least 1 L. of lost fluid. b. Some intake-output records require the nurse to estimate perspiration as +, ++, +++, or ++++ (+ represents sweating that is just visible, and ++++ represents profuse sweating).
14. Failure to estimate "uncaught" vomitus (Frequently, "uncaught" emesis is recorded merely as a lost specimen)	The amount of fluid lost as vomitus should be estimated, and recorded as an estimate—it is better to make a guess than to give no indication at all as to the amount.
15. Failure to estimate the amount of incontinent urine (Intake-output records often indicate the number of incontinent voidings but give no indication of the amounts; obviously, such records are of little value)	The amount of incontinent urine should be estimated—it is helpful to note the amount of clothing and bed linen saturated with urine.
16. Failure to estimate fluid lost as liquid feces	a. The patient should be encouraged to use the bedpan rather than the toilet so that the fluid loss can be directly measured. b. The amount of fluid lost in incontinent liquid stools should be estimated.

Table 12-20. *(Continued)*

Common Errors	Suggestions
17. Failure to estimate fluid lost as wound exudate	a. The amount of drainage on a dressing should be measured and charted—this can be done by measuring the width of the stained area and determining the thickness of the dressing. b. If extreme measures are necessary, the dressing can be weighed before application and again when removed.
18. Failure to check a urinary catheter for patency when there is decreased drainage of urine (It is sometimes too quickly assumed that decreased drainage from a catheter is due to decreased urine formation)	Decreased drainage from a urinary catheter is an indication to irrigate it and check for patency before charting the absence of, or decrease in, urinary output.
19. Failure to obtain an adequate measuring device for hourly or more frequent checks on urinary output (An error of even 10 ml. could be significant when dealing with small amounts of urine)	A handy device for frequent volume checks on urinary output is the Davol Uri-meter (see Figure 12-12). This device is calibrated to measure small amounts of urine —after the hourly amount has been measured, the petcock can be opened and the urine drained into a collecting bag.
20. Failure to record the amount of solution used to irrigate tubes and the amount of fluid withdrawn during the irrigation	a. One method for dealing with this problem is to add the amount of irrigating solution to the intake column, and to add the amount of fluid withdrawn to the output column. b. Another method is to compare the amount of irrigating solution used and the amount of fluid withdrawn during the irrigation—if more fluid was put in than was taken out, the excess is added to the intake column; if more fluid was taken out than was put in, the excess is added to the output column.

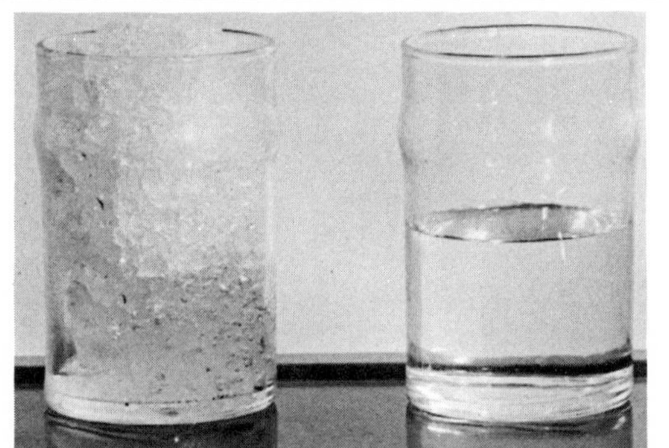

Fig. 12-11. Liquid volume of a glass of ice chips.

Body Weight

The daily weighing of patients with potential or actual fluid balance problems is of great clinical value because: (1) accurate body weight measurements are much easier to obtain than accurate intake-output measurements, and (2) rapid variations in weight closely reflect changes in fluid volume. A loss of body weight will occur when the total fluid intake is less than the total fluid output; conversely, a gain in body weight will occur when the total fluid intake is greater than the total fluid output. However, the nurse should recall that fluids can be lost to the body in the pooling that occurs, for example, with intestinal obstruction. Such losses, which can cause a serious fluid volume deficit, are not reflected by weight changes.

Daily weight measurement may be indicated in the same conditions listed earlier as indications for fluid intake-output measurement. At the minimum, all patients should be weighed on admittance, so that a baseline can be established for later comparison.

Ambulatory patients may be weighed on small portable scales; it is important that the same scale be used for repeated measurements, since any two portable scales seldom give the same reading. The daily variations in weight

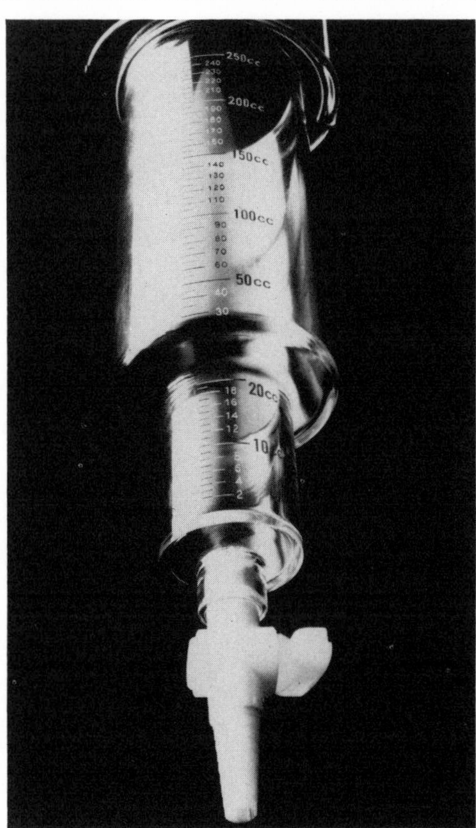

Fig. 12-12. Davol Uri-meter. (Davol Rubber Co., Providence, Rhode Island)

should reflect true body weight changes rather than variations between scales.

Seriously ill patients confined to bed can be weighed with a bed scale. (See Figures 12-13, 12-14.) The weighing procedure can be performed with a minimum of effort for both the patient and the nurse. The patient is turned on one side, making room for the scale board on the mattress. The scale is rolled under the bed, automatically positioning the weighing board over the mattress. The board is lowered until it rests on the mattress. The patient is turned onto the scale board with his body weight evenly distributed; the arms should be folded over the chest, if possible, to prevent them from hanging off the side of the board. The board is raised hydraulically a few inches above the mattress, the patient is weighed, and the board is lowered to the mattress; the patient is moved off the board and the scale is removed. The In-Bed scale is particularly safe, since the patient remains within the confines of the bed during the entire process.

It is useless to weigh the patient daily if the procedure is not performed the same way each day. The nurse should strive for accurate weight measurements, because the physician often bases the administration of fluids and diuretics on the recorded weight changes. The following practices should be followed:

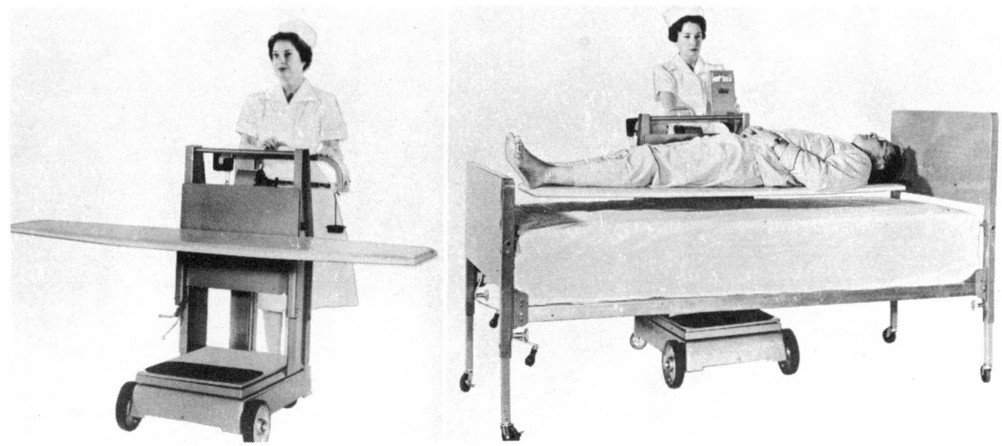

Fig. 12-13. (*Left*) In-bed Scale. (Acme Scale Co., Oakland, California)
Fig. 12-14. (*Right*) In-bed Scale in use. (Acme Scale Co., Oakland, California)

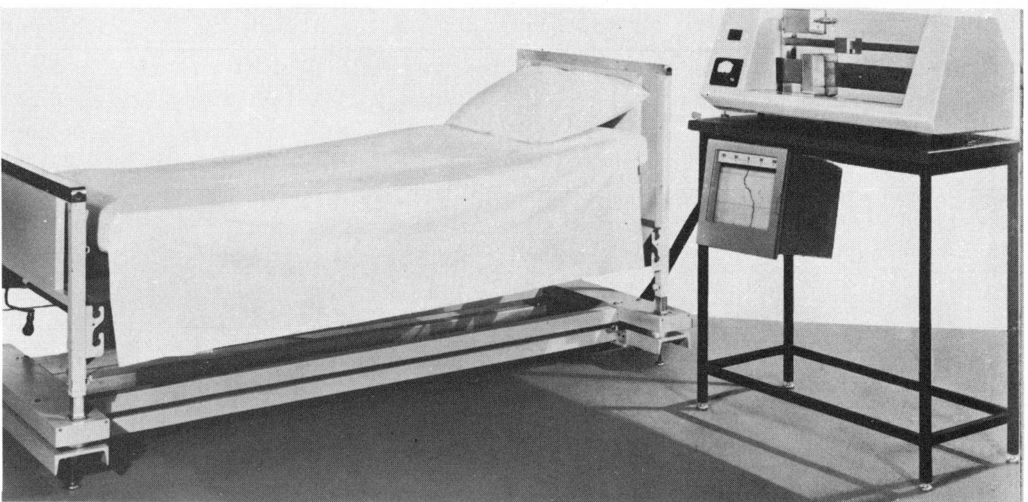

Fig. 12-15. Brookline Metabolic Scale, Model 100. (Brookline Instrument Co., Elmsford, New York)

The same scales should be used each time.

The weight should be measured in the morning before breakfast.

The patient should empty his bladder before each weight measurement.

The same or similar clothing should be worn each time (the clothing should be dry).

The patient may be weighed wearing his glasses and wristwatch, if desired—if so, they should be worn during each weight measurement.

A summary of all of the above points should be written on the cardex or the nursing care plan, so that a uniform weighing procedure is followed.

Brookline Scales

BROOKLINE METABOLIC SCALES The metabolic scales are available in adult and pediatric models. These scales have a sensitivity to one gram and are used primarily for research.

Pictured in Figure 12-15 is the Brookline Metabolic Scale, Model 100-A. This scale has a low weighing platform that fits directly under the bed or crib. A second part of the scale is a readout console which is placed on a balance table beside the bed and has a double balance beam. The bottom beam is calibrated in increments of 10 kg., the top beam in increments of 1 kg., and the micrometer adjusts the patient's weight to the nearest gram. The patient weight range is from 0 to 110 kg. and can be extended to 200 kg. with an accessory weight. In addition to measuring total body weight, changes in patient weight are shown on a console meter. An accessory strip chart recorder can be used to provide a continual record of weight changes.

The scale is set at zero with all the necessary equipment and bedclothes on the bed, thus eliminating them from consideration when the patient is weighed. The weight indicated on the scale is, therefore, the true weight of the patient, and pillows, linens and other equipment can be added or removed whenever necessary. The weight is checked prior to addition or removal; then the scale is readjusted to this reading after the equipment has been removed or added. Position changes of the patient do not affect the reading, as the scale has an automatic self-centering device which allows jolting of the bed without adverse effect on the instrument or even a change in the reading.

Usually fluid lost from the patient's skin into the bedding will not cause a significant error in weight measurement, because when the patient's fluid loss is not excessive, evaporation from the bedding to the room occurs as rapidly as water

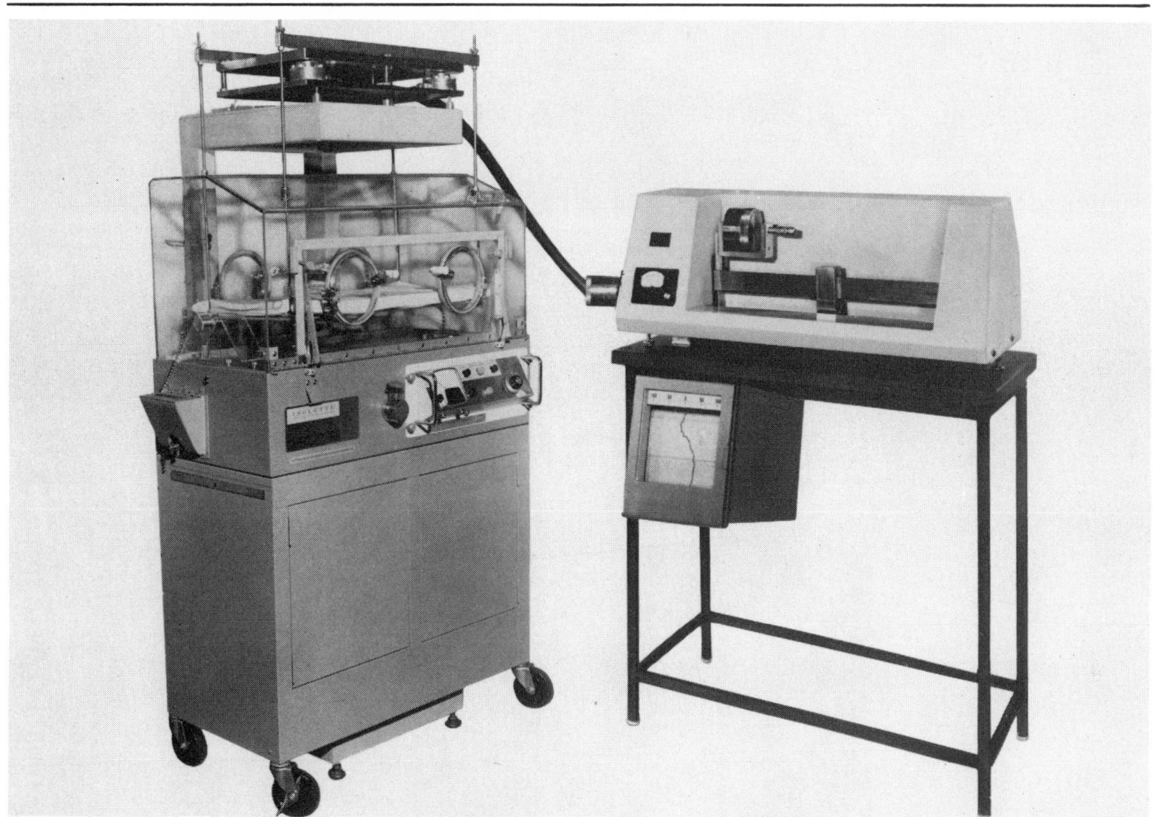

Fig. 12-16. Brookline Metabolic Scale, Model 80-A With Incubator. (Brookline Instrument Co., Elmsford, New York)

lost from the patient to the bedding. For insensible weight loss studies, the patient may be placed on a nylon net supported on top of the bed, allowing evaporation to take place from all surfaces of the body and eliminating absorption by the bedding.

When only evaporative water loss is being measured, all intravenous and catheter drainage apparatus are mounted on the bed. In this way, a change in weight reflects only evaporative water loss. On the other hand, if I.V. therapy is being controlled to maintain the patient's weight at a specific level, the I.V. bottles and urine bottles are kept off the bed, so that intake can be balanced against output.

Some of the clinical applications of the Brookline Metabolic Scale include the control of intravenous therapy and the management of patients with burns, cardiac failure, diabetic acidosis, open-heart surgery and hemodialysis.

A pediatric model of the Brookline Metabolic Scale is also available for continuous monitoring of an infant's weight. (See Figure 12-16.) This scale has a weighing platform which is designed to be mounted inside an incubator or on a table. Total patient weight up to 11 kg. is given to the nearest ¼ Gm., and the scale also provides a continuous record of weight changes when an accessory strip chart recorder is used.

BROOKLINE CLINICAL SCALES These scales have 25 gram accuracy and are used for fluid balance monitoring in dialysis, intensive care, coronary care and burn units.

Figure 12-17 pictures the Brookline Model 30N In-Bed Scale. The patient weight range of this model is from 0 to 150 kg. The scale is mounted on casters to roll from bed to bed or room to room. The scale platform is equipped with ramps to roll the bed on or off, and no

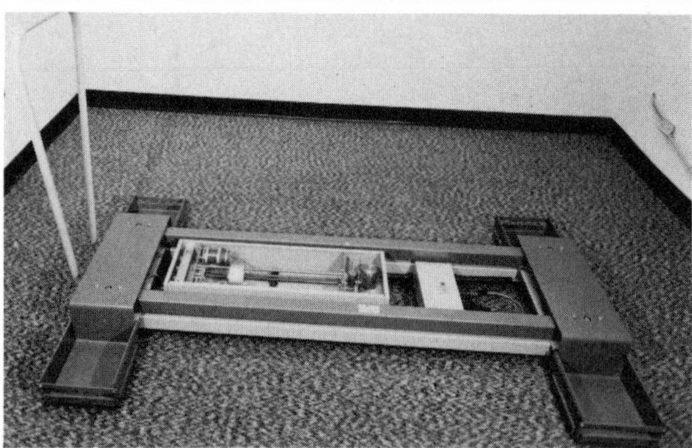

THE SCALE PLATFORM IS ROLLED IN FRONT OF THE BED, AND THE BED IS MOVED FORWARD ONTO THE PLATFORM. BEDS CAN BE MOVED ON AND OFF THE SCALE PLATFORM FROM EITHER END OF THE SCALE.

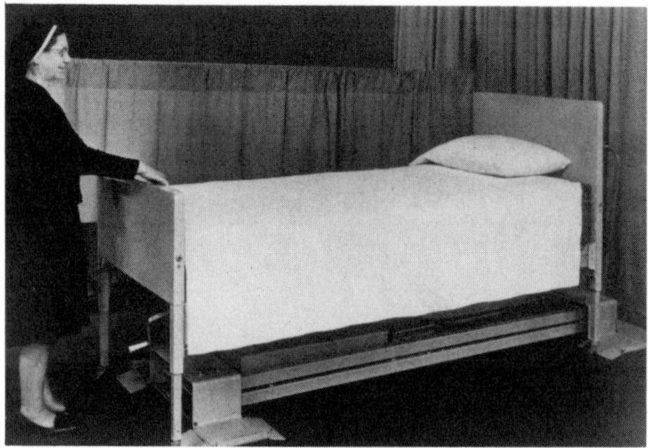

Fig. 12-17. Brookline In-Bed Scale, Model 30N. (Brookline Instrument Co., Elmsford, New York)

lifting of the bed or patient is required. All the nurse has to do is push a button on the console and the patient is automatically weighed. The weight and weight changes are continually monitored and numerically displayed on the readout console. (See Figure 12-18.) This console is light and portable and can be placed on a table near the bed or positioned at the nursing station for remote monitoring.

An accessory available with this scale is the Weight Change Indicator. (See Figure 12-18.) It automatically accumulates and displays the total weight change of the patient. One window displays weight loss; another window displays weight gain. This information is particularly valuable in dialysis units. Another accessory (Digital Printer, Model 313) provides a permanent record of the patient's weight and weight changes. The weight is printed in kg. to 0.1 kg. along with a reference number on a printed roll and can be pre-set to print automatically at 15, 30 and 60 minute intervals.

Table 12-21. Significance of Weight Changes

Symptom	*Imbalance Indicated by Symptom*
Acute weight gain (in excess of 5%)	Fluid volume excess
Acute weight loss (in excess of 5%)	Fluid volume deficit
Chronic weight loss	Protein deficit

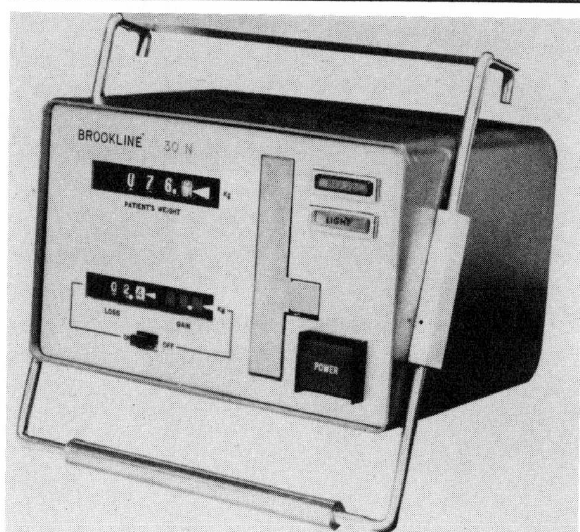

Fig. 12-18. Readout Console and Weight Change Indicator for Brookline 30N Scale. (Brookline Instrument Co., Elmsford, New York)

Frequency and Character of Stools

The nurse should record bowel movements, and any significant facts related to them, on the chart. The consistency of the stool (solid or liquid) and the frequency of evacuation should be noted.

Abnormal fecal losses and their causal relationship to fluid imbalances are discussed in a preceding section of this chapter.

Table 12-22 lists some of the fluid imbalances accompanied by changes in the character and the frequency of bowel movements.

Table 12-22. Significance of Stool Changes

Symptom	*Imbalance Indicated by Symptom*
Hard fecal mass	Fluid volume deficit
Abdominal cramping with diarrhea	Sodium deficit Potassium excess
Ileus, abdominal distention (little or no stool or flatus passed)	Potassium deficit

Blood Gases

While caring for certain acutely ill patients, the nurse may be required to observe blood gas changes and take appropriate actions (within the treatment regimen prescribed by the physician).

Some physicians leave an order to take samples for blood gas studies P.R.N. This requires the nurse to understand factors affecting blood gases and to recognize symptoms indicating a need to take a sample; such symptoms may include changes in respirations, color, level of consciousness, and restlessness. The nurse should recognize significant blood gas values and report them to the physician, as blood gas variations are early clues to changes in the patient's condition.

Blood gas analysis includes measurement of hydrogen, oxygen, and carbon dioxide tensions in arterial and venous blood and expressed, respectively, as pH, pO_2, and pCO_2. (See Table 12-23.)

Table 12-23. Blood Gas Values

Blood Specimen	*pH*	*pCO_2*	*pO_2*
arterial	(7.38-7.42) 7.41 average	35-38 mm Hg	95-100 mm Hg
venous	(7.35-7.45) 7.36 average	40-41 mm Hg	35-40 mm Hg

Arterial blood specimens are usually obtained from an indwelling catheter in the brachial, radial, femoral or temporal artery. If a catheter is not in place, a femoral punch may be performed to obtain an arterial blood sample. In some hospitals the nurse is not permitted to draw blood samples, particularly when an arterial punch is required; nevertheless, she may often obtain samples from indwelling catheters.

Venous samples are not as revealing as arterial samples, but when they are used, it is best to obtain the blood from a central vein. Blood from peripheral veins should not be used for blood gas studies because they do not indicate true values of pH, pO_2, and pCO_2. Unclotted blood is used to measure blood gases. Most blood gas analyzers require 2½ ml. of blood—some require only ½ ml. or less.

The changing blood gas values must be compared to each other and to previous readings and should be evaluated in relation to the patient's clinical appearance and medical history.

The nurse must understand the relationship between pH and pCO_2:

1. A fall in pH and a rise in pCO_2 indicates respiratory acidosis, often present in hypoventilation. Among the possible causes are emphysema, excessive secretions blocking the respiratory tract, heavy sedation, splinting due to pain in the chest area, tight dressings, and improperly regulated mechanical respirators (causing respirations to be too slow or shallow).
2. A low pH occurring with a low pCO_2 indicates metabolic acidosis. The pH is low because the body is deficient in base bicarbonate, and the pCO_2 becomes low when the lungs attempt to compensate by eliminating more CO_2 (hyperventilation).
3. A high pH and a low pCO_2 indicates respiratory alkalosis, the primary problem of which is hyperventilation. Possible causes include anxiety, fever, hypoxia, and improperly regulated mechanical respirators (causing respirations to be too fast or deep). If the hyperventilation is due to pain and anxiety, an appropriate analgesic should be administered.
4. A high pH and a high pCO_2 indicates metabolic alkalosis, of which the primary symptom is an excess of base bicarbonate. The lungs attempt to compensate by retaining more carbon dioxide and thus elevate the carbonic acid level.

Arterial pO_2 is naturally much higher than venous pO_2 because arteries carry oxygenated blood. (See Table 12-23.)

Hypoventilation results in a decreased pO_2 and an elevated pCO_2, indications for the nurse to try to improve pulmonary ventilation. Such actions may include (depending on the circumstance):

Turning the patient from side to side at frequent intervals to allow for gravitational drainage of mucus from the various lung segments

Placing the patient in Fowler's or Semi-Fowler's position to allow for greater chest expansion

Suctioning the patient as necessary to rid the respiratory tract of excessive secretions

Increasing activity, as outlined by the physician, to promote ventilatory and circulatory improvement

Performing other functions as prescribed by the physician, such as postural drainage, chest tapping and intermittent positive pressure breathing treatments

A low pO_2 with a normal pCO_2 is an indication to administer oxygen in a concentration, and by a route, prescribed by a physician.

A post-operative patient with a low pO_2 and a low central venous pressure probably has a blood volume deficit and requires replacement therapy.

A patient with poor tissue perfusion will also have a low pO_2. Such a patient displays poor color and a lower than normal body temperature. In this instance, the nurse should provide warmth with extra blankets.

CONCLUSION The preceding discussion of planned nursing observations has been quite general. The reader is encouraged to further explore and assimilate pertinent and detailed nursing observations (in context with appropriate nursing actions) in the chapters dealing with specific conditions (Chapters 17 through 27).

13 The Elements of Nutrition

Materials essential for nutrition can be divided into four categories: the "bulk" elements, which include protein, carbohydrate and fat; the vitamins; the minerals; and water.

THE "BULK" ELEMENTS

Protein, carbohydrate and fat make up the solid physical bulk of the diet and are broken down and converted in the course of digestion, absorption and metabolism.

PROTEIN Proteins have been defined as *organic compounds containing the element nitrogen.* Together with the carbohydrates and fats, they constitute the principal part of the solids of living matter. The name *protein* comes to us from a Greek word *proteios,* meaning *first,* coined by the Dutch chemist Mulder in 1839, reflecting his conviction of the importance of protein. Proteins are used principally for body building and maintenance rather than for energy purposes, and although protein foods are derived both from plants and animals, proteins from animal sources appear to predominate in the average American diet. Proteins are the distinguishing constituents of many important foods, such as meat, fish, poultry, eggs, dairy products, beans, peas and peanuts. Although milk contains protein, it is an exceedingly dilute source that also contributes large amounts of fat and carbohydrates.

Proteins have many essential functions, as described in Chapter 9. When protein foods are eaten, they are broken down in the digestive tract and absorbed into the blood as amino acids; in the liver and other manufacturing centers of the body, amino acids are reassembled into specific proteins to meet the diverse needs of the body.

CARBOHYDRATES The word carbohydrate means hydrated carbon—that is, the water and carbon combined. The hydrogen and oxygen atoms of carbohydrates are usually present in the same proportion as in water (HOH), so that the general formula of most carbohydrates can be expressed $C_n\ (HOH)_n$. The values for *n* can range from 2 to many thousands.

About 70 per cent by weight of the food in the average diet consists of carbohydrates, the distinguishing constituents of cereals, bakery products, confections, sugar, syrups, starch and fermentation products. They serve to provide calories for immediate use or, through the mechanism of storage, for delayed use. Carbohydrates not immediately used by the body for energy purposes are stored as fat.

FAT The term fat suggests such familiar substances as butter, lard, tallow, olive oil, cottonseed oil, cream and oleomargarine. In nature, fats exist in less obvious and less easily characterized combinations, as because of their complexity and variability, no satisfactory classification exists. Many protein foods, such as meat, fish and eggs, as well as dairy products, contain considerable quantities of fat, whereas carbohydrate foods are usually low in fat, if they contain any. The chief function of fat in the diet is to provide calories for energy.

THE CALORIE

In addition to being the unit of measure for heat, the calorie is also the unit of measure for energy. Since heat can be converted into energy, the two terms are interchangeable, and the calorie can be used to measure both. The calorie employed in nutrition is the large or *great calorie,* representing the quantity of heat needed to raise the temperature of 1 L. of water 1° C. Most adults expend about 70 calories per hour while resting, 105 calories per hour while standing, and several hundreds of calories per hour while exercising vigorously.

We use the calorie to express food values. A gram (about 1/28 of an ounce) of pure protein supplies 4 calories, as does a gram of carbohydrate. A gram of alcohol supplies about 7 calories, and a gram of fat, 9.

Most adults lose weight on a diet providing 1,600 calories per day, and all adults lose weight on a diet of 1,200 calories or less. Most office workers require upwards of 2,500 calories per day to maintain weight. Heat loss increases the caloric needs, so that an Eskimo requires more calories than a south sea islander, assuming that their activities are equal.

The human body is not indifferent to the nature of the food from which it derives its energy. For best health, it appears that about 15 to 20 per cent of the total calories should be derived from protein; 35 to 50 per cent from starch or carbohydrate; and about 35 to 50 per cent from fat foods. Some persons, who have been dubbed "carboholics," appear to have an inordinate tendency to transform the carbohydrate of the diet into body fat. Diets quite high in protein, limited to not more than 50 to 60 Gm. of carbohydrate a day, have been recommended for such persons.

When a person fails to receive his required quota of calories, he begins, unconsciously but literally, to consume himself; the internal chemical reactions of the body begin to metabolize body fat stores to generate needed calories. After the fat stores have been used up, the body converts solid tissues—chiefly muscles—into their constituent elements in order to obtain the desperately needed calories. When one is receiving an inadequate caloric intake, food entering the body is consumed for caloric purposes rather than for repair of damaged tissues or for new tissue growth.

We see the ominous effect of inadequate caloric intake in illness and injuries in the young. Tissue repair cannot proceed until the caloric intake is more than just adequate, a principle especially important in the growing individual. Naturally, the availability of generous quantities of fat helps ward off the evil day when the patient begins to cannibalize his own tissues. But that day inevitably comes sooner or later, unless one's daily demand for calories is met.

The symptoms of caloric deficit are easily recognized: hunger; mental depression; apprehension; jitteriness; loss of weight; and fatigue following even slight effort. There are more subtle and less obvious symptoms, such as a shortness of breath, especially on exertion.

Insidiously, as caloric deficit persists, the baleful symptoms of protein deficit have their onset. Under such circumstances, dietary proteins are consumed for energy rather than for tissue synthesis.

VITAMINS

Since vitamins differ from each other in composition, it is impossible to define them in terms of their chemical structure. However, vitamins can be defined from the physiologic standpoint as organic compounds that are essential constituents of the diet, yet are required only in minute amounts for the normal functioning of the body, since the role of vitamins in the chemistry of life processes is that of a catalyst.

The last of the basic nutritional essentials to be discovered, vitamins were at first believed to be amines. It was for this reason that they were designated as the *vital amines,* a term later shortened to vitamines, and still later to vitamins. We now know that vitamins differ widely from one another in their chemical nature and that they are not necessarily amines.

Vitamins cannot be manufactured within the body, at least not in quantities sufficient to meet the daily requirement. When they are ingested in excess of the need, they are usually excreted; more than enough does not appear to be better than enough. Vitamins are amazingly safe. Apparently only two vitamins, vitamins A and D, can cause harm, and then only in massive doses over a prolonged period. When the vitamin intake is inadequate, deficiency disease occurs. Governmental and industrial application of the new knowledge of vitamins has made vitamin deficiencies, almost universal a few years ago, now so unusual that many physicians have never seen them. Yet, in the developing areas of the world and in countries at war, vitamin deficiency disease still abounds.

Vitamin deficits arise not only from a decreased intake of vitamins, but from diseases of the digestive tract that impair the absorption of vitamins. Infectious diseases, burns, or injuries can help to bring on vitamin deficits by increasing the use of vitamins by the body. Deficiencies of the B vitamins, for example, are prone to occur in alcoholics.

Each vitamin deficit has its own characteristic clinical picture. Vitamin A deficit may be indicated by the inability to see in a dim light. Signs of deficits of B vitamins include cracking at the mouth corners, beefy red tongue, diarrhea, anemia, dermatitis, anorexia, nervous disorders, loss of coordination and even mental disease. Vitamin C deficit may be revealed by bleeding gums, bleeding under the fibrous covering of the bones, impaired wound healing and wound dehiscence. Clues to vitamin D deficit include bowed legs, prominences of the bony bosses of the head, growth failure, flabbiness of the muscles, and impairment in the use of calcium by the body. Vitamin B_{12} deficit, stemming from internal metabolic factors rather than inadequate intake, causes pernicious anemia.

Vitamin deficits are usually remedied by administering the appropriate commercial vitamin preparations by mouth, or by giving a concentrated natural source of vitamins, such as lemon juice or orange juice for vitamin C. More and more physicians are becoming convinced of the value of giving patients under the stress of illness, infectious disease, surgery, burns, injury and during convalescence, generous quantities of vitamins by means of a carefully formulated supplement.

MINERALS

Minerals are also called inorganic or ash elements. They are the chemical elements, exclusive of carbon, that remain wholly or partly in the ash when a food is burned. When minerals are dissolved in water, they develop electrical charges and are designated electrolytes. All minerals develop such charges when placed in an aqueous solution, except when they are part of a complex organic compound. The minerals usually listed in any table giving the mineral contents of foods include:

Sodium
Potassium
Calcium
Magnesium
Iron
Phosphorus
Sulfur
Chlorine

These minerals occur in important quantities in foods and have long been studied with respect to their functions in the body. During the past few years, additional chemical elements have been discovered in minute amounts in plant and animal materials. Some of these, including cobalt, copper, manganese, zinc and iodine, may play roles as important in animal nutrition as those elements that occur in larger quantities. Other minerals of common occurrence, but whose dietary properties have not been assessed, include aluminum, arsenic, bromine and fluorine. The latter has been found to be of definite value in preventing dental caries. Other chemical elements, including boron, molybdenum and silicon, have been found necessary for plants.

Clinical deficiencies of the following minerals have been observed:

Sodium
Potassium
Calcium
Magnesium
Iron
Copper
Iodine

Deficits of the first four minerals were covered in Chapter 9. Deficiency of iron or of copper is associated with anemia, whereas iodine deficiency results in endemic goiter. There is no specific deficit of fluorine.

WATER

Water is perhaps the most essential of all nutrients. Its role in the body was described in

Chapter 2. Although a generous intake of water is essential for health, and although water is usually regarded as completely innocuous, approximately seven times the usual daily intake of water can be harmful because it causes loss of the electrolytes from the body. For this reason, the syndrome resulting from excessive intake of water is called *water intoxication,* brought about by the dilution of the extracellular fluid and sodium deficit.

SOURCES OF INFORMATION

The National Research Council has set up Recommended Dietary Allowances for calories, protein, calcium, iron, vitamin A, thiamine, riboflavin, niacin, ascorbic acid and vitamin D (presented in the *Recommended Dietary Allowances,* 7th revised edition, National Academy of Sciences and National Research Council, 1968). The allowances are intakes designed for the maintenance of good nutrition in normal, healthy persons living in a temperate climate. They allow for the normal ranges of individual needs under the usual conditions of life, plus a moderate additional safety factor. They are *not* intended to cover the special requirements that may be created by illness, unusual exertion, or other stress.

The United States Food and Drug Administration has promulgated Minimum Daily Requirements in connection with the Federal Food, Drug, and Cosmetic Act. These requirements represent basic intakes deemed necessary for the actual prevention of deficiencies. The values are lower, in most instances, than the Recommended Dietary Allowances of the National Research Council.

For information and protection of consumers, the labels of special dietary foods and diet supplements are required to show the proportion of the Minimum Daily Requirement supplied by each nutrient listed. In case a Minimum Daily Requirement has not yet been set for a nutrient, or if the nutrient concerned has not been officially classified by the Food and Drug Administration as essential, this too should be stated on the label. In medical and dietetic literature, the Minimum Daily Requirements are referred to less frequently than are the Recommended Dietary Allowances.

An extremely helpful source for the evaluation of nutritional contributions of food portions is the book *Food Values of Portions Commonly Used* by A. Bowes and C. Church (edition 11, revised by Charles Frederick Church and Helen Nichols Church, Philadelphia, J. B. Lippincott Company, 1970). It is invaluable for the food and diet planner.

CONCLUSION It is indeed difficult to overestimate the importance of nutrition. The Germans have a saying *Das Essen macht den Mann* ("Eating makes the man"). We are, in more than a figurative sense, *what we eat.* This applies, of course, to sick as well as to healthy persons; eating in the broader sense includes not only the usual foods, but materials administered by nasogastric tube, rectal tube, or by the parenteral route.

14 The Nurse's Role in Preventing Imbalances of Water, Electrolytes, and Other Nutrients

INTRODUCTION

It is better to prevent disturbances of water, electrolytes and other nutrients than to have to treat them after they have developed. Any patient can develop a serious nutritional disturbance if his needs for nutrients are not considered and met; consequently, the practical application of the principles of nutrition is as much a part of nursing as is the administration of medications. Examples of common clinical events that can lead to nutritional disturbances include:

1. Inadequate intake
2. Excessive losses from such conditions as
   A. Fever
   B. Excessive perspiration
   C. Vomiting
   D. Gastric or intestinal suction
   E. Diarrhea
3. Medical therapy, such as the prolonged use of diuretics, laxatives, enemas, or steroids
4. Catabolic effects, such as those induced by
   A. Immobilization
   B. Draining decubitus ulcers
   C. Surgery (hemorrhage)
   D. Trauma

When one considers how frequently the nurse encounters situations such as these in her daily practice, the need for a carefully considered plan of action on her part becomes evident. Such a plan must include meticulous observation of the patient.

Compared to other healing disciplines, the profession of nursing is unique in that its ministrations are applied continuously to the hospitalized patient. The nursing staff is responsible for the intelligent execution of orders for solid foods and liquids during the entire 24-hour period. Far more is required than a rote performance of duties. Initiative is mandatory on the part of the nurse if the prescribed therapy is to produce optimal results.

In assuring the patient's nutritional welfare, the nurse functions in the framework formulated by the physician. At no time should she deviate from this framework without first consulting him. Nevertheless, much is left to her discretion. For example, the order "diet as tolerated" is frequently written on surgical services, and the physician assumes that the nursing staff understands the patient's condition so as to execute properly such a diet order. Indeed, it would be impossible for the physician to detail step-by-step exactly what should be done for every patient, even when the diet order is relatively specific. When the nurse knows the general purpose and scope of the diet, she can exercise her judgment in accordance with the individual patient's needs.

The nurse should be constantly aware of the problems that may be posed by medication. Suppose a thiazide diuretic has been ordered. Since the nurse knows that this medication will, in all probability, increase the patient's need for potassium, she can encourage the ingestion of high potassium foods and, in addition, alert the physician to the possible need for a potassium supplement.

In instances such as those cited above, the nurse can often institute action to meet the new situation, and on other occasions, she must report her findings to the physician and seek his direction. Among the valuable resource personnel available to the nurse for consultation is the dietitian, who can frequently provide helpful suggestions if she is given background information based on careful nursing observations. The wise nurse consults other members of the health team when confronted by problems that tax her knowledge. Obviously, the patient benefits from such coordination.

The busy physician can easily miss notations in the nursing notes concerning a patient's inadequate intake of food and liquids. Sometimes such notations are not made because of laxity in checking the patient's tray after meals, or in recording the findings on the patient's chart, which should always contain a meaningful summary of the patient's food and fluid intake by the members of the nursing staff.

The importance of accurate nursing observations is revealed in questions commonly asked by physicians when they evaluate the state of the patient's water and electrolytes balance:

1. Has the patient been eating and drinking normally? If not, for how long?
2. Have abnormal losses of body fluids occurred, as perspiration, vomiting, gastric or intestinal suction, drainage from enterostomy, colostomy, or fistulas, liquid stools, wound or burn exudate?
3. Has there been an acute weight loss or an acute weight gain?
4. Have therapeutic fluids been given by tube, rectum, or parenterally (if patient has been under treatment by another physician)?
5. Has the patient been on a restrictive diet (if patient has been under treatment by another physician)?
6. Has the patient been given medications that might cause body fluid disturbances?

Obviously, conditions that cause disturbances of water and electrolytes can also cause deficits of other nutrients, such as protein, carbohydrate, fat, or vitamins.

INADEQUATE INTAKE

Intake Via the Gastrointestinal Route

ORAL ROUTE With respect to the intake of water, electrolytes, vitamins, and other nutrients, the oral route has long been preferred for the prevention of deficits and the correction of mild deficits already present. It offers several advantages:

1. Because it allows gradual absorption, the oral route provides far greater efficiency in the utilization of administered nutrients.
2. Large quantities of water, electrolytes and other nutrients can be ingested over a short period without upsetting water and electrolyte balance.
3. The oral route is far less expensive.
4. The oral route appeals to the patient as being more natural.

(Naturally, the gastrointestinal tract must be functional if the oral route is to be used.)

The ingestion of nutrients is so commonplace that its significance is frequently overlooked, possibly because the oral route lacks the dramatic impact of parenteral or nasogastric feedings. Yet, oral administration can frequently prevent serious disturbances of the body fluids.

Since the oral route is the normal way to obtain nutrients, it possesses a distinct psychologic appeal, as a patient frequently feels he is quite ill simply because he is denied food by the oral route.

Nursing Measures to Promote Eating

Illness or imposed dietary restrictions may greatly decrease the desire to eat, and offering an adequate diet does not guarantee that the patient will accept it. The real test of nursing skill is not to order and serve a diet; rather, it lies in getting the patient to eat it. The dietitian must usually individualize the diet if she is to motivate the patient to eat it. In some institutions, the patient can receive individual attention from the dietitian; unfortunately, this is frequently not possible. In such instances, it is especially important that the nurse study the patient's eating habits, his food likes and dislikes, as well as the cultural and religious beliefs that influence his eating habits.

Whenever possible, the patient should be permitted choices, since this will increase the acceptability of the diet. The nurse must remember that dietary restrictions are often difficult for the patient, and unless steps are taken to make the restrictions tolerable, the patient will either cease eating or fail to adhere to the diet. The patient will be more likely to follow the diet if the nurse explains why it has been ordered.

The nurse can help the patient accept his diet if she displays a sincere interest and makes it clear that she understands how difficult it is to be placed on a restricted diet after years of freely choosing foods. A forceful, goading, or heckling approach may turn the patient against the diet.

A pleasant environment encourages eating, but the establishment of such an environment is not always easy. The wise nurse makes every effort to eliminate unpleasant sights and odors. Naturally, this cannot be done in ward rooms with seriously ill patients, but, at least, unpleasant sights such as drainage bottles and parenteral infusion apparatus can be screened. Soiled dressings can be changed before meals, and ileostomy bags can be changed or emptied. Ambulatory patients can eat their meals outside the ward.

Since strong emotions affect both appetite and digestive processes unfavorably, the nurse should attempt to minimize such feelings. Emotional comfort is as important as physical comfort, but it is often more difficult to achieve; incidents that irritate the patient should be noted on the nursing care plan and avoided, if possible, in the future. Unpleasant procedures should be avoided in the vicinity of mealtime, since what may appear minor to the nurse may be quite irritating to the seriously ill patient. Sometimes the presence of a member of the family may help to relax the patient at mealtime; sometimes he may prefer to eat alone.

Many patients like to have their hands and face washed before each meal. Patients having unpleasant mouth tastes such as occur with oral surgery or bronchiectasis can be given a mouthwash before mealtime.

Since unpleasant symptoms, such as pain and nausea, greatly decrease the patient's interest in eating, every possible nursing measure should be taken to alleviate these and similar sources of discomfort. If simple comfort measures fail, it may be wise to administer p.r.n. medications in preparation for the meal.

A patient in need of a cleansing enema or a bladder catheterization is not apt to eat or drink well.

Nothing should interfere with the patient's eating his food while it is still warm. The tray should be kept neat and attractive; spilled liquids decrease the appeal of food, hence deter the patient's appetite.

The nurse should give any assistance required to prepare the food for eating or to arrange the eating utensils for easy access.

The patient should be placed in a comfortable position. (All too frequently, the tray is placed unthinkingly out of reach, or no provision is made to help the patient cut his food or pour his coffee.) If the patient must be fed, it should be done in a considerate and unhurried manner. The patient who might be embarrassed by his eating habits (for example, the patient who drools because of a stroke) should be tactfully provided with privacy.

The size of the serving should be appropriate for the patient's appetite, as a patient with a small appetite can be repelled by large portions of food. Serving the meal in courses may help such persons eat more.

Unnecessary interruptions during meals should be avoided, because the not-too-eager appetite can be easily discouraged by the poor planning of nursing activities. Sufficient time should be allowed for eating; the patient must never be rushed. Frequently, a patient will stop eating when he sees other trays in the ward being removed or when he is asked repeatedly if he is finished. The patient should be convinced that he can eat at his own pace—*careful explanation is frequently required to accomplish this.* Above all, the nursing staff should not become so wrapped up in routine that they unthinkingly subject the patient to time stress.

Every effort should be made to prevent nausea and vomiting after meals, and so the patient should not be turned quickly or subjected to excessive physical activity. On the other hand, mild exercise should not be condemned, for it may aid digestion. If nausea should occur, appropriate medication may be given in accord with medical orders, and in the absence of a p.r.n. order for

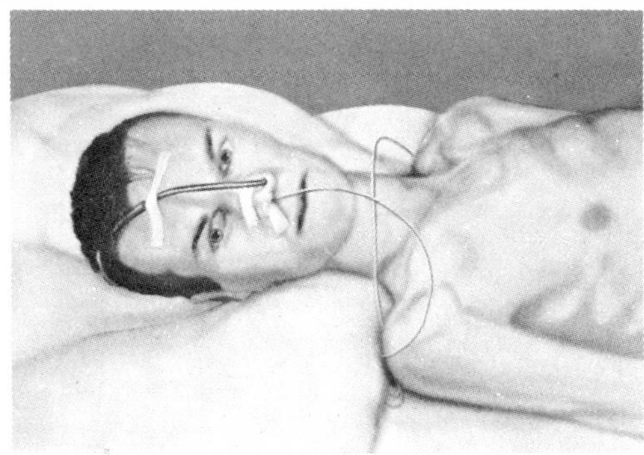

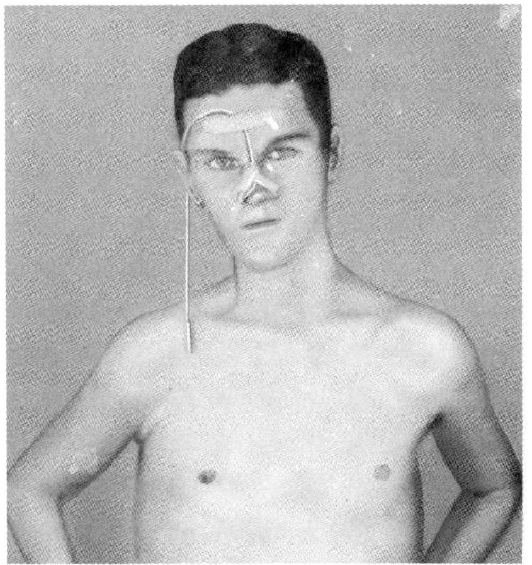

Fig. 14-1. Improvement in nutritional status as a result of tube feedings. (Barron, J.: Tube feeding of postoperative patients. Surg. Clin. N. Am., p. 1489, December, 1959)

nausea, the nurse might seek a medical order. The cause of the nausea can be sought and noted on the chart.

Although the points just enumerated are well-known to most nurses, *we are convinced that they cannot be overemphasized.* One does well to remember that any program of diet therapy is worthless if the patient does not eat! Conversely, any measure capable of promoting food and liquid intake contributes to the patient's welfare. The nurse should impress the importance of these facts on the auxiliary staff members, who are frequently charged with important responsibilities associated with feeding the patients.

Nasogastric Tube Feedings

INDICATIONS FOR TUBE FEEDINGS Oral intake might be impossible, even though adequate gastrointestinal function is present, in such situations as:

1. Semiconsciousness or unconsciousness
2. Oral surgery
3. Extreme anorexia
4. Swallowing problems
5. Weakness caused by chronic debilitating conditions
6. Disorientation
7. Serious mental diseases, such as major psychoses

The nurse must be aware of these conditions and report inadequate intake when any of them are present. The patient should not be permitted to develop malnutrition before another route for intake of nutrients is adopted. One solution to the problems posed by such patients is the use of nasogastric tube feedings, which have many advantages, especially when the problems requiring them are likely to be of long duration.

When oral intake is inadequate, tube feedings are used to administer the protein and calories necessary for tissue healing in such conditions as fractures, decubitus ulcers and burns. An intake of at least 1,600 to 2,000 calories must be provided if the protein is to be used for tissue repair; otherwise, it will be used to meet energy needs.

Disorders of the gastrointestinal tract, such as biliary or pancreatic fistulas, or delayed emptying of the stomach, may necessitate passing a feeding tube beyond the affected area in order to administer nutrients. One of the few contraindications for tube feedings is the complete obstruction of the lower gastrointestinal tract.

Even if the underlying disease process cannot be corrected, the patient can live more comfortably during the weeks and months remaining if he is adequately nourished. The incidence of trophic ulcers, wasting and debilitation is decreased by adequate nourishment.

Anorexia and malnutrition create a vicious cycle: anorexia leads to malnutrition; malnutrition promotes anorexia. The use of tube feedings for several weeks improves the patient's nutri-

Table 14-1. Nutrient Contents of Tube Feeding Mixtures*

Type of Feeding	*Calories*	*Protein Gm.*	*Fat Gm.*	*CHO Gm.*	*Ca Gm.*	*Fe mg.*	*Vit. A I.U.*	*Ascorbic Acid mg.*	*Thiamine mg.*	*Riboflavin mg.*	*Niacin mg.*
Sustagen 500 Gm. Water 1,000 Gm.	2,035	118	18	323	3.5	8	2,778	167	5.5	5.5	50
Whole Milk 1,000 Gm. Egg Yolks (4) Heavy Cream 40% 240 cc. Karo Syrup 100 Gm. Yeast: 2 cakes dissolved in 200 cc. hot water—mix altogether and cook in a double boiler. Cool, strain, and add orange juice 200 Gm. Cod Liver Oil 16 Gm.	2,321	54	158	183	1.5	7	7,270	110	0.9	2.9	10.2
Water 100 Gm. Powder Skim Milk 225 Gm. Powder Whole Milk 200 Gm.	1,798	132	56	193	4.8	3	2,890	28	1.4	7.3	2

* *Above are recommended by the Commission on Nutrition of the Medical Society of the State of Pennsylvania.*
Goodhart, R., and Wohl, M.: Manual of Clinical Nutrition, pp. 92-93. Philadelphia, Lea & Febiger, 1964.

tion, as well as his appetite, thus interrupting the cycle. Many anorexic patients request permission to "eat around the tube" after several weeks of tube feedings. Visual evidence of the general improvement brought about by tube feedings is presented in Figure 14-1.

TUBE FEEDING MIXTURES Any tube feeding mixture should provide all the required solid nutrients—protein, carbohydrate, fat, minerals and vitamins—and should incorporate generous quantities of water; however, additional water must be supplied if the daily requirement is to be met. It is especially necessary to provide adequate water for the elderly, the confused, the lethargic and the comatose, since these patients frequently do not experience or express normal thirst. The physician should prescribe the contents of the tube feeding and should designate the quantity and the times when it should be given.

A commercial feeding preparation, Sustagen, is easy to use since it requires only the addition of water; when supplemented by adequate water, Sustagen has maintained a state of adequate nutrition in comatose patients for years. It has also been found to be tolerated when administered directly into an enterostomy. (See Table 14-1.) Sustagen represents the end product of a long period of research at the Homer Phillips Hospital in St. Louis.

Also used for tube feedings are powdered milk, and mixtures of milk, eggs, cream, syrup, yeast and other ingredients. (See Table 14-1.)

Whole foods can be liquefied in a blender and administered by means of a tube, providing the ingredients of a natural diet with all known and unknown dietary essentials, relatively inexpensively, and sometimes causing less diarrhea and other untoward symptoms than commercial preparations. The content of such mixtures is readily varied if diarrhea should occur. Commercial strained baby foods can be administered as tube feedings. (See Table 14-2.)

TUBE FEEDING METHODS Every nurse should thoroughly understand both the role and the method of tube feedings, which can be administered by gravity flow or by mechanical pump.

Table 14-2. Composition and Nutritive Value of Blenderized Tube Feeding Mixture

	Amount	*2,000 ml.**	*1,000 ml.*
Strained peas	Jars	1	½
Strained carrots	Jars	1	½
Strained beets	Jars	1	½
Strained applesauce	Jars	1	½
Strained beef	Jars	3	1½
Strained liver	Jars	1	½
Eggs	(Number)	2	1
Strained orange juice	ml.	200	100
18% cream	ml.	180	90
Milk	ml.	700	350
Glucose	Gm.	60	30
Salt	Gm.	5	2

* 2,000 ml. contain approximately 1,977 calories, 11 Gm. of sodium chloride, 120 Gm. protein, 89 Gm. fat and 174 Gm. of carbohydrate. Each 500 ml. would contain about 495 calories and 30 Gm. of protein.

Artz, C., and Hardy, J.: Complications in Surgery and Their Management, p. 352. Philadelphia, Saunders, 1961.

Many variations have been devised for administering tube feedings by gravity flow:

1. An **Asepto syringe** can serve as a funnel; it is frequently used to administer the feeding mixture. The syringe attaches directly to the nasogastric tube, and flow rate is regulated by the height at which the nurse holds the syringe. (See Figure 14-2.)

   Advantages of this method:
   A. The equipment is simple and easy to care for.
   B. The patient can be observed closely for untoward symptoms because the nurse is present during the entire feeding.

   Disadvantages of this method:
   A. The flow rate can be only crudely adjusted by raising or lowering the syringe.
   B. The tube feeding mixture is often administered too rapidly because the nurse lacks sufficient time to remain at the bedside for a slow delivery of the feeding.
   C. The syringe usually has to be refilled several times to give the desired amount of the feeding mixture.

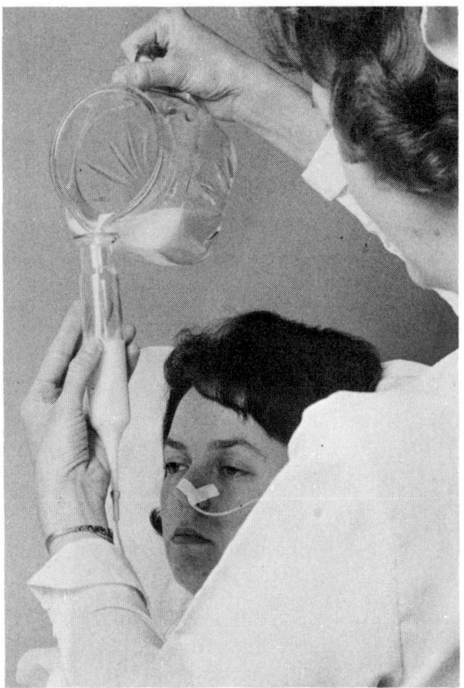

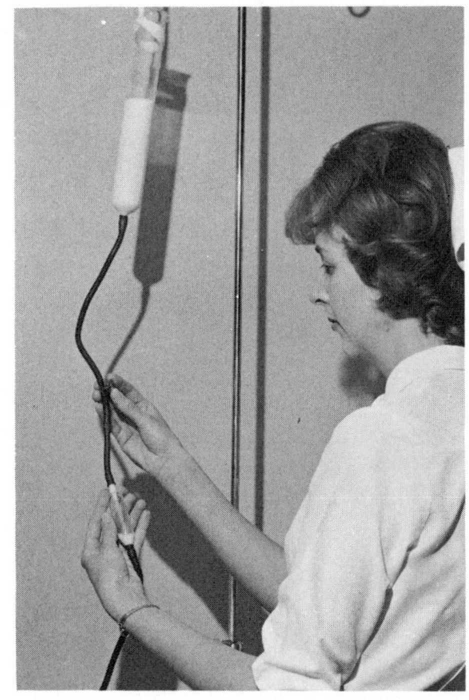

Fig. 14-2. (*Left, top*) Tube feeding with a syringe.

Fig. 14-3. (*Right, top*) Tube feeding with a flask and a Murphy-drip apparatus.

2. Another commonly used apparatus consists of a **Murphy drip tube** used in conjunction with a Kelly flask or a Vitex Salvarsan tube (pictured), rubber tubing and a screw clamp. The flask or tube can be suspended from an I.V. standard. (See Figure 14-3.)

   Advantages of this method:

   A. The flow rate can be regulated as desired by adjusting the clamp and counting the drip flow in the Murphy drip tube.

   B. The nurse does not have to be constantly present during the feeding.

   C. The reservoir is calibrated for easy measurement, and holds several hundred ml., depending on the type of flask used.

   Disadvantages of this method:

   A. Resterilized rubber tubing often cracks and can harbor pathogenic organisms.

   B. The mixture is not in a closed container.

3. Some hospitals use **resterilized parenteral fluid bottles** and disposable intravenous tubing to administer tube feedings slowly by the drip method. The disposable tubing attaches directly to the nasogastric tube, and the bottle is suspended from an I.V. standard. (See Figure 14-4.)

   Advantages of this method:

   A. The flow rate can be adjusted as desired—when necessary, a large amount of the feeding mixture can be delivered over a long period of time.

   B. The nurse does not have to be constantly present.

   C. The plastic tubing is disposable; the bottle can be resterilized often.

   D. The mixture is in a closed container.

   Disadvantages of this method:

   A. During prolonged administration, the

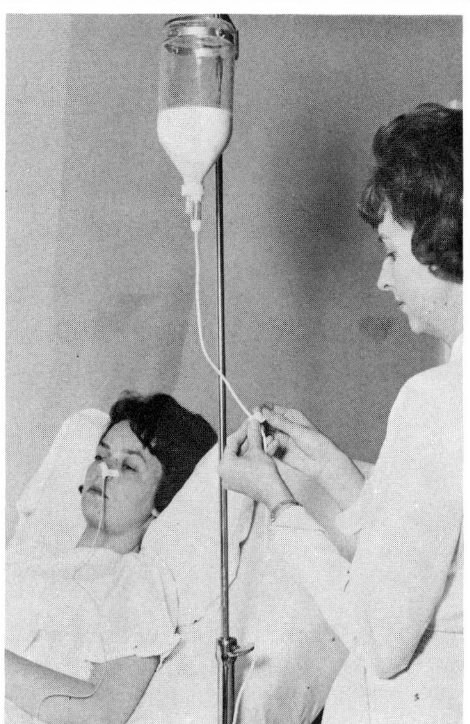

Fig. 14-4. Tube feeding with a resterilized I.V. bottle and disposable I.V. tubing.

mixture may be exposed to room temperature too long, causing bacterial multiplication in the mixture.

B. A thick mixture may clog the narrow tubing.

4. The **Davol disposable gastric feeding unit** consists of a graduated polyethylene bag, pet-cock shut-off for measurement of flow, drip chamber, wide plastic tubing, and a Sims connector for attachment to the gastric or the duodenal tube. The unit is suspended from an I.V. standard. (See Figure 14-5.)

   Advantages of this method:

   A. The flow rate can be adjusted as desired—when necessary, a large amount of the feeding mixture can be delivered over a long period of time.

   B. The apparatus will accommodate both light and heavy fluids; the flexible drip chamber may be used to assist the flow of viscous fluids.

   C. The equipment is entirely disposable—it may be used more than once, as a one-patient item, if rinsed well after each feeding.

   Disadvantages of this method:

   A. During prolonged administration, the mixture may be exposed to room temperature too long, causing an increased bacterial count.

   B. The cost to the patient can be a disadvantage if the set-up is used only once or twice.

5. The **mechanical pump method** is more dependable than the gravity drip method for slow constant delivery of tube feedings. Factors that may cause an uneven flow rate in the gravity drip method include:

   A. A change in the patient's position after the flow rate has been adjusted; almost invariably the patient will desire to change his position during the feeding, especially when the mixture is given slowly.

   B. Failure to adjust the flow rate as frequently as necessary; frequent checks are indicated to assure maintenance of the desired flow rate.

   C. A viscous mixture may clog the tube, especially when the flow has been disrupted by a position change.

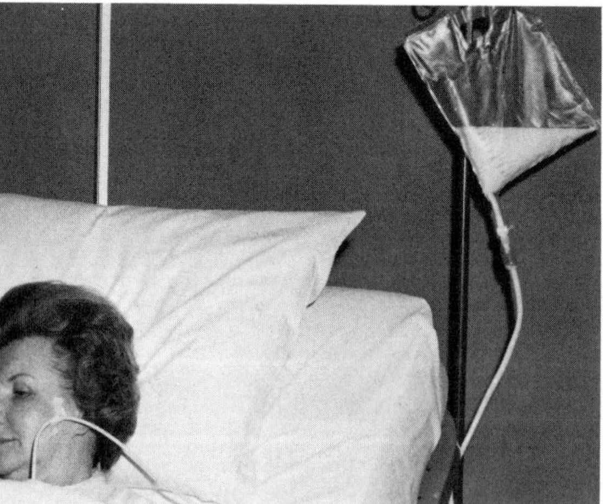

Fig. 14-5. Tube feeding with Davol Gastric Feeding Unit. (Davol Rubber Co., Providence, Rhode Island)

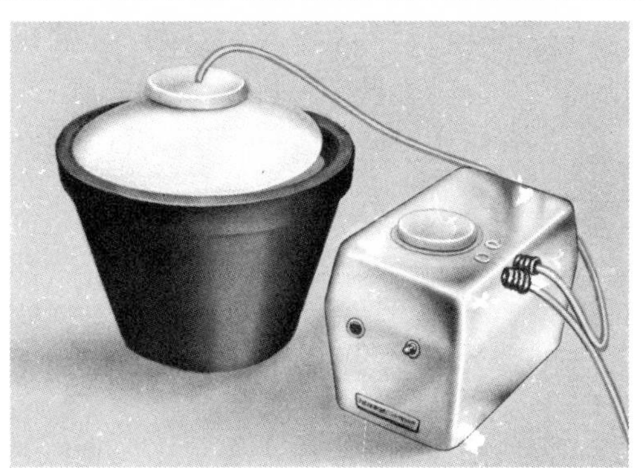

Fig. 14-6. Barron food pump. (Friedrich, H.: Oral feeding by food pump. Am. J. Nurs., p. 63, February, 1962)

A food pump, on the other hand, assures a constant flow rate regardless of the patient's position.

An example of a commercial food pump is the Barron food pump. (See Figure 14-6.) This device is the result of extensive work done by James Barron, M.D., of the Henry Ford Hospital, and the Engineering and Medical Departments of the Chrysler Corporation. The pump can be used to deliver intermittent or continuous feedings.

The equipment includes the pump mechanism, the food container, an outer insulated container for ice and the latex tubing. (See Figure 14-7.) To prevent spoilage, the feeding solution is cooled by placing the food bottle in the non-drip insulated ice container.

The speed of the feeding, determined by the physician, is controlled by a pulley on the underside of the pump. (See Figure 14-8.) There are four speeds for delivery of the solution:

1. First speed (low)— 43 ml./hr.
2. Second speed — 65 ml./hr.
3. Third speed —113 ml./hr.
4. Fourth speed —200 ml./hr.

The slowest speed is usually necessary when the patient is first started on tube feedings, to minimize nausea, vomiting, cramping and diarrhea; the speed is gradually increased to the desired rate.

When used properly, food pumps conserve the nurse's time. The instructions accompanying the pump should be carefully studied before the feedings are started; otherwise the results will not be satisfactory.

Selection of the Feeding Method When the tube feedings are ordered, the physician may indicate a specific method for administering the feeding solution. If he has no preference, the nurse may decide which method is best for the patient.

Factors to be considered in determining the best method to use include: (1) the patient's con-

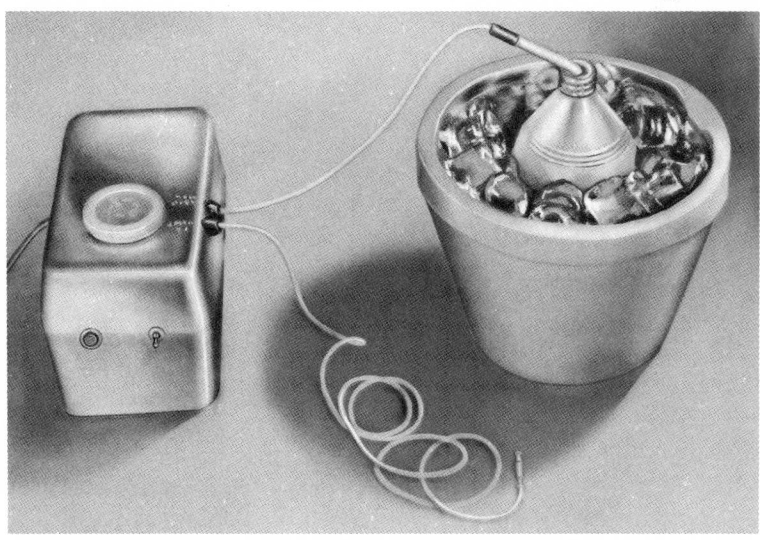

Fig. 14-7. Pump mechanism, food container, insulated ice container, and tubing of the Barron food pump. (Barron, J.: Tube feeding of post-operative patients. Surg. Clin. N. Am., p. 1488, December, 1959)

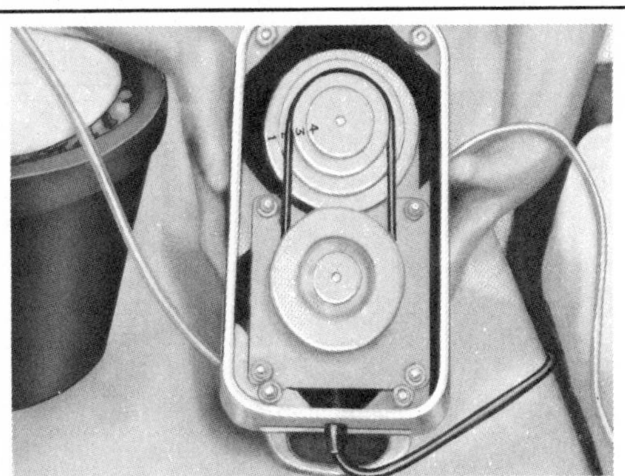

Fig. 14-8. Pulley for regulating speed of Barron food pump. (Friedrich, H.: Oral feeding by food pump. Am. J. Nurs., p. 63, February, 1962)

dition; (2) the viscosity of the feeding mixture; (3) the type of equipment available.

The patient's condition is an important factor. For example, comatose patients must have a slow delivery of solution to prevent gastric distention and vomiting, with possible tracheal aspiration. A food pump set at a slow speed or a gravity drip method suitable for slow delivery of the mixture should be used. Patients receiving duodenal or upper jejunal feedings require a slow, constant feeding rate; best results are obtained with a mechanical food pump set at a low speed. All patients, however, do not require a constant, slow delivery of the feeding mixture. Many alert patients, free of gastrointestinal problems, can tolerate fairly rapid feedings if the amount given each time is small; any of the feeding methods described earlier can be adapted for their needs.

Failure to consider the viscosity of the feeding mixture can result in clogging the apparatus. A thick mixture is best given with a mechanical food pump, or with a gravity drip apparatus having wide diameter tubing.

The type of equipment available greatly influences the method chosen; most hospitals have their own routine set-ups for tube feedings.

PREVENTION OF TUBE FEEDING COMPLICATIONS Although tube feedings have proved to be of immense value, they can cause trouble if given incorrectly. Complications of tube feedings include:

1. Diarrhea
2. Nausea
3. Vomiting
4. Aspiration pneumonia
5. Inadequate provision for water requirements
6. Metabolic alkalosis (primary base bicarbonate excess)

In order to avoid untoward reactions from tube feedings, the nurse should keep the following in mind:

1. The feeding mixture and the apparatus used to administer it are excellent culture sites for bacteria, and proper precautions should be taken so that neither the tube feeding mixture nor the equipment used for administration will become contaminated.
   A. Whatever the set-up used for administering tube feedings, it should be carefully cleaned prior to use. Glass receptacles should be washed in hot, soapy water and rinsed well following each feeding. Between feedings, equipment should be stored in a closed container or wrapped in a clean towel. Equipment should be resterilized often, even though tube feeding is not a sterile procedure. As mentioned earlier, disposable equipment may be used. One should always keep in mind possible sources for contamination of equipment; for example, uncovered equipment stored at the bedside in the summer attracts flies, especially if it has not been thoroughly cleaned.
   B. In order to discourage bacterial growth, the tube feeding mixture should be refrigerated until at least one hour before use. Diarrhea frequently occurs when the feeding mixture is improperly stored.
   C. Only enough tube feeding mixture for a 24-hour period should be made up in advance.
   D. From 20 to 50 ml. of lukewarm water should be administered through the tube after each feeding when the inter-

mittent method is used. This will force the remaining mixture into the stomach and clean the tube.

E. When continuous feedings are necessary, the equipment should be changed often. Because of the danger of spoilage, the reservoir should not be filled to capacity and exposed to room temperature until emptied. Instead, small amounts of fresh solution should be added at regular intervals. Occasionally, when the gravity drip method is used, ice bags are wrapped around the mixture reservoir to retard spoilage.

F. As mentioned earlier, the Barron food pump has its own provision for cooling the mixture. When the food pump tube is to be disconnected for more than several minutes, the end of it should be placed in the food container and the motor turned on, to prevent spoilage of food and obstruction of the tube.

2. The tube feeding mixture should be given slowly and in small amounts in order to avoid distention, nausea and excessive peristalsis.

   A. When the intermittent feeding method is used, the amount given at each feeding is determined by dividing the total 24-hour dose by the number of feedings. Frequently, 2,000 ml. is given over a 24-hour period. Divided feedings may be given at intervals of 2, 3, or 4 hours, and individual feedings frequently vary between 150 to 300 ml. (The individual feeding should not exceed 400 ml. unless it is to be given quite slowly.)

   B. If the patient should experience difficulty, then the feeding can be diluted with water, to be administered by slow drip or by a slow speed setting on the mechanical pump.

   C. If the patient has trouble with abdominal distention, it may be necessary to aspirate trapped air from the stomach prior to giving the tube feeding mixture.

3. The tube feeding mixture should be neither too hot nor too cold, since such temperature extremes cause nausea and discomfort, especially if the feeding is given quickly.

   A. Feedings should be warmed to body temperature—but not to exceed 100° F.—by placing the container in a pan of warm water. The mixture should not be overheated, however, since this would curdle the protein and clog the tubing.

   B. The fact that the mixture fed by the Barron food pump is not warm presents no difficulty, since the amount entering the stomach over any given period is small.

4. Measures should be taken to prevent gastric distention due to the introduction of excessive amounts of air during the feeding.

   A. The feeding mixture reservoir should not be allowed to empty completely before more mixture is added, and when the last of the feeding is about to flow into the tube, a small amount of water should be added to the reservoir and the tube clamped off.

   B. Small quantities of air cause no difficulty; if care is used during the feeding, excessive air will not enter.

5. Unpleasant stimuli can be minimized to prevent nausea.

   A. The esthetic factors for patients taking food by mouth apply also to patients receiving nasogastric tube feedings. Unpleasant stimuli inhibit the flow of digestive juices needed for food utilization.

   B. Even though the patient is not taking nourishment orally, one should respect his need for a clean mouth. Regurgitation can occur in patients receiving tube feedings, and when it does, the patient should be given a mouthwash. Even the semi-alert patient can taste tube feedings. The nares should be cleaned and lubricated often in order to minimize the discomfort caused by the nasogastric tube.

6. If nausea should occur, the feeding should be stopped and the patient given a rest period until further medical orders are received. A p.r.n. medication for nausea may be necessary. After the nausea subsides, a small amount of the feeding can be given slowly while the nurse observes the patient's reaction. The following can be tried when nausea occurs:
   A. Decrease the fat content of the mixture
   B. Dilute the mixture
   C. Administer the mixture more slowly
7. If diarrhea occurs, the feeding should be discontinued until further medical orders are received.
   A. The order may involve a modification of the feeding, most frequently a decrease in its carbohydrate content.
   B. Medication, such as Kaopectate or paregoric, can be ordered and given through the tube to relieve the diarrhea.
   C. Addition of applesauce or of Kanana Banana Flakes to the mixture frequently controls the diarrhea.
8. Precautions should be taken to prevent the aspiration of gastric contents if vomiting or regurgitation occurs. Aspiration of the feeding mixture can cause pneumonia or strangulation.
   A. If possible, the patient should be in a sitting position when receiving nasogastric feedings. If this is not possible, the head of the bed should be elevated to a 45° angle, unless this position is contraindicated. The head of the bed should remain elevated for 30 minutes to one hour following feeding.
   B. If vomiting occurs, the patient's head should be turned to the side and lowered to promote drainage of the vomitus.
   C. A suction machine should be available for immediate use when the patient is semiconscious, unconscious, or otherwise unable to control the expulsion of vomitus. A nurse should remain with such patients throughout the feeding to cope with vomiting or regurgitation.
9. The amount of the feeding taken should be recorded, as should the amount of water added before, between, and after feedings.
10. Urine output should be recorded, and unless abnormal fluid losses are occurring, the amount of water taken by mouth should roughly equal the urinary output.
11. The nurse will do well to watch for signs of inadequate water intake, particularly when the feedings are high in protein content. Otherwise, uremia may develop.
   A. Often, tube feeding mixtures are rich in protein, which cannot be properly metabolized without generous quantities of water. Should insufficient water be provided, water will be drawn from the tissues to supply the needed volume for urinary excretion of the increased solute load. Eventually, dehydration (sodium excess) will occur, along with an accumulation of nitrogenous waste product in the bloodstream.
   B. The nurse should be alert for the untoward effects of excessive protein in relation to water, including nausea, vomiting, diarrhea, and eventually, ileus. If the condition is allowed to go uncorrected, it will result in a high fever and accompanying disorientation. Laboratory tests will reveal an elevated blood urea nitrogen (BUN) level.
   C. Malfunctioning kidneys require more water to excrete a given amount of solute than do normal kidneys, and because aged patients frequently have impaired renal function, they require more water than do the young.
   D. Early in protein overloading, the urine volume is large even though the water intake is inadequate; this can easily lead the staff to think that the water intake is adequate. In such instances, however, output actually exceeds intake. By the accurate recording of careful observations, the nurse can unmask the true situation.
   E. Confused or unconscious patients

should be observed carefully for inadequate water intake, since they are not aware of thirst.

12. A check commonly used to determine if the nasogastric tube is in the stomach is the withdrawal of a small quantity of gastric juice prior to each feeding. Gastric juice which has been withdrawn should be gently forced back into the stomach rather than discarded.
    A. While it is essential to check the position of the tube before giving a feeding, aspiration of even small amounts of stomach juices before each feeding can add up to an important quantity over the course of 2 or 3 days' tube feeding therapy.
    B. Metabolic alkalosis can easily result when small amounts of gastric juice are repeatedly removed over several days. Gastric juice is rich in potassium, chloride and hydrogen ions. The loss of chloride causes the bicarbonate of the body to rise in compensation. Loss of potassium further contributes to the alkalosis, since the kidneys of the potassium-deficient patient excrete hydrogen preferentially.
    C. Other methods can be used to check if the tube is properly situated. For example, the tip of the tube can be placed in a glass of water and if many bubbles appear as the patient exhales, the tube is probably in the respiratory passage. However, trapped air in the stomach can produce occasional bubbles. The nurse can also ask the patient to hum—if the tube is in the trachea, he will be unable to do so.
13. Measures should be taken to prevent nausea following the feeding.
    A. Avoid movements that might contribute to nausea for 2 to 3 hours after the feeding.
    B. Again, consider the esthetic factors discussed above.
14. Constipation may sometimes be a problem when liquefied natural foods are administered very slowly into the stomach. These measures can be taken to prevent constipation and fecal impactions:
    A. The frequency of bowel movements and the character of the stools should be observed and charted so that constipation can be detected before a fecal impaction forms.
    B. The nurse who is familiar with the symptoms of constipation and fecal impaction will report their presence to the physician. Thus, if the patient fails to have a bowel movement for 3 successive days, the physician can be notified. Some patients may require attention before 3 days; a few may normally have bowel movements no oftener than every 3 or 4 days. Other reportable signs include: dry, hard feces expelled with difficulty or watery stools following a prolonged period without a bowel movement. The nurse should recall that a fecal impaction can manifest itself with diarrhea, since the bowel may become irritated by the impacted fecal bolus and force liquid feces around the impaction and out the anus.
    C. A change in the content of the feeding mixture may correct the constipation.
    D. Laxatives may be added through the feeding tube to correct and eliminate the constipation.
    E. Adequate quantities of water are beneficial.

Intake Via the Parenteral Route

The nurse's role in administering parenteral nutrients is discussed in Chapter 16.

MODIFYING THE DIET TO PREVENT OR MINIMIZE BODY FLUID DISTURBANCES

Fever

An increased metabolic rate accompanies fever, and each degree Fahrenheit the temperature is elevated causes a 7 per cent increase in metabolic rate, whereas each degree of Centigrade elevation causes a 13 per cent increase. Prolonged fever, particularly if it is high, can easily lead to body fluid disturbances, especially when the body's requirements for water and electrolytes are neglected; fever causes an increased loss of water and electrolytes from lungs, skin and kidneys. The increased metabolism that accompanies fever depletes the body stores of glycogen and causes an increased catabolism of protein. The increased solute load resulting from protein breakdown places an extra burden on the kidneys, and losses of sodium, chloride and potassium are increased.

The patient suffering from prolonged fever needs to have his intake of all nutrients augmented, and yet the feverish patient usually has anorexia. Moreover, there appears to be decreased intestinal motility and subnormal absorption of nutrients during fever. Catabolism of body tissues can easily lead to metabolic acidosis (primary base bicarbonate deficit).

The patient with prolonged fever requires increased water up to 3,000, 4,000 or more ml. daily. His intake of the bulk nutrients—protein, fat and carbohydrate—should be increased; so should his intake of the water soluble vitamins, including members of the B complex and C. Adequate electrolytes, too, should be provided, particularly sodium and potassium. The effort to increase the patient's nutritional intake should not, of course, overtax his ability to ingest and digest food. Small, frequent servings will help avoid overtaxing the gastrointestinal tract. If the patient is unable to ingest adequate nutrients by mouth, then feedings by nasogastric tube or by the parenteral route should be considered.

Sweet concentrated liquids can cause abdominal distention and loss of appetite. Carbonated beverages, on the other hand, are usually well tolerated, as are fruit juices, tea, coffee and water. The fat of fluid whole milk tends to slow down the emptying time of the stomach; skim milk is probably preferable for most patients.

Often a liquid diet is indicated for the acutely ill patient, providing 800 to 1,200 calories, and meeting water and calorie needs to prevent severe depletion. The patient should be returned to a full diet as soon as he is able to ingest it.

If possible, the daily intake of protein for the febrile patient should be 60 to 100 or more Gm. High protein drinks, such as powdered or liquid commercial protein concentrates, or eggnog, are frequently useful. Fats are an excellent source of calories and can be given in the form of egg yolk, milk, cream, ice cream, margarine and butter, provided they are tolerated, but when fats are not tolerated, carbohydrates can be used to provide generous quantities of calories.

While the patient is convalescing from a febrile illness, a diet generous in all essentials should be administered in order to repair deficits.

Excessive Perspiration

Sensible perspiration, or sweat, is a hypotonic liquid containing sodium, potassium, chloride, and small amounts of magnesium, ammonia, and urea. Insensible perspiration consists of water only and is lost through evaporation from body surfaces, including the skin and the lungs.

High environmental temperatures can cause the loss of large quantities of body water and electrolytes. In hot surroundings some workmen have been found to lose 8 to 10 L. of sweat a day. The bedfast patient must be given additional fluid if the environmental temperature is elevated.

Patients under heavy drapes in operating rooms that are not air conditioned can lose large volumes of fluid in the form of perspiration; heatstroke and death have occurred in excessively hot operating rooms.

Perspiration losses can be recorded both on the intake-output sheet and on the nurse's notes. The saturation of pajamas and bed linen should be recorded, as should the number of times it has been necessary to change them. Because it is difficult to estimate the amount of perspiration, some persons tend to ignore it altogether.

Insensible loss equals approximately 1,000 ml./m.^{2} of body surface/day in the hospitalized patient, but when respiration is hyperactive or fever is present, this loss may be greatly increased. Sweat losses (sensible perspiration) depend chiefly upon temperature, humidity, metabolic rate and fever and in disease, may equal 1,000 or more ml./m.^{2} of body surface/day. Sweat losses can be roughly measured by weight changes if one considers other gains and losses of fluids.

Liquids should be given freely to the heavily perspiring patient and should contain both water and electrolytes. If sweat losses are replaced by water alone, sodium deficit (low sodium syndrome, hyponatremia, heat exhaustion) can easily occur. Among the sources of salt are the salt content of foods, salty broths, salt added at the table, and commercial salt tablets. Naturally, one should guard against producing a sodium excess by the administration of excessive quantities of sodium chloride. The patient on a low sodium diet often develops excellent sodium conservation. This applies only to patients not receiving diuretics, since diuretics counteract the body's sodium conserving action.

When the heavily perspiring patient is unable to take fluids by mouth, parenteral fluid orders should be requested from the physician.

Vomiting

One should know when to advise against oral intake, as well as when to encourage it. For example, the patient who is vomiting persistently should not drink water, since vomited water will carry with it gastric electrolytes.

Since persistent vomiting calls for parenteral administration of fluids, the nurse should report its presence to the physician, as untreated vomiting can lead to metabolic alkalosis and superimpose ketosis of starvation. Under such circumstances, alkalosis is more likely to occur than acidosis. One cannot depend upon them neutralizing each other.

When vomiting ceases or decreases in frequency, the patient can be given bland foods in small amounts. Toast, crackers, ginger ale and, in some instances, milk—especially skim milk—are tolerated well, but orange juice tends to increase peristalsis.

Recall that vomitus consists of water, hydrogen, chloride, sodium, potassium and other chemicals, and as much as 6 L. of gastric secretion can be lost in a 24-hour period.

The reinstitution of a normal diet can repair mild deficits, particularly if the diet is supplemented with between-meal feedings of potassium-rich foods, such as meats, fruits, vegetables, milk and fruit juices. Excellent commercial potassium supplements are available and have the advantage that they can be given in doses containing known quantities of potassium. Examples are K-Lor, Kaon, and K-Lyte.

Gastrointestinal Suction

The patient receiving gastrointestinal suction should never be given water or ice chips by mouth, since water washes electrolytes from the stomach, causing metabolic alkalosis. Statland cited a patient who was receiving suction and was permitted to ingest 21 L. of water. The water was drawn back from the suction tube, leaving the patient in profound alkalosis, which proved fatal. Ice chips made with appropriately constituted electrolyte solutions are permissible, but a specific solution should be prescribed by the physician. A commercial oral electrolyte solution (Lytren) can be used to make chips for this purpose.

Sometimes the order is given to permit ice chips sparingly; the term "sparingly" can readily be stretched by well-meaning but ill-advised persons to the point where the intake of plain ice is excessive.

Diarrhea

Diarrhea results in the loss of water, electrolytes and partially digested nutrients. Prolonged diarrhea frequently results in potassium deficit, as well as in metabolic acidosis, and prolonged watery diarrhea can result in sodium excess, since water is lost in excess of electrolytes. During the acute stage of diarrhea, the gastrointestinal tract is usually put at rest through parenteral alimentation. Food is given by mouth as soon as it can be tolerated, and some physicians institute oral feedings by the use of oral electrolyte solutions; others use skim milk. Some doctors employ tea and toast.

Liberal fluid intake should be encouraged with frequent, high caloric feedings. Such foods as puddings, custards and milk supply calories

Table 14-3. Diuretic Drugs

Nonproprietary Name	*Trade Name*	*Usual Daily Dosage Range*
Thiazide Diuretics		
Bendroflumethiazide	Naturetin	2.5 to 5 mg. orally
Benzthiazide	Exna; Aquatag	25 to 100 mg. orally
Chlorothiazide N.F.	Diuril	500 to 1000 mg. orally
Cyclothiazide	Anhydron	2 mg. (1 mg. 2 or 3 times a week)
Hydroflumethiazide	Saluron	25 to 200 mg. orally
Hydrochlorothiazide U.S.P.	Esidrix; HydroDiuril; Oretic	25 to 200 mg. orally; maintenance, 75 to 100 mg.
Methyclothiazide	Enduron	2.5 to 10 mg. orally
Polythiazide	Renese	1 to 4 mg. orally
Trichlormethiazide	Naqua; Metahydrin	2 to 8 mg. orally
Mercurial Diuretics		
Chlormerodrin N.F.	Neohydrin	55 to 110 mg. orally
Meralluride U.S.P.	Mercuhydrin Sodium	1 to 2 ml. parenterally
Mercaptomerin sodium U.S.P.	Thiomerin	0.2 to 2 ml. parenterally
Carbonic Anhydrase Inhibitors		
Acetazolamide U.S.P.	Diamox	250 to 375 mg. orally
Dichlorphenamide U.S.P.	Daranide	100 to 200 mg. orally initially; 25 to 150 mg. maintenance
Potassium-Conserving Diuretics		
Spironolactone U.S.P.	Aldactone	25 mg., 2 to 4 times daily
Triamterene	Dyrenium	100 to 200 mg. orally; maintenance, 100 mg.
Other Diuretics		
Ethacrynic acid	Edecrin	25 to 200 mg. orally
Sodium ethacrynate	Sodium Edecrin	0.5 to 1.0 mg. per kg. body weight, I.V.
Furosemide	Lasix	40 to 80 mg. orally 20 to 40 mg. parenterally

Adapted from Rodman, M. and Smith, D.: Pharmacology and Drug Therapy in Nursing, pp. 301-302. Philadelphia, J. B. Lippincott Company, 1968.

and protein and are well tolerated, provided the patient does not have a special sensitivity to them. The diet is gradually changed to normal.

MEDICAL THERAPY CAUSING NUTRITIONAL DISTURBANCES

Diuresis

The primary purpose of diuretics is to promote the excretion of sodium and water from the body. In varying degrees, most diuretics tend also to promote the excretion of potassium. Diuretics associated with hypokalemia include the thiazides, the mercurials, furosemide (Lasix), ethacrynic acid (Edecrin) and the carbonic anhydrase inhibitors, such as acetazolamide (Diamox). (See Table 14-3.)

Although the usual diet provides potassium in amounts ranging from 75 to 125 mEq. per day, losses of potassium by patients receiving any of the above diuretics can amount to several times this amount. Failure to eat well should be reported to the physician, because potassium deficit is even more apt to occur when the dietary intake is inadequate or when there are other abnormal losses of potassium from the body. Unfortunately, the body apparently has no adequate mechanism for the conservation of potassium, and indeed, the patient dying of a potassium deficit may lose 30 to 40 or more mEq. a day in the urine in spite of his dire need.

Determination of the daily urinary excretion of potassium through analysis of the potassium content of the 24-hour urine specimen helps guide potassium replacement. A useful rule of thumb suggests that the patient receive a daily quota of potassium equal to his daily urinary excretion plus 10 per cent. Thus, if a patient was found to be excreting 160 mEq. of potassium in the urine each day, the total potassium intake for prevention of a deficit would be 176 mEq. daily. If the dietary intake of potassium was estimated at 75 mEq.—a frequent average intake—then one would administer about 100 mEq. of potassium as a supplement. A pharmaceutical supplement such as K-Lyte provides 25 mEq. of potassium in each effervescent tablet, and one tablespoon of Kaon Elixir supplies 20 mEq., whereas approximately 15 mEq. is contained in one tablespoon of Potassium Triplex. A 5 Gm. packet of K-Lor furnishes 20 mEq. of potassium. The need for potassium supplementation of the diet of patients receiving diuretics becomes more pronounced when the diuretic has been taken for a long period.

When possible, diuretics should be administered intermittently rather than daily, allowing the patient to partially restore his potassium supply by dietary means. Regardless of the methods used to reduce the possibility of potassium deficit, the patient should be observed closely for undue fatigue, weakness, anorexia, flaccid muscles, and gaseous abdominal distention, and all patients receiving diuretics associated with potassium loss should have occasional plasma potassium determinations.

The patient should be encouraged to consume adequate quantities of potassium rich foods, such as bananas, oranges, dried fruits, fruit juices, meats and nuts. (See Table 14-4.)

An excellent source of the potassium content of foods, as well as other dietary values, is *Bowes and Church's Food Values of Portions Commonly Used*, Philadelphia, J. B. Lippincott Co., 1970. This book is particularly helpful to the nurse because food contents are expressed in terms of common servings rather than in portions of 100 Gms.

Potassium-conserving diuretics include spironolactone (Aldactone) and triamterene (Dyrenium). Aldactone is an aldosterone blocking agent and thus promotes sodium loss and potassium retention, whereas Dyrenium has a unique mode of action, interfering with the exchange of sodium ions for potassium and hydrogen ions. Hyperkalemia can occur when potassium-conserving diuretics are used in patients with renal insufficiency since such patients already have a tendency for potassium retention. Symptoms to be alert for include paresthesias of the extremities, nausea, weakness and intestinal cramping with diarrhea, and if hyperkalemia is severe, cardiac arrest can occur. Only patients with adequate renal reserve should receive potassium-conserving hormones. Periodic plasma potassium determinations should be obtained. Diuretics that allow retention of potassium are often used in conjunc-

Table 14-4. Potassium Content of Various Foods in Common Portions

Food, Amount	*mEq. of K*
Beverages:	
Whole Milk, 240 ml.	9.11
Non-Fat or Skim Milk, 240 ml.	5.11
Instant Coffee, Folgers (2 Gm. in 240 ml. water)	6.14
Tomato Juice, ½ cup (canned)	7.29
Orange Juice, ½ cup (fresh)	5.68
Grapefruit Juice, ½ cup (canned)	4.41
Grape Juice, bottled, ½ cup	3.84
Apple Juice, ½ cup	3.20
Coca-Cola, 180 ml.	2.25
Pepsi-Cola, 240 ml.	0.18
Ginger-Ale, 240 ml.	0.03
Fruits:	
Banana, raw, 1 medium	16.12
Figs, dried, 7 small	19.96
Grapefruit, raw, ½ medium	10.24
Orange, 1 medium	9.21
Peaches, dried, uncooked, ½ cup	28.16
Raisins, dried seedless, 2 tbsp.	3.68
Apricots, raw, 2-3 medium	7.06
Cereals:	
Oatmeal, cooked, 1 cup	3.32
Corn Flakes, 1 cup	1.02
Meats and Meat Substitutes:	
Canadian Bacon, cooked, 1 slice	2.32
Frankfurter, cooked, 1 average	2.72
Ham, cooked, 2 slices	13.31
Hamburger, cooked, 1 patty	9.77
Rib Steak, cooked, 1 serving (½ lb. raw)	9.93
Pink Salmon, ½ cup (canned)	7.42
Cheese, American Cheddar, 1 piece (2 x 2 x 1)	2.96
Egg, whole, 1 medium	1.23
Others:	
Brazil Nuts, shelled, ⅓ cup	17.15
Bre'r Rabbit Syrup, 1 tbsp.	6.91
Bar Candy, chocolate covered, average 10¢ size, 2½ oz.	14.84

Adapted from Bowes, C., and Church, H.: Food Values of Portions Commonly Used. Philadelphia, Lippincott, 1966.

tion with diuretics that cause potassium loss, as their combined use reduces the possibility of hyperkalemia. Ordinarily, no potassium supplementation should be given with potassium-conserving diuretics.

Frequently, the sodium intake of patients receiving diuretics is restricted, reducing the need for large doses of potentially harmful diuretics. Usually, sodium restriction will not involve less than 1,000 mg. of sodium a day, because the use of low sodium diets containing lower levels of sodium in patients receiving diuretics can cause acute sodium deficit.

Low sodium diets and diuretics may be used to treat a variety of conditions, such as congestive heart failure, nephrosis, hepatic cirrhosis and toxemia of pregnancy. Because low sodium diets are commonly used, the nurse should know what constitutes such diets and be able to instruct patients in their use.

An average daily diet not restricted in sodium contains approximately 5,000 mg. or more of sodium, whereas low sodium diets can range from a mild restriction to as low as 200 mg. of sodium a day, depending on the patient's needs. The American Heart Association has prepared booklets describing mild, moderate and strict sodium-restricted diets. The moderate sodium-restricted diet allows 1,000 mg. of sodium daily; the strict diet allows only 500 mg. of sodium daily. The booklets are available to patients on request of their physicians.

Patients requiring only a mild sodium restriction have a great deal of freedom in planning their meals and may salt most foods lightly (about half as much as usual) during preparation. Because most canned and processed foods are already salted, no additional salt should be added. Salt should not be used at the table. (One level teaspoon of salt contains about 2,300 mg. of sodium!) Foods high in sodium content should be avoided. Examples of such foods include:

Sauerkraut and other vegetables prepared in brine
Bacon
Luncheon meats
Frankfurters
Ham
Salt pork
Sardines
Processed cheese
Bouillon cubes
Peanut butter
Catsup
Mustard
Kosher meats
Sausage
Meat tenderizers
Relish
Horseradish
Olives
Pickles
Worcestershire sauce
Potato chips
Pretzels

Patients on a low sodium diet must limit their intake of commercially processed foods which contain sodium benzoate, monosodium glutamate, and baking powder. Baking soda (sodium bicarbonate) should not be used as an antacid, since one level teaspoon of baking soda contains 1,000 mg. of sodium! Baking soda used in excessive amounts can produce metabolic alkalosis, particularly in the aged.

Tooth pastes, tooth powders, and mouth washes may be high in sodium content, and, therefore, patients on sodium restricted diets should be instructed not to swallow these products and to rinse their mouths well with water after their use. Medicines not prescribed by the physician should be avoided, as some medicines contain enough sodium to interfere with the desired intake. Among these are certain laxatives, pain relievers, sedatives, cough syrups and antibiotics.

Prolonged Use of Laxatives and Enemas

The abuse of laxatives and enemas in our society is appalling. One reason for their widespread use is misunderstanding of the term constipation, which really refers to a hard, dry stool, difficult to evacuate. Even though the patient may not have a bowel movement for several days, *he is not constipated unless his stools are hard, dry and difficult to evacuate.* Some persons normally have bowel movements every day; others may have them every 3, 4, or 5 days. If the latter individuals have soft stools, they are not regarded as constipated.

It is the compulsion to have a daily evacuation that has led to the frequent use of laxatives and enemas. Many patients feel they must be "cleaned out" daily or their health will be impaired, a misconception which should be corrected by the nurse at every opportunity; otherwise, patients will continue to use laxatives and enemas unnecessarily. Reliance on laxatives and enemas decreases the natural reflex activity of the colon; hence, *stronger* laxatives and *more* enemas are required.

The repeated administration of plain water enemas causes electrolytes to be drawn into the bowel, since the body always tries to make any collection of fluid isotonic with extracellular fluid. Therefore, when the enema is evacuated, it carries not only water, but electrolytes with it. Sodium deficit, potassium deficit, or both can be produced by repeated water enemas.

Should the patient actually be constipated, he should be provided a diet with these characteristics:

1. Generous quantities of fruits, vegetables, and bran cereals
2. Increased water intake
3. Regular meal hours

Stool softeners, such as Colace (dioctyl sodium sulfosuccinate) are useful physiologic tools for increasing the softness of the stools, and a glass of warm water or hot coffee first thing in the morning can stimulate the evacuation reflex.

Because roughage is often useful, C. H. and J. A. Ross have suggested the following dried fruit recipe, which provides a supply for several breakfasts and does not necessarily require added sugar:

½ lb. dried apricots
½ lb. dried figs
½ lb. dried prunes
½ lb. dried raisins

Soak overnight in 2 pints of water. Bring to a boil in the morning. Reduce heat and simmer 45 minutes. Do not boil the fruit bodies out of shape. Cool and refrigerate. Serve 2 ounces for breakfast covered with a fruit juice different from day to day.

Adrenocorticosteroids

Administration of adrenocorticosteroids may cause sodium and water retention and excretion of potassium, particularly when prolonged high doses are employed. For patients on such doses, the potassium intake should be increased and the sodium intake restricted, because if potassium loss is not replaced, metabolic alkalosis and potassium deficit may result.

The nurse should be alert for signs of fluid volume excess, such as weight gain, edema and increased blood pressure and should also observe for signs of potassium deficit, such as weakness, fatigue, anorexia, flaccid muscles and gaseous abdominal distention. The newer synthetic steroids, such as triamcinolone (Aristocort or Kenacort), do not have a strong influence on electrolytes and thus are associated with fewer fluid balance problems.

Prolonged administration of cortisone encourages negative nitrogen balance, and dietary treatment includes a generous intake of protein, a potassium supplement, and an adequate caloric intake to prevent weight loss. The use of cortisone can also cause decreased tolerance to carbohydrates, with hyperglycemia and glycosuria.

The effect of adrenocorticosteroids on fat metabolism is not clearly understood, but prolonged administration tends to deposit fat in the subcutaneous tissues, producing the "moon face" and "buffalo hump" associated with steroid therapy. The hydrochloric acid and pepsin contents of the stomach are increased, a fact which may be related to the occurrence of ulcers in patients on steroid therapy.

CATABOLIC EFFECTS CAUSING NUTRITIONAL DISTURBANCES

Immobilization

All patients subjected to long periods of bedrest develop metabolic disturbances, one of which is the increased excretion of calcium. As pointed out by Kottke and Blanchard,

> The long bones of the lower extremities are designed to bear weight, and as long as weight is being borne by them, the calcium is maintained in the matrix of the bones. When the stresses of weight bearing have been removed, the calcium is very soon mobilized and enters the blood stream with the resulting increased concentration of circulating calcium in the blood. This increased calcium is filtered out through the kidneys, where it is deposited as calcium salts to form kidney and bladder stones.*

* Kottke, F., and Blanchard, R.: Bedrest Begets Bedrest. Nursing Forum, 3:71, No. 3, 1964.

Table 14-5. Acid-Base Reaction of Foods

Potentially Acid or Acid Ash Foods	*Potentially Basic or Alkaline Ash Foods*
Breads, all types	Fruits, all types (except cranberries, plums, and prunes)
Cakes and cookies, plain	Jams and jellies, honey
Cereals and crackers	Milk, cream, and buttermilk
Cheese, all types	Molasses
Eggs	Nuts: almonds, coconut, chestnuts
Fish and shellfish	Vegetables, all types except corn and lentils
Fruits: cranberries, plums, and prunes	
Macaroni, spaghetti, noodles	
Meats and poultry	
Nuts: Brazil, filberts, peanuts, walnuts	
Vegetables: corn and lentils	

Neutral Foods		
Butter or margarine	Cooking fats and oils	Starches, corn and arrowroot
Candy, plain	Syrups	Sugars

Cooper, L., *et al.*: Nutrition in Health and Disease. ed. 14, p. 542. Philadelphia, Lippincott, 1963.

Pathologic fractures can occur due to bone rarefaction. Increased calcium excretion begins in the first week of immobilization and continues for a period of 4 to 8 weeks. After this period, the calcium drops back to normal or subnormal levels.

Some authorities feel that when calcium is being lost from the body, the intake should be increased over normal, and others believe that only the amount of calcium required for maintenance of body stores should be permitted.

Ordering the diet modification lies within the province of the physician, and the nurse should consult him before making any modifications other than water intake. When calcium is restricted, the patient is permitted only one pint of milk a day; of course, other foods high in calcium, such as cheese and salmon, should be excluded from the diet. In addition to losing calcium, the immobilized patient loses nitrogen and may develop negative nitrogen balance unless his intake of protein is adequate.

The nurse can help to prevent the development of stones in the urinary system by encouraging a daily fluid intake of 3000 ml. or more, in order to increase urinary volume, since small crystals have less tendency to accumulate mass when urine flow is continuous and great. (Some physicians want patients with stone-forming tendencies to take oral fluids at regular intervals around the clock; they feel there is no point in pushing urine flow for only two-thirds of the 24 hours.) Other preventive nursing measures include turning the patient frequently, elevating the head of the bed, having the patient sit up, if possible, to prevent stasis of urine, plus frequent active and passive exercises.

Adjusting the pH of urine can help prevent stone formation. An acid urine increases the solubility of calcium and magnesium phosphates and carbonates. The commonly occurring calcium phosphate stone, apatite, will not form when the urine pH is below 6.6. The use of cranberry juice, ale, beer and meats helps acidify the urine, and urine acidifying drugs, such as ammonium chloride or methenamine mandelate (Mandelamine), are commonly used in conjunction with dietary modifications. Table 14-5 shows how the diet can be modified to yield an acid or alkaline ash.

Decubitus Ulcers

A draining decubitus ulcer can quadruple the body's need for protein, as the ulcer exudate is high in protein content. The fact that most patients with decubiti are immobilized further contributes to the increased protein need.

It is often difficult for the patient to consume sufficient protein, since his appetite is usually poor. The nurse must use all her ingenuity to find foods rich in protein but acceptable to the patient. Usual food sources of protein can be supplemented by commercial high protein supplements or by skim milk powder. Both can be added to food without changing the bulk or flavor appreciably. Two tablespoons of dry skim milk powder supplies 6 Gm. of protein and can be added to cereal, scrambled eggs, pudding, soup, hamburger and other foods.

The increased protein need must be considered as important as turning the patient often and keeping the skin clean and dry.

Hemorrhage

The well-nourished person can usually regenerate red blood cells following one episode of hemorrhage. Chronic blood loss, however, depletes the red cell stores and results in anemia. The body compensates for the decrease in circulating blood volume that accompanies hemorrhage by drawing fluid from the tissue spaces into the vascular compartment—an interstitial fluid-to-plasma shift of water and electrolytes. The total extracellular fluid volume is unchanged; only the distribution of the fluid is affected.

The patient who has suffered chronic hemorrhage should be provided a diet rich in protein, iron and vitamin C. Up to 100 Gm. of protein a day should be given; excellent sources of protein are meat, eggs, cheese and fish. Protein supplements can also be employed, between meals or at bedtime or both. Iron can be supplied as meat, liver, prunes, apples, grapes, spinach, beans, enriched cereals and eggs. In addition, it is well to give an additional source of iron, preferably ferrous sulfate, by mouth. Vitamin C intake can be increased by generous servings of citrus fruits. Lastly, the fluid intake should be generous.

Trauma

Trauma, such as burns, fractures, wounds and crushing injuries, causes loss of protein through direct destruction of tissues. It contributes further to the loss through the so-called toxic destruction of protein, an increased catabolism brought on mysteriously by the trauma. It also promotes the accumulation of protein-rich fluid at the site of the injury, which contributes further to possible protein depletion. Immobilization made necessary by the injury also causes losses of protein and, in addition, of electrolytes.

Because of these losses and because of the requirements for optimal healing, the protein, electrolyte and vitamin C intake of the injured patient should be increased; as much as 150 Gm. of protein daily is frequently administered. The diet should be high in calories to prevent ingested protein from being consumed for energy purposes.

15 The Treatment of Body Fluid Disturbances

PRELIMINARY TESTING

In planning therapy for the patient with an actual or potential disturbance of the body fluids, the first step is to determine the status of the kidneys. Various types of solutions, particularly those containing potassium, can be hazardous if renal function is not adequate. The presence of any one of the following criteria indicates suppressed kidney function:

1. Specific gravity of urine above 1.030
2. Less than 3 voidings in 24 hours
3. No urine in the bladder

Renal depression almost invariably occurs in patients who have suffered massive acute losses of extracellular fluid, and so many patients with fluid imbalances have oliguria or even anuria. Before administering fluid therapy, it is necessary to determine if the suppression of urination is due simply to an extracellular fluid volume deficit, or whether it is due to serious renal impairment. If urinary suppression is caused simply by volume deficit, the therapeutic test will reveal that fact by re-establishing urinary flow, making it safe to proceed with the fluid therapy program, including the administration of potassium-containing solutions.

The therapeutic test consists of administration of a special solution, frequently called an initial hydrating solution or a pump-priming solution. Such a solution often provides sodium, 51 mEq./L., chloride, 51 mEq./L., and glucose, 50 Gm./L. It actually represents a solution containing one part of isotonic solution of sodium chloride in 5 per cent glucose, and two parts of 5 per cent glucose in water. The solution is administered at the rate of 8 ml./m.^{2} of body surface/minute for 45 minutes. When the kidneys begin to function, as shown by the restoration of the flow of urine, then the initial hydrating solution is discontinued and therapy is started with other types of solutions. If the urinary flow is not restored, the infusion rate is reduced to 2 ml./m.^{2} body surface/minute and continued for another hour. If urination has not occurred at the end of this period, the physician assumes he is dealing with renal impairment rather than functional depression, thus demanding a battery of laboratory tests plus careful management by specialists.

THE GOALS OF FLUID THERAPY

In planning day-to-day therapy for the individual patient, including what type of solution is needed in what amount, the physician considers the three goals of therapy:

1. Any pre-existing deficits of water and electrolytes must be repaired.
2. Water and electrolytes must be provided to meet the patient's maintenance requirements.
3. Continuing abnormal losses of water and electrolytes through such routes as vomiting, diarrhea, tubal drainage, wound drainage, burn drainage, diuresis, and the like, must be replaced.

There are various, widely different methods for achieving these goals. Rather than describe several methods, we will present one simple method that has worked out well in practice, that will help give the nurse a basic understanding of the principles involved in fluid therapy. From the standpoint of clinical results, this method is no better than other methods of fluid therapy and certainly has its drawbacks and limitations—we have chosen it for pedagogical reasons. The method that we shall briefly describe is that developed by Butler and his co-workers at the Massachusetts General Hospital, which has, since that time, been used with great success in many parts of the world.

ADMINISTERING FLUID THERAPY

In perhaps 90 per cent of patients with fluid imbalances, a single solution of the type devised by Butler can be used to provide water and electrolytes for maintenance and repair. Such a solution is so designed that *when used to meet the patient's fluid volume requirement, it supplies electrolytes in quantities balanced between the minimal needs and the maximal tolerances of the patient.* The Butler-type solution is actually one-third to one-half as concentrated as plasma, providing free water for urinary formation and metabolic activities and, in addition, both cellular and extracellular electrolytes. It incorporates 5 or 10 per cent of carbohydrate to minimize tissue destruction, reduce ketosis and spare protein. The Butler-type solution utilizes the body homeostatic mechanisms, which select the electrolytes that are required and reject those that are not needed. Butler-type solutions, when used properly, have a great margin of safety and are enormously useful in managing body fluid disturbances that result from acute differences between intake and output of water and electrolytes not controllable by the body homeostatic mechanisms. Probably 90 per cent of all body fluid disturbances are of this nature and include extracellular fluid volume deficit, sodium excess, potassium deficit, and the four acid-base disturbances.

EXTRACELLULAR FLUID VOLUME DEFICIT The goal of therapy in this imbalance is to provide both cellular and extracellular electrolytes to compensate for losses without altering the composition of the extracellular fluid. While a treatment solution containing water and electrolytes in the proportions present in extracellular fluid may appear to be the logical choice, it is not, since such a solution would not provide the water needed for urinary excretion and for replacement of plain water lost from the skin and lungs. A balanced solution provides the body homeostatic mechanisms not only with free water for these purposes, but also with the materials they need to restore volume and at the same time maintain the normal composition of the extracellular fluid.

SODIUM EXCESS OF EXTRACELLULAR FLUID In sodium excess, which is often accompanied by volume deficit, the goal of therapy is to provide water to dilute the concentration of electrolytes both in the extracellular fluid and in the cellular fluid while supplying maintenance amounts of electrolytes to re-establish the normal composition of the body fluid. The free water in balanced solutions dilutes the electrolyte concentration excess, and the body homeostatic mechanisms are also supplied with the electrolytes they may need to re-establish the normal water-to-electrolyte ratio.

POTASSIUM DEFICIT OF EXTRACELLULAR FLUID The purpose of therapy in potassium deficit is to repair the deficit while providing adequate amounts of potassium for maintenance needs. Balanced solutions contain sufficient potassium to repair both cellular and extracellular deficits and at the same time provide potassium and other electrolytes for maintenance.

PRIMARY BASE BICARBONATE DEFICIT OF EXTRACELLULAR FLUID (METABOLIC ACIDOSIS) In this imbalance, one needs to provide bicarbonate ions to replace acid ions, to promote excretion of nonbicarbonate anions, and to counteract the processes responsible for producing ketosis. Balanced solutions contain at least 20 mEq. of lactate/L., which the liver converts into base bicarbonate, to be broken down by the kidneys into bicarbonate ions, which are conserved, and acid ions, which are excreted. Balanced solutions also contain free water to promote urinary excretion, thus speeding up the washing out of acid ions, and carbohydrate to reduce ketosis by providing the body with a nonfat energy source, thus decreasing the burning of body fat. Since metabolic acidosis usually causes a loss of water and electrolytes—especially sodium, potassium, and chloride—culminating in fluid volume deficit, a balanced solution also supplies the water and electrolytes needed to maintain fluid volume and to prevent secondary electrolyte deficits from developing.

PRIMARY BASE BICARBONATE EXCESS OF EXTRACELLULAR FLUID (METABOLIC ALKALOSIS) The goal of therapy in this imbalance is to provide nonbicarbonate anions, such as chloride, to replace bicarbonate ions. Because metabolic alkalosis is almost always accompanied by potassium deficit and will not respond to therapy unless potassium is also supplied, balanced solutions must contain adequate amounts of both chloride and potassium. When such a solution is administered, the body homeostatic mechanisms will selectively retain the chloride ions to replace bicarbonate ions, as well as potassium to correct the potassium deficit.

PRIMARY CARBONIC ACID DEFICIT OF EXTRACELLULAR FLUID (RESPIRATORY ALKALOSIS) Parenteral therapy is of secondary importance in this imbalance, since the chief effort should be directed toward managing the condition that initially caused hyperventilation. The function of fluid therapy in this disturbance is to complement the efforts of the kidneys as they attempt to compensate, by excreting bicarbonate and retaining acid. Therefore, the object of fluid therapy in respiratory alkalosis is to provide chloride ions that can be used to replace bicarbonate ions and at the same time provide free water to replace water lost through the lungs in overbreathing. Balanced solutions contain adequate amounts of both chloride and free water, so they are useful for supportive therapy.

PRIMARY CARBONIC ACID EXCESS OF EXTRACELLULAR FLUID (RESPIRATORY ACIDOSIS) Fluid therapy is also of secondary importance in managing this disturbance, because the function of parenteral fluids in respiratory acidosis is to support the corrective efforts of the homeostatic mechanisms by supplying them with ions such as lactate or acetate that can be converted into bicarbonate. Balanced solutions are useful here since they contain lactate ions.

In all the imbalances just described, balanced solutions can be used both for repair and for maintenance. Dosage is relatively simple and is based primarily on the patient's fluid volume, which is assessed mainly by acute changes in body weight. A moderate fluid volume deficit is indicated by weight loss up to 5 per cent in a child or adult, up to 10 per cent in an infant, and by symptoms moderate in degree, whereas a severe fluid volume deficit is indicated by an acute weight loss of over 5 per cent in a child or adult, and over 10 per cent in an infant, with symptoms and laboratory findings severe in degree.

In the patient whose fluid volume is normal at the time therapy is started, his maintenance requirements can be met by the administration of 1,500 ml. of a Butler-type solution/m.^{2} body surface/day. In the patient who has a moderate pre-existing deficit, 2,400 ml./m.^{2} body surface/day will both correct this deficit and meet maintenance needs. If the patient has a severe pre-existing deficit, then one can correct the deficit and provide maintenance by giving 3,000 ml. of a Butler-type solution/m.^{2} body surface/day.

The Butler-type solution is given intravenously, by mouth, or by nasogastric tube, but *not subcutaneously*. The dose should be calculated carefully, regardless of what route is used; in giving the solution intravenously, the usual rate of administration is 3 ml./m.^{2} of body surface/minute.

Various modifications of the Butler-type solution are made available by manufacturers of parenteral solutions. The usual solution for older children and adults contains 75 mEq. of total cation (and hence of total anion), and that used for infants and small children contains 48 mEq. of total cation (and hence of total anion). Manufacturers gladly provide information concerning available solutions and their proper use.

For replacing continuing abnormal losses (concurrent losses) from vomiting, drainage from an intestinal tube or fistula, severe diarrhea, and so on, replacement solutions with a composition resembling the body fluid lost are added to the daily fluid ration. Thus, to replace gastric juice, one administers a gastric replacement solution intravenously and to replace intestinal or duodenal juices, he uses an intestinal replacement solution intravenously. For replacing concurrent losses of hypotonic fluids, such as perspiration and watery diarrheal fluids, additional amounts of balanced solution are added to the amount the patient is already receiving for repair and maintenance. Concurrent losses are replaced on a volume for volume basis at a flow rate of 3 ml./m.^{2} body surface/minute.

CALCULATING DOSAGE

Among the most beautiful passages in the medical literature are these from the clinical reports of early physicians who used parenteral fluid therapy. Latta, of Leith, Scotland, thus described the effect of an intravenous solution administered to a patient suffering from cholera in 1832:

> . . . Like the effects of magic, instead of the pallid aspect of one whom death had sealed as his own, the vital tide was restored and life and vivacity returned . . .

Cantini, who practiced in Naples, Italy, and died in 1893, wrote as follows:

> The cold, cyanotic, dehydrated, comatose patients, lying pulseless and almost lifeless, became animated after the subcutaneous infusion of warm salt water. Remarkably their pulse and voice often returned in a few minutes and they are even able to sit alone in bed . . .

Neither Dr. Latta nor Dr. Cantini felt much need for precise knowledge of parenteral fluid dosage, nor was a great need experienced for many decades to come, for as long as it remained an emergency measure, to be performed only as a last resort, the clinical response of the patient—if respond he did—was regarded as gauge enough for proper dosage. Now, with striking advances in the knowledge of clinical fluid disturbances during the past four decades, there has been a great extension in the use of parenteral fluids. The medical profession has, therefore, felt a mounting need for simple, widely applicable dosage gauges suitable for assisting the physician in determining the volume and the rate of administration of parenteral fluids.

The gauges for dosage most frequently used have been body surface area and body weight related to age; caloric requirement has been employed to a lesser extent. Some authorities feel that body weight related to age possesses an important shortcoming: requirements for water and electrolytes determined on the basis of body weight are different for patients of different ages. However, when using body surface area, expressed in terms of square meters of body surface per day, requirements for water and electrolytes are approximately the same for patients of all age groups, as shown in the figure 1 for approximate water requirement and for approximate sodium requirement. (See Figure 15-1.)

Body surface area is proportional to many essential physiologic processes, including heat loss, blood volume, glomerular filtration rate, organ size, respiration, blood pressure and nitrogen requirement. Alan Butler and his co-workers at the Massachusetts General Hospital were the first to emphasize that the basic water and electrolyte requirements are also proportional to body surface area, regardless of the age or size of the patient. They pointed out that since body surface area provides a quantitative index of our total metabolic activity, it also provides us with a remarkably useful gauge for determining doses and proper rate for parenteral administration of water and electrolytes in fluid therapy. In addition, body surface area can provide nurses with a simple, rapid method of checking the correctness of parenteral fluid orders, especially in regard to volume and rate of administration, and in particular to determine if orders for sodium and potassium in parenteral solutions are within the realm of safety.

There are various methods of measuring body surface area, including the covering method, geometric method, skinning method, and other investigational methods. Clinicians employ simple nomograms that enable one to rapidly estimate body surface area from height and body weight. Actually, one can quickly obtain the approximate surface area from weight alone, as shown in Table 15-1.

The table is simple to use: an infant weighing 10 lbs. would have an approximate surface area of .27 m.^{2}; a child weighing 50 lbs. would have an approximate surface area of .87 m.^{2}; an adult weighing 150 lbs. would have an approximate surface area of 1.75 m.^{2}.

APPROXIMATE WATER REQUIREMENT

ML./LB.
70
65
60
55
50
45
40
35
30
25
20
15
10
5
Infant
10-year-old
Adult

ML./M2
1500
1400
1300
1200
1100
Infant
10-year-old
Adult

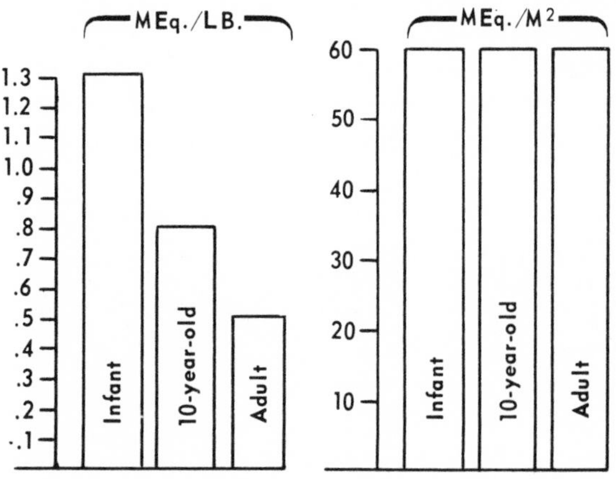

Fig. 15-1. We can use the same values for water and sodium requirements for persons of all ages if we use body surface area, rather than weight, as the dosage criterion.

The body surface areas arrived at by use of the weight chart are approximate only, and apply to individuals of average body build. In general, obese or stocky individuals have less surface area than tall lanky persons of the same weight (just as a long, low one-story ranch house has more external surface than a two- or three-story house of equal floor space). For example, our 10-lb. infant would have a surface area of .2 m^2 if he were only 16 inches tall, but he would have .3 m^2 of surface area if he were 28 inches in height. Our 50-lb. child would have .68 m^2 of surface area if he were 2 feet, 10 inches tall and .84 m^2 if his height were 3 feet, 10 inches. Our 150-lb. adult would have 1.47 m^2 of surface area if he were only 4 feet, 4 inches tall and 1.86 m^2 if he had a height of 6 feet.

The body surface area gauge for dosage is especially useful for checking the correctness of water and electrolytes ordered for patients with body fluid disturbances. Remember the following rules:

1. For maintenance, administer 1,500 ml./m^2 body surface/day.
2. For correction of a moderate deficit in extracellular fluid volume plus maintenance, administer 2,400 ml./m^2 body surface/day.
3. For correction of a severe deficit in extracellular fluid volume plus maintenance, administer 3,000 ml./m^2 body surface/day.
4. Concurrent losses are replaced with an appropriate replacement solution on a volume for volume basis.
5. Rate of administration should be 3 ml./m^2 body surface/minute, except when giving initial hydrating solution.

By applying these rules, the nurse can quickly check the correctness of an order for fluid therapy. Let us suppose that the physician has written an order for a liter of solution to be given over a 24-hour period to an infant weighing 20 lbs. with a moderate fluid volume deficit. A quick check of the conversion chart shows that a 20-lb. baby would have .45 m^2 of body surface; the volume of fluid for correction of a moderate fluid volume deficit in such a baby should be .45 times 2,400 ml., or about 1,080 ml.

Let us suppose, on the other hand, that a large man with a severe fluid volume deficit is to receive 3 L. of solution for the first 24 hours. Reference to the conversion chart shows that a 175-lb. man would have a body surface area of 2.0 m^2; 2.0 times 3,000 ml., the requirement per m^2 of body surface per day for a severe fluid

Table 15-1. Chart for Converting Weight to Surface Area

(Figures are approximate and apply only to individuals of average build.)

Pounds	*Surface Area in Square Meters*
4	.15
6	.20
10	.27
15	.36
20	.45
30	.60
40	.72
50	.87
60	.97
70	1.10
80	1.21
90	1.33
100	1.4
125	1.6
150	1.75
175	2.0
200	2.2
250	2.7

volume deficit, is 6 L., or 6,000 ml.; 3 L., therefore, is grossly inadequate.

Suppose that a 12-year-old boy with no fluid imbalance is to be given water and electrolytes for maintenance for a few days following abdominal surgery. The physician orders 3 L. of his favorite maintenance solution. The boy's body surface area is 1.33 m.^{2} and maintenance should call for 1,500 ml. times 1.33, or 1,995 ml., approximately 2 L. of fluid. The extra liter ordered might embarrass the boy's homeostatic mechanisms, and the physician should appreciate having the order questioned. Of course, in the presence of fever or heavy sweating, the extra fluid might well be entirely proper.

Using the above information, the rate of administration for the infant with .45 m.^{2} of body surface would be $.45 \times 3 \times 60 = 81$ ml./hr.; for the 2.0 m.^{2} man, $2 \times 3 \times 60 = 360$ ml./hr.; for the 1.33 m.^{2} boy, $1.33 \times 3 \times 60 = 240$ ml./hr.

The quantity of sodium or potassium being administered parenterally can quickly be checked by recalling that the average daily maintenance requirement for sodium is 50 to 70 mEq./m.^{2} of body surface/day, also valid for potassium. The minimal need for each of these cations is 10 mEq./m.^{2} of body surface/day, and the maximal tolerances, 250 mEq./m.^{2} of body surface/day.

IMBALANCES REQUIRING SPECIFIC TYPES OF THERAPY

The simple plan of therapy described above is not suitable for treating the remainder of our 16 basic imbalances, including extracellular fluid volume excess, sodium deficit, potassium excess, calcium deficit, calcium excess, magnesium deficit, protein deficit, and the two shifts involving the water and electrolytes of plasma and interstitial fluid. These imbalances require specific therapy.

In extracellular fluid volume excess, calcium excess, and potassium excess, the object of therapy is to remove from the extracellular fluid excesses of a single electrolyte or of a combination of water and electrolytes.

EXTRACELLULAR FLUID VOLUME EXCESS

Fluid therapy usually is not indicated in this imbalance; rather, therapy is directed toward the causative factors. Symptomatic treatment consists of restriction of fluids, administration of diuretics, or both. When the excess has resulted from excessive administration of isotonic solutions, discontinuing the infusion may be all that is required in the patient with functional homeostatic mechanisms. Administration of a balanced solution at the rate of 1 ml./m.^{2} body surface/minute will provide free water to aid in excretion of excess electrolytes and at the same time will provide potassium and other electrolytes that may be deficient. If the excess has developed over a long period of time, as may occur in the patient with chronic kidney disease, chronic liver disease, or congestive heart failure, withholding of fluids is not indicated. The homeostatic mechanisms do not function normally in patients with these conditions and treatment is directed toward the underlying condition. The volume excess may also be corrected by use of a low sodium diet. Finally, the patient with chronic malnutrition may develop a volume excess, largely because of plasma protein deficit; in this case, treatment is directed toward improving the patient's nutritional status.

CALCIUM EXCESS OF EXTRACELLULAR FLUID This imbalance is always secondary to a metabolic disease, so primary treatment is directed toward correcting the underlying cause. The patient should be placed on a low calcium diet, and those requiring therapy for other imbalances should be given only calcium-free solutions. Hypercalcemic crisis is the most critical syndrome of calcium excess, and it represents an emergency situation requiring urgent therapy lest the patient die of cardiac arrest. Unfortunately, medical management of hypercalcemic crisis has generally been unsatisfactory, and none of the regimens tried has been consistently successful because of slow action or inherent toxicity. Inorganic phosphate appears to be effective in rapidly lowering serum calcium levels, beginning within 3 minutes of the start of the infusion, with return to normal calcium values within 24 hours. Despite their effectiveness, phosphate solutions produce several undesirable side effects; nevertheless, the urgency of the situation appears to justify their use. Sulfate solutions are also effective and do not produce the widespread side effects associated with phosphate solutions, but they take longer to act and tend to produce magnesium deficit; consequently, magnesium supplements should be available when a sulfate solution is being used.

POTASSIUM EXCESS OF EXTRACELLULAR FLUID The method used to treat this imbalance depends upon the status of the patient's homeostatic mechanisms. An uncomplicated potassium excess can be corrected simply by avoiding additional potassium intake, either orally or parenterally. If the homeostatic mechanisms are functioning normally, a 5 per cent solution of sodium bicarbonate is the preferred solution in treatment of severe potassium excess, since the kidneys retain sodium in preference to potassium, which causes increased urinary excretion of potassium. In patients whose homeostatic mechanisms are impaired, insulin and dextrose is useful in forcing potassium from extracellular fluid back into the cells, the most satisfactory method of producing a temporary fall in the extracellular fluid potassium level. Carbonic anhydrase inhibitors and ion exchange resins can also be used in treating this imbalance, but they tend to produce metabolic acidosis, an undesirable side effect. When potassium excess is accompanied by severe kidney disease, peritoneal dialysis or hemodialysis may be necessary.

Patients suffering from severe disruptions in electrolyte concentration or composition of the extracellular fluid often need immediate replacement therapy. The patient may have functional homeostatic mechanisms, but the magnitude of the deficit is so severe, or the deficit has developed so rapidly, that balanced solutions cannot provide adequate electrolytes to correct the imbalance. Therefore, specific repair solutions are required for sodium deficit, calcium deficit, and magnesium deficit.

SODIUM DEFICIT OF EXTRACELLULAR FLUID In treating this imbalance, one must administer sodium chloride in such concentration as to return the sodium level to normal without subsequently producing a fluid volume excess. If fluid volume is normal or excessive, a 3 or 5 per cent solution of sodium chloride is used, dosage being based on the deficit of sodium in the plasma. Hypertonic solutions of sodium chloride should be administered only intravenously; they are given at a rate of 1 ml./m.^{2} body surface/minute. When the sodium deficit is accompanied by extracellular fluid volume deficit, an isotonic solution of sodium chloride, or normal saline, is used to correct the sodium deficit, and when the sodium deficit has been repaired, the volume deficit can be corrected with a balanced solution. Isotonic solution of sodium chloride is administered intravenously at a flow rate of 3 ml./m.^{2} body surface/minute.

CALCIUM DEFICIT OF EXTRACELLULAR FLUID The accepted mode of therapy for this disturbance is administration of a 10 per cent solution of calcium gluconate combined with an isotonic solution of sodium chloride, particularly important if severe muscle spasms or convulsions have occurred. The recommended dose for children is 1 ml. of the 10 per cent solution of calcium gluconate/kg. body weight, diluted with two volumes of isotonic solution of sodium chloride administered over a 10-minute period; the total dose of 10 per cent calcium gluconate solution should not exceed 10 ml. in any one infusion. Older children and adults can be given a dose of 10 ml. of 10 per cent calcium gluconate solution diluted with two volumes of isotonic solution of sodium chloride. If the disease process that originally caused the hypocalcemia cannot be immediately controlled, it may be necessary to repeat the infusion. In the patient with hypoparathyroidism, administration of a phosphorus-free balanced solution promotes absorption of calcium and thus helps maintain the normal levels of calcium and phosphorus in the plasma.

MAGNESIUM DEFICIT OF EXTRACELLULAR FLUID Magnesium sulfate either by mouth or intravenously is the treatment of choice in magnesium deficit. Parenteral treatment includes intravenous administration of a 10 ml. ampule of 50 per cent magnesium sulfate solution combined with 1 L. of a balanced solution containing no calcium or phosphorus; this is necessary because the symptoms of magnesium deficit are exaggerated by high intakes of calcium and, particularly, of phosphorus. Flow rate should be no faster than 6 ml./m.^{2} body surface/minute. Response is usually comparatively rapid, and tetanic symptoms often disappear within a matter of hours. However, since a significant percentage of the administered magnesium will be lost in the urine, supplemental doses may be necessary. It is important to keep in mind that tetany caused by magnesium deficit cannot be corrected by administration of calcium, and vice versa.

PROTEIN DEFICIT OF EXTRACELLULAR FLUID The goal of therapy in protein deficit is to help prevent the vicious circle of nutritional deficiency, which goes from anorexia to malnutrition to still further anorexia. The only way to break the circle is to provide protein and adequate calories to prevent amino acids from being used for energy purposes, plus potassium and magnesium for effective utilization of protein. The most desirable therapy is high-protein foods or supplements orally or by nasogastric tube, but if the patient cannot tolerate such therapy, or if his condition contraindicates such feedings, administration of protein hydrolysate solutions containing essential amino acids, adequate calories in the form of dextrose or alcohol or both, and electrolytes for maintenance requirements will prevent further development of protein deficit in most patients.

PLASMA-TO-INTERSTITIAL FLUID SHIFT Therapy of this imbalance is directed toward limiting the shift, if possible, maintaining plasma volume, treating vascular collapse and heart failure if they occur, and preparing for the possibility of a secondary interstitial fluid-to-plasma shift. Unfortunately, massive plasma-to-interstitial fluid shifts often cannot be restricted except by correcting the primary cause. For localized shifts, a tight binder around the affected part may effect relief; if a massive shift involves loss of plasma, plasma volume can be restored or maintained by administering plasma or a plasma expander, such as dextran, intravenously. An electrolyte replacement solution with a composition resembling extracellular fluid should be used if the shift involves only water and electrolytes. A gastrointestinal replacement solution or lactated Ringer's solution is ideal if the kidneys are functioning normally, but if kidney function is depressed, isotonic solution of sodium chloride may be given. The amount of plasma, dextran, or electrolyte solution needed varies with the weight of the patient and the magnitude of the shift. Vascular collapse and heart failure are usually fatal complications following prolonged lack of oxygen during shock; treatment includes administration of oxygen and stimulants such as caffeine, nikethamide (Coramine), epinephrine, and norepinephrine. Lastly, to help limit the severity of the secondary interstitial fluid-to-plasma shift that occurs with remobilization of edema fluid, unnecessary administration of fluids during the plasma-to-interstitial fluid shift should be avoided.

INTERSTITIAL FLUID-TO-PLASMA SHIFT The rapid interstitial fluid-to-plasma shift that occurs with remobilization of edema fluid following the reverse shift or following excessive intravenous administration of hypertonic solutions is unpreventable and may be so severe as to overload the renocardiovascular system. When this occurs, the goal of therapy is to reduce the amount of fluid returning to the heart, accomplished by placing tourniquets around the extremities in such a way that they block venous return but do not interfere with arterial circulation. Phlebotomy may be necessary. If the shift occurs as a compensatory measure following internal or external loss of whole blood, it can be halted by transfusion of whole blood.

WHOLE BLOOD DEFICIT A whole blood deficit should be repaired by giving whole blood, but if the extracellular fluid volume is excessive, red cells should be given alone.

COMPLEX COMBINED IMBALANCES The severe burn is an excellent example of a complex combination of body fluid imbalances. Therapy of this condition requires knowledge of the hazardous aftermaths of the burn, which include losses of body fluid, shock, renal depression and remobilization of edema fluid. Carefully controlled therapy must be directed at the correction of the imbalances secondary to these aftermaths.

Types of Solutions

Solutions vary greatly from hospital to hospital. The nurse is urged to become familiar with the solutions employed in the hospital in which she works, information which can be gained by talking with the hospital pharmacist or with knowledgeable physicians and by carefully reading the excellent literature provided by the pharmaceutical company that supplies the parenteral solutions for the hospital.

16 Parenteral Fluid Administration—Nursing Implications

INTRODUCTION

The nurse plays a major role in the administration of parenteral fluids. Her exact responsibilities are not uniformly defined and vary with geographical areas and individual hospitals. For example, the nurse in a large medical center does not usually start intravenous fluids; the nurse in a small hospital starts them routinely because resident physicians are not available. Many hospitals have organized intravenous therapy teams to start infusions; nevertheless, regardless of who starts the fluids, the nurse shares in the responsibility of assuring their safe and therapeutic administration. To ably assume this responsibility, she must understand basic principles of safe fluid administration and become familiar with parenteral fluids. If intelligent observations are to be made during their infusion, the purposes, contraindications and complications associated with their use must be known.

ROUTES AND TECHNIQUES OF PARENTERAL FLUID ADMINISTRATION

Intravenous

INDICATIONS FOR USE Veins provide an excellent route for the quick administration of water, electrolytes and other nutrients. Fluids administered intravenously at the proper rate and in the proper dose pass directly into the extracellular fluid. They are rapidly acted upon by the body homeostatic mechanisms and hence do not, in proper doses, produce abnormal changes in volume or electrolyte concentration of extracellular fluid. The intravenous route is essential when nutrients are needed in a hurry, such as glucose in severe hypoglycemia, 5 per cent sodium chloride in severe sodium deficit, or calcium gluconate in acute calcium deficit. Relatively large volumes of fluids can be given by the intravenous route, provided due care is exercised.

GENERAL PSYCHOLOGICAL CONSIDERATIONS Few persons are without some fear or dread of a needle being introduced into their veins; normal fears are exaggerated in illness, since many patients associate intravenous fluids with critical illnesses and are disturbed when such therapy is employed. It is the nurse's responsibility to explain away as much of the fear as possible and point out that I.V. fluids are commonly used until oral intake is again possible.

Because all patients are individuals, the nurse must plan her approach on an individual basis. Some patients feel less singled out if they are allowed to observe others on the ward receiving I.V. fluids. A detailed explanation of why and how the fluids are given is indicated for some; others want only a brief account. In any event, the patient should *never* be approached with no explanation at all; the fear of not knowing what is to happen can be worse than the most painful venipuncture. Some patients will not ask questions for fear of learning something too unpleasant to accept; yet, their imaginations may run wild during the infusion. Some patients have heard of fatalities during an intravenous infusion, for example, due to an air embolus. The nurse must always remember that although I.V. therapy is commonplace to her, it is far from routine to the patient.

Only persons capable of skillful venipuncture should start fluids on anxious patients; just one traumatic experience may make I.V. therapy totally unacceptable to them. The nurse starting fluids must always appear confident—patients sense insecurity and are understandably upset by it. An I.V. therapy department with competent therapists provides many advantages, one of which is the skill developed by such therapists in performing venipuncture.

Not only must the nurse dispel the patient's fears; she must also dispel the fears of the family, because it is not uncommon for a relaxed patient to become upset after observing the obvious anxiety of his relatives. The need for intravenous therapy should be explained to the family and any misconceptions cleared up.

SELECTION OF SITE

Suitable Superficial Veins A number of superficial veins are available for venipuncture. (See Figure 16-1.) Those most commonly used include:

- Veins in and around the cubital fossa (antecubital, basilic, and cephalic veins)
- Veins in the forearm (basilic and cephalic veins)
- Veins in the radial area of the wrist
- Veins in the hand (metacarpal and dorsal venous plexus)
- Femoral and saphenous veins in the thigh
- Veins in the foot (dorsal venous plexus, medial and lateral marginal veins)
- Scalp veins in infants and the aged

Criteria for Selection Selection of a vein depends upon a number of factors:

- Availability of sites (depends upon condition of veins)
- Size of needle to be used
- Type of fluids to be infused
- Volume, rate and length of infusion
- Degree of mobility desired
- Skill of operator

Hand Veins The early use of hand veins is important if parenteral therapy is to be prolonged. This allows each successive venipuncture to be made above the previous site, eliminating pain and inflammation caused by irritating fluids passing through a vein injured by previous venipuncture. Because of their small diameter, hand veins do not accommodate large needles—a small gauge scalp vein needle is sometimes used for venipuncture in the hand.

Small veins cannot accept large volumes or rapid administration of fluids, due to the fact that an irritating solution is more traumatic in small veins because less blood is present to dilute it. These peripheral veins collapse sooner in the presence of shock than do more centrally located veins. And finally, extravasation of blood may occur on venipuncture in this area, particularly when there is thin skin and inadequate connective tissue.

Forearm Veins The cephalic vein flows upward along the radial border of the forearm and is an excellent site for venipuncture; the size of the vein will accommodate a large needle. The accessory cephalic vein joins the cephalic vein below the elbow, and it too is a good site for venipuncture. Both veins are frequently used for blood administration. When prominent, the median antebrachial vein can be used for venipuncture, although the location of superficial veins of the forearm is somewhat variable and not always well-defined.

Venipuncture in a forearm vein allows the patient some arm movement without the risk of puncturing the posterior venous wall.

Elbow Veins The median cephalic and median basilic veins are found in the antecubital fossa, both veins readily accessible to venipuncture because they are large and superficially located. In addition, they are kept from rolling and sliding by surrounding tissues. They will accommodate large needles, large volumes of fluids, and all but the most irritating intravenous fluids.

Because arteries in the antecubital area, though usually more deeply located, lie in close proximity to veins, it is easy to mistake an artery for a vein in this area. Aberrant arteries are not uncommon in the cubital fossa. (These arteries, more superficially located than usual, are found in 1 out of 10 persons.) Injection of fluids into an artery usually causes the patient to complain of sudden severe pain in the arm and hand, caused by arteriospasm; this is an indication to stop the infusion immediately.

When frequent blood specimens are necessary, it is wise to save the veins in the antecubital area for this purpose; large quantities of blood can be obtained from them. These veins can be used many times without damage if good technique is used. (It is extremely difficult to get sufficient blood from small veins.)

A disadvantage in using veins in the antecubital area is the restriction of elbow flexion during the infusion. Therefore, when long-term

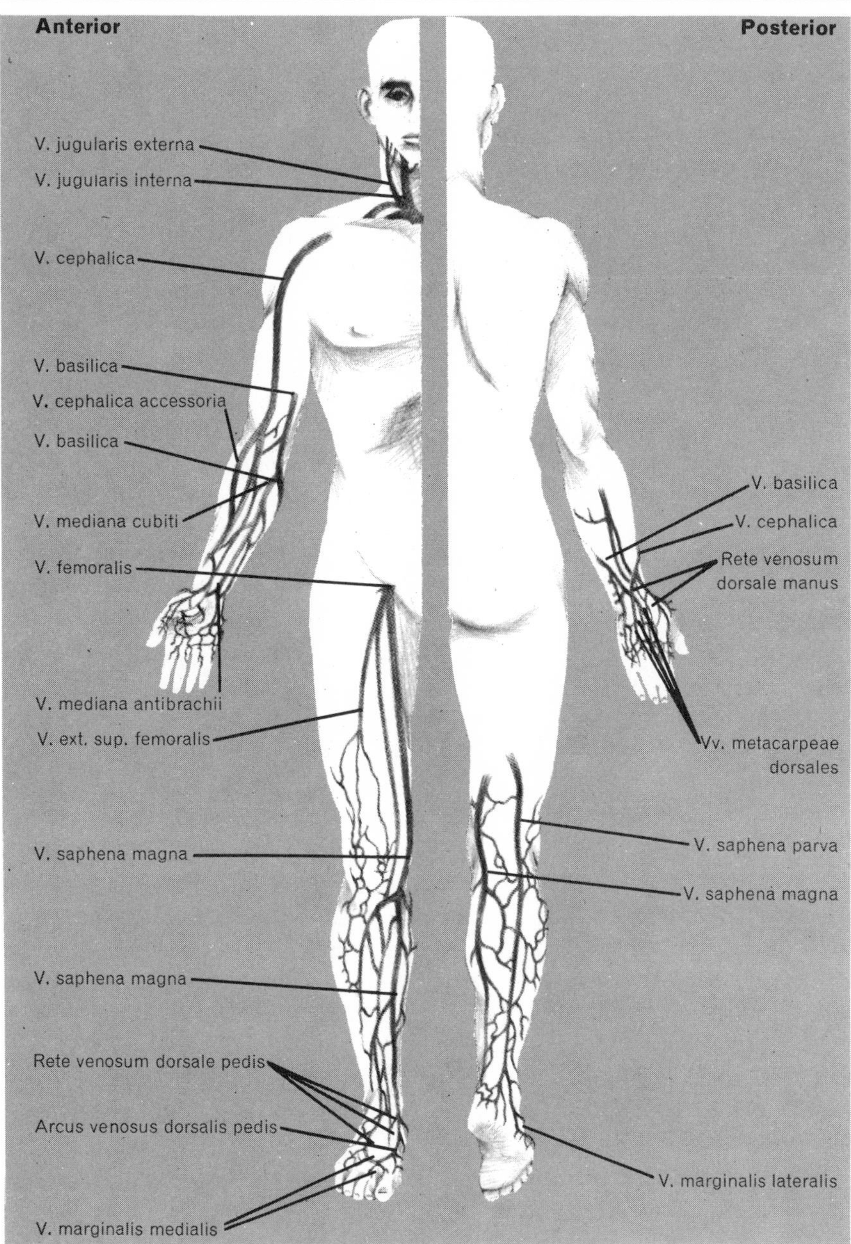

Fig. 16-1. Superficial veins available for venipuncture.

infusions are anticipated or the patient is uncooperative, it is best to use the veins in the forearm, because the patient can be moved and ambulated with less danger of dislodging the needle. The nurse should remember that damage to veins in the antecubital area can limit the use of sites below.

A right-handed person has more freedom if the infusion is given in the left arm; however, the need for multiple venipunctures is an indication to employ alternate sites in both arms.

Lower Extremity Veins Veins in the dorsum of the foot are sometimes used when other veins are not available or desirable; larger veins are found in the ankle, even though the use of these can be dangerous. Thrombus formation at the venipuncture site occurs to some degree in all venipunctures, but when ankle veins are used, the thrombus can extend to deep veins and may result in pulmonary embolism.

Venipuncture should not be performed on a varicose vein or at a site below a varicosity, as such veins do not readily transport fluids into the general circulation, and they may cause a pooling of fluid in veins around the injection site. Pooling of infused medications can cause an untoward reaction when a toxic concentration reaches the general circulation. Varicose veins are easily traumatized, and moreover, they are difficult to enter because they tend to roll; moreover, the blood flow in them is frequently reversed.

GENERAL CONSIDERATIONS

1. When feasible, it is best to use veins in the upper part of the body.
2. When multiple punctures are anticipated, it is best to make the first venipuncture distally and work proximally with subsequent punctures.
3. Avoid venipuncture in the affected arm of patients with axillary dissection, as in radical mastectomy.
4. Avoid checking the blood pressure on the arm receiving an infusion because the cuff interferes with fluid flow, forces blood back into the needle, and may cause a clot to form.
5. When the patient is on his side, the upper arm should be used for venipuncture. The lower arm has increased venous pressure which interferes with fluid flow and may cause clot formation in the needle.
6. Restraints should not be placed on or above the infusion site.

METHODS FOR VENOUS ENTRY Fluids may be introduced into a vein by means of:

- A metal needle
- A plastic needle (catheter mounted on a needle) (See Figure 16-2)
- A plastic catheter threaded through a metal needle (See Figure 16-3)
- A plastic catheter introduced by means of a cut-down (minor surgical procedure)

SELECTION OF METHODS Short-term infusions are usually given through metal needles, and either a regular straight needle or a scalp vein needle may be used. The scalp vein needle is approximately ¾ of an inch long and has attached plastic wings, used for holding the needle during venipuncture. (See Figure 16-4.) This needle has a thin wall and provides a larger lumen with a smaller needle diameter and because the bevel is short, there is less danger of accidentally puncturing the posterior wall of the vein. The size of the needle to be used depends on the vein as well as on the type of solution. Most commonly used are 19 or 20 gauge, one or one-and-a-half inch long needles; an 18 gauge needle is indicated for blood administration. (The smaller the gauge number, the larger the internal diameter of the needle.) If possible, the gauge of the needle should be appreciably smaller than the lumen of the vein to be entered, as when a large needle occludes the flow of blood, irritating solutions may produce chemical phlebitis. If a small needle is used, irritating fluids can mix readily with blood, decreasing the chance of phlebitis.

A plastic needle is a catheter mounted on a metal needle. When the venipuncture is made, the catheter is slipped off the needle into the vein and the metal needle is removed—useful for long-term fluid therapy.

An intracatheter is a catheter inserted through a metal needle and used when a longer catheter

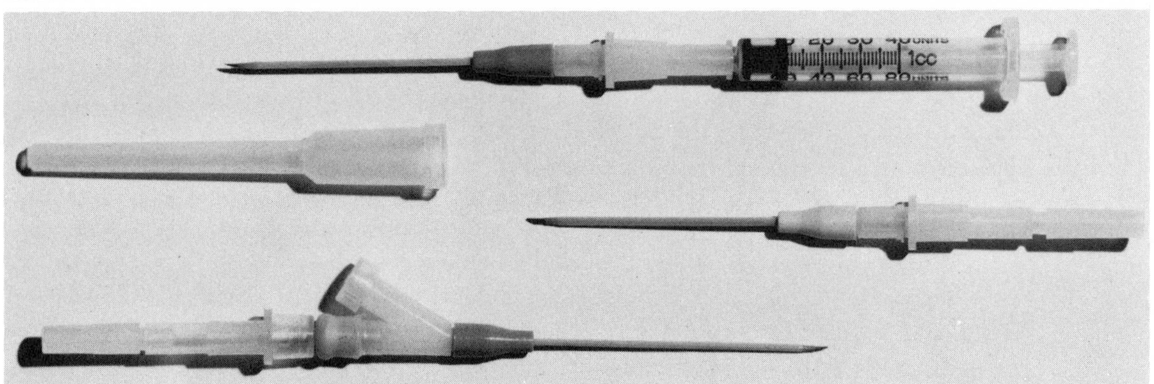

Fig. 16-2. Deseret Angiocath. (Deseret Pharmaceutical Co., Inc., Sandy, Utah)

is desired. Often it is used to administer drugs or irritating solutions that may cause tissue necrosis if infiltration occurs.

A cut-down may be performed when veins become exhausted from prolonged therapy and when peripheral veins have collapsed from shock. Some physicians perform cut-downs at the beginning of fluid therapy if it is to be prolonged. (Obese patients and infants frequently require cut-downs.)

TECHNIQUES OF INSERTION

Venipuncture with a Metal Needle After a suitable site has been located, the next step is to distend the vein, usually accomplished by a tourniquet; it also helps to steady the vein when the tourniquet is placed no higher than 2 inches above the site of injection. It should be tight enough to impede venous flow while arterial flow is maintained, but never too tight—a common error. Occasionally, other methods are necessary to distend the vein, such as placing the part in a dependent position for several minutes, or applying heat by means of a warm towel, immersion in warm water, or the use of an electric hair dryer or electric blanket. (See Figure 16-5.) Heat does little good if it is applied only to the immediate area of the injection site—the entire extremity must be warmed. Sometimes a light flap over the proposed site of venipuncture helps; so does exercising the muscles distal to the site of puncture. However, exercising should not be done

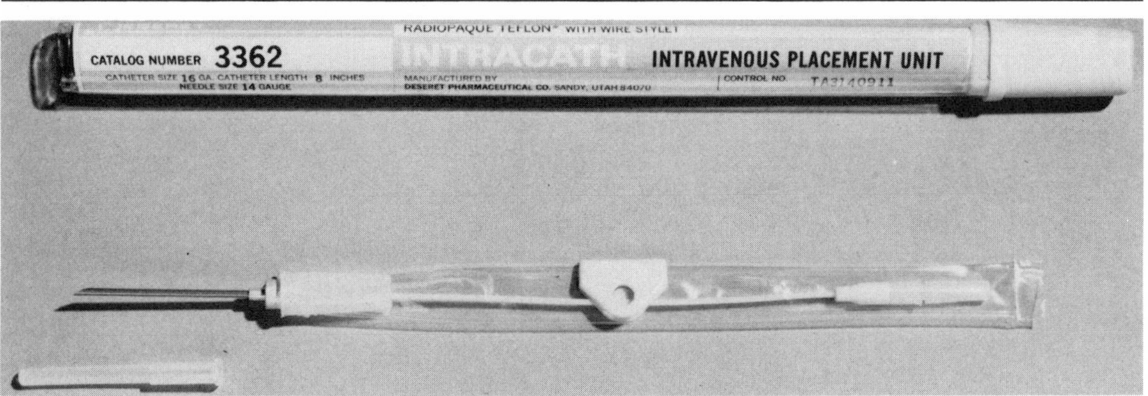

Fig. 16-3. Deseret Intracath. (Deseret Pharmaceutical Co., Inc., Sandy, Utah)

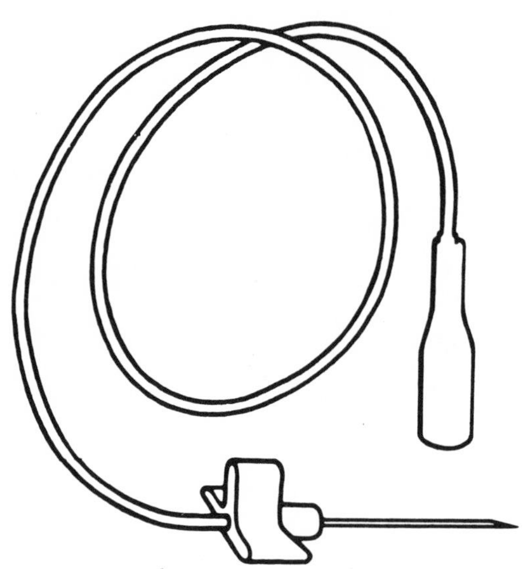

Fig. 16-4. Pediatric Scalp Vein Infusion Set. (Cutter Laboratories, Inc., Berkeley, California)

when blood is being drawn for determination of serum electrolytes, since a false reading may result.

A large gauge needle always causes pain; its insertion may be preceded by locally injecting a small amount of 1 per cent procaine. This should be done only by order of the physician; in addition, the patient should be questioned about a possible allergy to procaine. The injection of procaine tends to obscure landmarks and should be done intradermally, in only extremely small amounts. Sometimes it is advantageous to insert the procaine above the proposed site for venipuncture since distal anesthesia occurs after a short wait. Frequently, the operator does not wait a sufficient time for the full anesthetic effect of the procaine, which results in a tendency to use larger amounts of procaine than are necessary.

Usually only alcohol is used to prepare the site for insertion of the needle, but sometimes the area is cleaned with a detergent prior to the use of alcohol. If heat has been applied to the site, the alcohol sponge should be at room temperature —a cold solution causes vessels to contract. If the injection site is hairy, the area should be shaved, taking care to prevent nicks; this eliminates much of the discomfort associated with the removal of adhesive tape after the infusion.

Generally, the bevel of the needle should be facing upward during insertion. (See Figure 16-6.) However, the introduction of a large needle into a small vein may require the bevel to face downward; otherwise, the needle would pierce the posterior wall of the vein when the tourniquet is removed.

With the tourniquet in place, the needle should pierce the skin to one side of, and approximately one half to one inch below, the point where the needle will enter the vein. As the needle enters the skin it should be at about a 45° angle; after the skin is entered, the needle angle is decreased. Although it seems more logical to enter the vein from above, there seems to be less flattening of the vein when a lateral approach is used. The free hand is used to palpate the vein while the needle is being introduced. An experienced operator can feel a snap as the needle enters the vein; after this, less resistance is offered to the needle. At this point, one should proceed very slowly with the insertion of the needle,

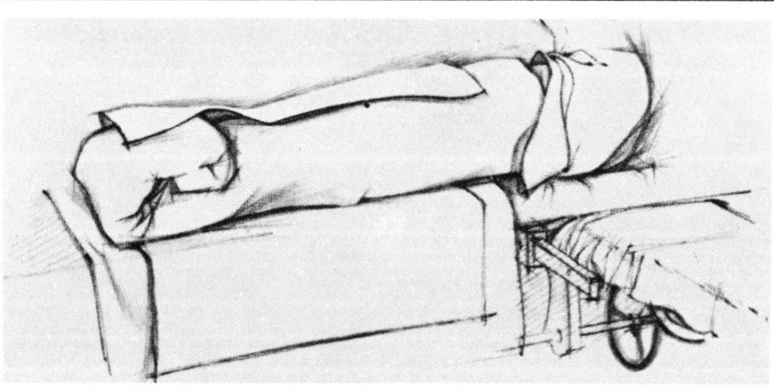

Fig. 16-5. Use of a warm towel to distend veins prior to venipuncture. (Abbott Laboratories: Parenteral Administration, p. 7, North Chicago, Illinois, 1965)

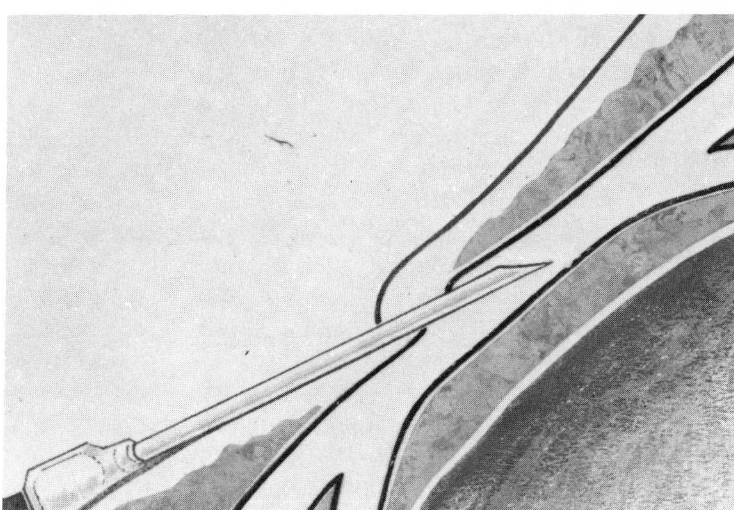

Fig. 16-6. Needle bevel position for venipuncture. (Pfizer Laboratories: Intravenous technique. Spectrum, September-October, 1961)

threading it into the lumen approximately one-half to three-fourths of an inch. The tourniquet is then released. Frequently a thin stream of blood is seen in the tubing when the needle enters the vein. To be sure the needle is in the vein, the infusion bottle can be lowered below the site of injection; the negative pressure causes blood to enter the tubing.

The next step involves anchoring the needle comfortably and safely. A sterile cotton ball or a small gauze pad should be placed under the hub of the needle and fixed in place with adhesive tape and another strip of tape should be placed over the needle to help hold it steady. A loop should be made in the tubing and taped in place; this allows some slack in the tubing and minimizes pull on the needle when the patient moves. (See Figure 16-7.) The fluid should be allowed to run in and the proper flow rate established. The area should be observed for swelling; its presence indicates that the needle is not in the vein and fluid is entering the subcutaneous area. The infusion should be discontinued immediately when swelling is noted; a venipuncture must then be made in another area. If a hematoma develops during an unsuccessful venipuncture attempt, the needle should be immediately removed and pressure applied to the site.

Plastic Needle A venipuncture is performed in the usual manner, with the needle inserted far enough to ensure entry of the catheter into the vein. After the catheter is slid into the vein to the desired length, the needle is carefully removed. If the venipuncture is not successful, withdraw the catheter completely from the puncture site before reinserting the needle. (The manufacturer's direc-

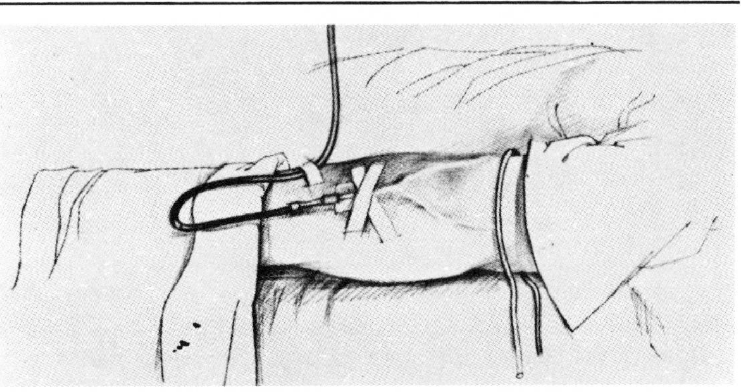

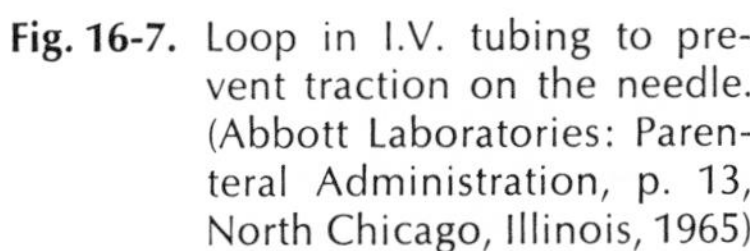

Fig. 16-7. Loop in I.V. tubing to prevent traction on the needle. (Abbott Laboratories: Parenteral Administration, p. 13, North Chicago, Illinois, 1965)

tions should be followed closely.) A small sterile dressing should be applied to the puncture site after the catheter is anchored securely with tape.

Plastic Catheter Inserted Through a Needle After performance of a normal venipuncture, the catheter is inserted into the vein through the needle. If venipuncture is not successful, pull out the needle and catheter together. The catheter should not be pulled out first because the sharp edges of the needle could sever it as it is being withdrawn. (The manufacturer's directions should be followed closely.)

An antibiotic ointment is sometimes applied to minimize the occurrence of catheter sepsis. The catheter should be anchored securely with tape and a sterile dressing should cover the area; sometimes the dressing is changed daily and more ointment applied. The date of insertion and the size and type of catheter used should be noted. Finally, all catheter placement sets should be inspected periodically for placement and security of dressing.

Hypodermoclysis

Hypodermoclysis, the administration of a solution subcutaneously, compares unfavorably with the intravenous route and is used less and less because of its many problems.

The types of fluids that can be given subcutaneously are few, since they must closely resemble the electrolyte content and tonicity of extracellular fluid if they are to be absorbed. Some of the fluids generally considered reasonably safe for subcutaneous administration include:

Isotonic saline (0.9%)
Half-isotonic saline (0.45%) with 2½% dextrose
Ringer's solution
Half-strength Ringer's with 2½% dextrose
Lactated Ringer's solution
Half-strength lactated Ringer's with 2½% dextrose

Fluids that are contraindicated for subcutaneous administration include electrolyte-free solutions, hypertonic solutions, alcohol, amino acids, fat emulsions, and solutions that differ significantly from body pH (such as the gastric replacement solutions). Orders for the subcutaneous administration of any of these solutions should be questioned.

The subcutaneous administration of a 5 per cent dextrose in water solution attracts electrolytes from the surrounding tissues and from the plasma, which enter the pool created at the infusion site. (This electrolyte movement occurs to make the solution absorbable.) Often the pool remains at the infusion site for some time before it is absorbed, and the subsequent decreased plasma volume can cause hypotension and even shock. If the patient is already suffering from sodium deficit, the ultimate result can be death. Hospitalized aged patients may already have low plasma sodium levels secondary to extracellular fluid losses, and since such patients develop sodium deficit more readily than younger adults, they should certainly not receive electrolyte-free solutions subcutaneously.

Probably the only advantage hypodermoclysis has over the intravenous route is that it is easier to start. It is most often used for obese patients, infants, and the aged, for all of whom intravenous fluids are difficult to start. Suitable sites include the subcutaneous tissues on the lateral aspect of the thigh or abdomen. Infections are not uncommon with hypodermoclysis and are usually proportionate to the distention that occurs (because of tissue ischemia) and to the length of time required for the infusion.

Most often, two needles are used and the fluid is infused into two sites at once; the inverted Y-tubing from the solution bottle separates and goes to two sites. (See Figure 16-8.) The rate of infusion depends upon how well the fluid is absorbed from the injection site. When the fluid is absorbed well, 250 to 500 ml. can be given at one site in 1 hour to an adult, but after a short while, fluid is not this readily absorbed and the tissues become hard and swollen. To hasten absorption, hyaluronidase (Wydase), may be injected into the tissues at the injection site. The patient must be checked often when this route is used; a large amount of swelling can develop unless the flow rate is adjusted carefully. A small sterile gauze pad should be placed under the needle hub and another should cover the injection site. Following the removal of the needle, a light sterile dressing should be applied, as edematous injection sites are fertile fields for infections.

COMMENT Much discomfort is usually associated with hypodermoclysis. This route is undependable, especially when large amounts of fluids are needed in a hurry. Fluids are not absorbed well from the subcutaneous tissue when blood volume is severely reduced because of accompanying peripheral collapse. The fluids that can be given safely are quite limited, and ironically, the patients for which hypodermoclysis is most often used (infants, the aged, and the obese) are the ones most prone to be harmed by them. Most authorities feel that a cut-down carries less risk than does hypodermoclysis.

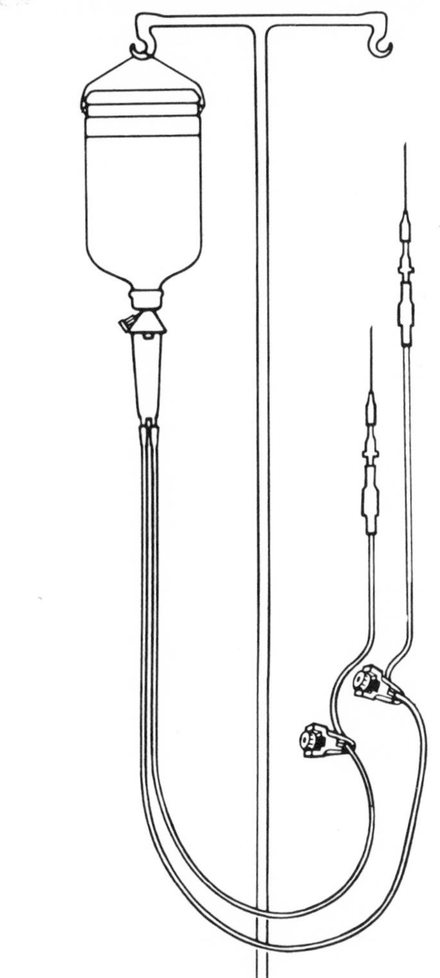

Fig. 16-8. Hypodermoclysis Setup (Saftielysis™ Longleg Set). (Cutter Laboratories, Inc., Berkeley, California)

GENERAL CONSIDERATIONS IN FLUID ADMINISTRATION

Determining Flow Rate

PHYSICIAN'S ORDERS Ideally, when the physician writes an order for intravenous fluids he also should designate how fast they are to be given; however, very few actually do this. Physicians in university hospitals are more prone to give the desired rate of flow than those practicing in non-teaching hospitals, where most merely list on the order sheet the type and the amount of fluids to be given. The nurse should encourage the physician to write more specific orders; it is highly desirable that he determine infusion rates because of his deeper understanding of the patient's condition as well as of the fluids to be administered. Unfortunately, attempts to obtain specific orders from the physician are not always fruitful. Although poorly prepared to do so, the nurse is often left with the task of deciding how fast to give fluids. If the nurse is to intelligently assume this responsibility, she must learn more about parenteral fluids and their safe administration.

FACTORS INFLUENCING THE DESIRED RATE OF ADMINISTRATION Factors considered in determining the best flow rate for the infusion include:

Type of fluid
Need for fluids
Cardiac and renal status
Body size
Age
Patient's reaction during the infusion
Size of the vein

The desired rate for the infusion varies with the type of fluids used. For example, a 5 per cent dextrose in water solution can be administered faster than a 10 per cent dextrose in water solution or a 5 per cent alcohol solution. Although the other variables must also be considered, it is helpful for the nurse to know the usual infusion rates for various solutions. They are given in the descriptions of parenteral fluids in the next section of this chapter.

The patient's need for fluids influences the desired rate of administration; for example, a patient in hypovolemic shock needs fluids in a hurry. The infusion in this instance is much faster than usual. The presence of cardiac or renal damage can greatly alter the desired infusion rate, because the heart and kidneys both play a major role in the utilization of fluids introduced intravenously. If the pumping action of the heart is inadequate, a rapid infusion of fluids could cause a dangerous fluid excess. The failure of the kidneys to excrete unneeded water and electrolytes can also result in excessive amounts of these substances in the body.

Body surface area is an important criterion for fluid infusion rate. As mentioned in Chapter 15, the usual flow rate is 3 ml./m.^{2} of body surface/minute. This rate does not apply to all types of fluids and must at times be altered. Generally speaking, however, it is logical that a large individual can tolerate a greater amount of fluid per minute than a smaller individual, if other factors are equal.

The aged almost always have some degree of cardiac and renal impairment; therefore, fluids are administered more slowly to them than to younger adults.

One of the best guides to safe flow rate is the patient's reaction to the infusion; the fact that individuals respond differently to parenteral fluid infusions, just as they do to other medications, must never be forgotten. For this reason, the patient should be checked at least every 15 minutes during an infusion. The nurse should be aware of symptoms associated with the improper administration of various solutions so that she can know what to look for. Reactions associated with different parenteral fluids are described later in the chapter.

VARIATIONS OF DROP SIZE WITH DIFFERENT COMMERCIAL SETS Most nurses think in terms of "drops per minute" when considering rate of fluid flow. It must be remembered that commercial parenteral administration sets vary in the number of drops delivering 1 ml. (See Table 16-1.) Unless one knows which administration set is to be used, it is more practical to consider the number of milliliters to be infused in 1 minute. From this figure, the number of drops per minute can be computed when the drop size of the administration set is learned.

Formula:

Drop Factor × ml./min. = drops/min.

For example, to deliver 3 ml./minute using a set with 10 drops to 1 ml., a flow rate of 30 drops/minute would be necessary. To administer the same amount using a set with 15 drops to 1 ml., a flow rate of 45 drops/minute would be necessary.

CALCULATION OF FLOW RATE If the nurse knows the amount of fluid to be given in a prescribed time interval, plus the drop factor of the administration set to be used, she can easily compute the desired number of drops/minute. The following formula is used:

$$\text{Drops/min.} = \frac{\text{Total volume infused} \times \text{Drop factor (drops/ml.)}}{\text{Total time of infusion in minutes}}$$

Sample Problem:

Infuse 1,000 ml. of 5% D/W in 2 hours (Assume an administration set with 10 drops to 1 ml. is to be used)

Total volume = 1,000 ml.
Drops/ml. = 10
Total time of infusion in minutes = 120

$$\frac{1{,}000 \times 10}{120} = \text{approximately 80 drops/min.}$$

To save the nurse time, some handy calculators* have been devised by manufacturers of parenteral fluids to determine the desired flow rate when the above factors are known, directions for which are included with the calculators.

---

* Abbott Laboratories—(Normosol Calculator)
Baxter/Travenol Laboratories—(Minislide Calculator)
McGaw Laboratories—
(Solution-Administration Set Conversion Chart)

Table 16-1. Variation in Size of Drop in Commercial Administration Sets—Approximate No. of Drops to Deliver 1 ml.

Company	"Regular" Set	"Special" Sets
Abbott Lab.	15	60 (Microdrip) 10 (Blood Set)
Baxter/Travenol Lab.	10	50 (M-50 Minimeter) 60 (Metal Drip System)
Cutter Lab.	20	60 (Saftiset Sixty Set)
McGaw Lab.	13	60

Adapted from Weisberg, H.: Water, Electrolyte and Acid-Base Balance, ed. 2, p. 286. Baltimore, Williams & Wilkins, 1962.

MECHANICAL FACTORS INFLUENCING FLOW RATE After the desired flow rate has been regulated, there are several mechanical factors that may alter it:

1. Change in needle position: A change in the needle position may push the bevel against or away from the venous wall. An adequate flow rate becomes diminished when the needle is pushed against the vein, whereas it is increased when the needle moves away from the venous wall. Care must be taken to prevent speed shock by making sure the solution is flowing freely before adjusting the rate.
2. Height of the solution bottle: Because infusions flow in by gravity, a change in the height of the infusion bottle or bed can increase or decrease the rate—the greater the distance between the patient and the bottle, the faster the rate.
3. Patency of the needle: A small clot may occlude the needle lumen and decrease or stop the flow rate—when released, the rate increases. Clot formation may occur when an increase in venous pressure in the infusion arm forces blood back into the needle, causes of which can include lying on the infusion arm or constriction with a blood pressure cuff.
4. Venous spasm: A cold or irritating solution may retard flow rate by producing venous spasm. A warm pack placed proximal to the infusion site will help relieve this condition.
5. Plugged air vent: A plugged air vent can cause an infusion to stop. Thus, patency of the air vent should be checked when no other cause is apparent for the stopped infusion.
6. Crying in infants: This problem raises venous pressure and thus slows the rate of flow.

PARENTERAL FLUIDS—SPECIAL CONSIDERATIONS

Parenteral Nutrition

Parenteral nutrition is frequently lifesaving. As Dr. Robert Elman said, "Parenteral alimentation does not compete with oral alimentation; it competes only with death." Substances that can be given intravenously include:

Carbohydrates
Protein hydrolysates
Alcohol
Vitamins
Water
Electrolytes

Provision of nutrients intravenously is indicated when it is desired to put the gastrointestinal tract at relative rest, as in the presence of nausea, vomiting, diarrhea, peritonitis, ileus, or fistula. Intravenous nutrition is also indicated when the patient cannot take nutrients by an enteral route. In considering the nutritional needs of the patient exclusively on parenteral feedings, it should be borne in mind that the recommended energy need of an adult at bedrest is 1,600 calories; this is a basal figure and does not allow for fever, high environmental temperatures, or other causes of increased metabolism. Although under usual circumstances it is difficult to restore the nutritionally depleted patient by the intravenous route, it is possible to maintain the state of nutrition fairly well for limited periods.

In recent studies at the University of Pennsylvania's Harrison Department of Surgical Research, it was found that complete parenteral nutrition could be given to promote wound healing and weight gain in adults and normal growth in children. Researchers used a solution of 20% dextrose and 5% fibrin hydrolysate (amino acids), along with added vitamins and electrolytes; one liter of this solution contains approximately 1,000 calories and 6 grams of nitrogen. Frequently, a unit of albumin was added to supplement the protein intake. Because of the solution's hypertonicity, it was infused continuously at a constant slow rate into the superior vena cava via an indwelling subclavian catheter. Patients have been maintained in positive nitrogen balance on this regimen for prolonged periods, and more than 1,000 patients with various conditions precluding adequate enteral nutrition have been supported exclusively by vein with 2,000 to 5,000 calories per day for 10 to 365 days.

The goal of parenteral nutrition is chiefly to pinch-hit until the patient can again take nutrients by mouth. Every effort should be made to restore a patient receiving parenteral feedings to the oral or tube route as soon as possible. The nurse can contribute to this restoration by reporting signs of improvement, such as the absence of nausea and vomiting, and by encouraging the patient to take materials by mouth as soon as permissible. This, of course, does not apply when parenteral alimentation is necessitated by the urgent need for a nutrient, such as glucose in severe hypoglycemia, 5 per cent sodium chloride in severe sodium deficit, or calcium gluconate in acute calcium deficit. In such instances, the use of the intravenous route is essential.

CARBOHYDRATES Included in the carbohydrates that can be administered and absorbed intravenously are glucose, fructose, and invert sugar. These are all monosaccharides and therefore ready for utilization by the body cells. Disaccharides and polysaccharides cannot be utilized when given by the intravenous route. Table 16-2 presents an analysis of various parenteral carbohydrate solutions.

To provide the patient with sufficient calories through the administration of carbohydrate alone would necessitate giving a large quantity of a dilute solution, or a smaller quantity of a concentrated solution. To supply 1,600 calories with a 5 per cent dextrose solution would require 9 L., a volume exceeding the tolerance level of most patients. Mixtures of carbohydrate and alcohol are useful because of their rich caloric contribution and limited bulk.

Table 16-2. Parenteral Carbohydrate Solutions

Types of Solutions	*Calories/L.*	*Tonicity*
Dextrose		
2½% Dextrose in water	85	Hypotonic
5% Dextrose in water	170	Isotonic
5% Dextrose in saline	170	Hypertonic
10% Dextrose in water	340	Hypertonic
10% Dextrose in saline	340	Hypertonic
20% Dextrose in water	680	Hypertonic
50% Dextrose in water	1,700	Hypertonic
Fructose		
5% Fructose in water	187.5	Isotonic
10% Fructose in water or saline	375	Hypertonic
Invert Sugar		
5% Invert sugar in water	187.5	Isotonic
5% Invert sugar in saline	187.5	Hypertonic
10% Invert sugar in water or saline	375	Hypertonic

Concentrated solutions, such as 20 per cent or 50 per cent dextrose, are useful for supplying calories for individuals with renal insufficiency or who for other reasons are unable to tolerate large volumes. In order that the glucose be utilized, concentrated solutions must be administered slowly and intermittently. When administered rapidly, such solutions act as a diuretic and pull interstitial fluid into the plasma for subsequent renal excretion. Such hypertonic solutions damage veins in direct proportion to their tonicity, and when used, they should be injected into large functioning veins so that they will be diluted by the relatively large blood volume. A functioning vein is soft to the touch; moreover, it fills when compressed proximally—that is, on the side toward the heart. However, the site of injection should be alternated to avoid repeated irritation of one vein.

Carbohydrate is often administered parenterally to minimize the ketosis of starvation, because when ingestion of carbohydrate and fats is inadequate, the body burns its own fats to supply caloric needs. As a result of this process, ketone bodies are formed and since these are acids, they neutralize bicarbonate and produce metabolic acidosis (primary base bicarbonate deficit). Ketones require water for renal excretion and thus cause an increased demand for renal water expenditure. Administration of 100 Gm. of carbohydrate daily can prevent the ketosis of starvation by supplying readily accessible carbohydrate.

One advantage of carbohydrate as a source of calories lies in the fact that following its utilization, there remains only water and carbon dioxide to be used by the body or excreted. Nevertheless, when solutions of carbohydrate are administered too rapidly, the body cannot utilize all the carbohydrate and part of it is excreted in the urine. The body receives no benefit from the excreted glucose, and further, the glucose may carry with it other important nutrients. If a hypertonic carbohydrate solution is infused too rapidly, hyperinsulinism may occur, because the pancreas secretes extra insulin to metabolize the infused carbohydrate; discontinuance of the administration may leave an excess of insulin in the body. Symptoms include nervousness, sweating and weakness. It is not uncommon for small amounts of isotonic carbohydrate solution to be given after hypertonic solutions to "cover" for the extra insulin and allow the return to normal secretion. The nurse should be familiar with the usual rates of administration of carbohydrate solutions.

Rates of Administration The maximal speed for administration of glucose to normal adults without producing glycosuria is approximately 0.5 Gm./kg./hr. At this rate, it would take 3 hours for the injection of 1 L. of 10 per cent dextrose. Some people maintain that fructose can be administered more rapidly than glucose, and that invert sugar's optimal rate of administration lies somewhat between the two. Whether fructose and invert sugar offer real advantages from the standpoint of rate of administration appears open to question.

It is, of course, the province of the physician to specify the rate of administration of parenteral fluids. Factors unknown to the nurse could well alter average infusion rates in the case of a particular patient. Nevertheless, it is wise for the nurse to keep infusion rates in mind as guidelines for what is usually safe. (See Table 16-3.)

Table 16-3. Maximal Rates of Infusions for Carbohydrate and Water Solutions

Solution	Time
Dextrose 5% 1,000 ml.	1½ hours
Dextrose 10% 1,000 ml.	3 hours
Dextrose 20% 1,000 ml.	6 hours
Invert Sugar 5% 1,000 ml.	1½ hours
Invert Sugar 10% 1,000 ml.	2 hours
Fructose 10% 1,000 ml.	1½ hours

PROTEIN HYDROLYSATES* Protein is necessary for cellular repair, wound healing, growth, and for the synthesis of certain enzymes and vitamins. One cannot supply enough carbohydrate parenterally to prevent burning of some body protein for energy purposes. Hence, one should supply the minimal requirements for protein by parenteral administration of protein hydrolysate solutions, if the patient is to be maintained exclusively on parenteral nutrition for more than a limited period of time. Protein hydrolysates are usually given in conjunction with other substances, such as glucose or alcohol, or both, in order to supply sufficient calories so that the protein will be used for tissue repair rather than for caloric purposes. (See Table 16-4.)

Starvation causes a breakdown of protoplasm, largely a protein substance, and since protein contains nitrogen, there is an increased excretion of nitrogen. In starvation, there is little or no intake of nitrogen; therefore, more nitrogen is lost than is taken in—hence, the patient is said to be in *negative nitrogen balance*. It has become customary to use the measurement of nitrogen balance as an indication of the state of the patient's protein metabolism, just as water balance is used to

* Amigen—Baxter/Travenol Laboratories
C.P.H.—Cutter Laboratories
Aminosol—Abbott Laboratories
Hyprotigen—McGaw Laboratories

Table 16-4. Parenteral Amino Acid Solutions

Type of Solution	*Calories/L.*	*Tonicity*
5% Amino Acids	175	Isotonic
5% Amino Acids 5% Dextrose	345	Hypertonic
5% Amino Acids 12.5% Fructose 2.4% Alcohol	778	Hypertonic

Adapted from Weisberg, H.: Water, Electrolyte and Acid-Base Balance, ed. 2, p. 297. Baltimore, Williams & Wilkins, 1962.

measure the degree of water exchange. Approximately 1 Gm. of nitrogen is contained in 6.25 Gm. of protein.

Positive nitrogen balance can be achieved by supplying protein, or the elements of protein, plus sufficient calories to prevent protoplasmic breakdown. A healthy adult requires approximately 1 Gm. of protein/kg. (2.2 pounds) of body weight daily to replace normal protein losses. Nitrogen balance can be maintained either by vegetable or animal protein; the latter is, in general, a far more efficient source of protein nutrition than the former. Nevertheless, some vegetable proteins, such as soybean, peanut and yeast, closely approach animal protein in nutritional value. Clinically, protein hydrolysates are useful for a wide variety of patients who are unable to ingest sufficient food to maintain positive nitrogen balance; for adult patients, two to three liters each 24 hours is the average dosage.

Rates of Administration The first few milliliters of the protein hydrolysate should be given slowly, since some patients have what might be termed as *pharmacologic sensitivity* to certain amino acids. If any untoward symptoms occur, the infusion should be stopped.

Sometimes excessively rapid administration causes nausea, a feeling of warmth, flushing of the face, and vomiting. These symptoms usually disappear when the rate of administration is retarded. Other patients experience unpleasant effects, such as peculiar sensations of taste and smell.

If complications do not occur, a reasonable administration time for 1 L. of a 5 per cent protein hydrolysate solution is 1½ to 2½ hours. Individual variation in rate tolerance is great; the patient's reaction to the infusion should be checked often.

Protein hydrolysate solutions have a high NH_4^+ level and should be administered with especial care to patients with hepatic insufficiency or emaciation; a rate slower than usual for other I.V. solutions should be employed. Seriously impaired renal function constitutes a contraindication to the administration of protein hydrolysate or amino acid solutions, since the seriously impaired kidney cannot normally excrete nitrogenous wastes.

Supplemental medications should not be added to the solution or injected into the administration tubing without first checking their compatibility with both the physician and the pharmacist. Every protein hydrolysate solution should be examined carefully before it is infused into the patient. Either particulate matter or cloudiness should call for discarding the solution. *Once a bottle is opened, it should be administered at once; it should never be placed in a refrigerator for later use.* Deaths have occurred from this unwise practice.

PARENTERAL HYPERALIMENTATION The infusion of large amounts of basic nutrients sufficient to achieve tissue synthesis and growth is known as parenteral hyperalimentation. Commercial sets are available for mixing varying quantities of protein hydrolysate and hypertonic dextrose solutions. One set provides for mixing 750 ml. of 5% fibrin hydrolysate in 5% dextrose in water (D/W) with 350 ml. of 50% D/W. The resulting solution contains approximately 1,000 calories, and because it is very hypertonic, it is best infused through an indwelling catheter directed into a large vein, such as the superior vena cava. Initially, 1 or 2 L. is administered daily; this is gradually increased according to the patient's tolerance to a maximum of 4 or 5 L. daily. The flow rate must be slow and constant over the 24-hour period, for too rapid administration may cause osmotic diuresis and, untreated, can lead to dehydration and convulsions. Early signs of too rapid administration include lassitude, headache and nausea. The nurse must keep a close check on fractional urines and report any glycosuria. Because potassium is needed for the transport of glucose and amino acids across the cell membrane, as much as 200 mEq. of potassium may be given with 4,000 calories. (Magnesium, calcium and phosphorus are included when necessary.) Because of the possible interaction of drug additives with protein hydrolysate, the nurse should check with both the physician and the pharmacist before adding parenteral medications to the solution—a precipitate can form which may not always be visible. Sometimes parenteral medications are administered through an alternate infusion.

ALCOHOL SOLUTIONS One Gm. of absolute ethyl alcohol yields 6 to 8 calories. Obviously an excellent source of calories, alcohol has been combined with carbohydrate and with both carbohydrate and protein hydrolysates to provide a high calorie repair solution. When alcohol is infused with carbohydrate, it is apparently burned preferentially, thus permitting the glucose to be stored as glycogen. Alcohol spares body protein by providing readily accessible calories, and its sedating effect is highly desirable for patients with pain. *Sedation can be achieved in the average adult without symptoms of intoxication by giving 200 to 300 ml. of a 5 per cent solution per hour.*

The nurse should be aware of the physiologic and psychologic effects of alcohol parenterally administered; these include dulling of memory, loss of ability to concentrate, an improved sense of well-being, increased respiration and pulse, and vasodilation. Alcohol solutions should *not* be employed in shock, impending shock, epilepsy, severe liver disease, or in patients with coronary thrombosis. Nausea and vomiting do not occur as frequently when alcohol is given parenterally as when a comparable amount is taken orally. However, whenever the rate of administration of alcohol given parenterally exceeds its metabolic destruction by the body, restlessness, inebriation and coma can occur. The lethal dose of alcohol is approximately 500 ml. of pure alcohol. The amount of alcohol contained in a liter of 5 per cent alcohol solution, 50 ml., is thus quite safe. Nevertheless, the rate at which alcohol solutions are administered obviously influences the patient's reaction to the alcohol.

Table 16-5. Parenteral Alcohol Solutions

Type of Solution	*Calories/L.*	*Tonicity*
Alcohol 5% Glucose 5%	450	Hypertonic
Amino Acids 5% Fructose 12.5% Alcohol 2.4%	778	Hypertonic

The parenteral administration of alcohol, particularly of hypertonic solutions, can cause phlebitis. Tissue necrosis can occur if the needle accidentally leaves the vein and permits solution to perfuse the surrounding tissue spaces. Table 16-5 shows the caloric values and the tonicity of various solutions of alcohol.

PARENTERAL VITAMINS Vitamins should be administered parenterally when there is inadequate oral intake or when parenteral therapy is necessary for longer than 2 or 3 days. Although not food in themselves, vitamins are essential for the utilization of other nutrients. The need for vitamins is increased during periods of stress, such as acute illness, infection, surgery, burns, injury and convalescence. Some parenteral fluids have vitamins incorporated, and special vitamin preparations designed for injection with parenteral fluids are also available.

The vitamins most frequently needed in parenteral alimentation are vitamin C and members of the B complex, all of which are water soluble and stored by the body only in small amounts; they serve as co-enzymes in the essential metabolic processes of the cells. Vitamin deficiency has been observed after only one week of parenteral administration of glucose and water alone. However, since most patients are on parenteral therapy for only limited periods, they do not require the fat soluble vitamins A and D.

Because there is some waste of parenterally infused vitamins through urinary excretion, it is necessary to administer generous amounts to assure an adequate intake. Hence, the patient who is on exclusive parenteral alimentation is usually given more than the daily vitamin requirement—sometimes as much as ten times the minimal requirement. A basic formula of parenteral vitamins is as follows:

Thiamine	10 mg.
Riboflavin	5 mg.
Niacinamide	50 mg.
Calcium Pantothenate	20 mg.
Pyridoxine Hydrochloride	20 mg.
Folic Acid	5 mg.
Vitamin B_{12}	15 μg.
Vitamin C	up to 1 Gm. as indicated

Vitamin C is particularly important in surgical patients to promote wound healing, whereas the B complex vitamins provide factors to aid carbohydrate metabolism and the maintenance of normal gastrointestinal function. (An occasional patient may show extreme sensitivity to the B complex vitamins.) Sometimes vitamin K is given; flushing, sweating, and a constricted feeling in the chest may follow the intravenous injection of vitamin K.

WATER The patient on parenteral fluids exclusively can be provided with water by means of solutions of carbohydrate or electrolytes or both, the most common of which is 5 per cent dextrose in water. Also useful are the various hypotonic electrolyte solutions, which supply glucose or fructose, electrolytes, and water. However, they must be used with caution. For example, isotonic solution of sodium chloride has the same tonicity as body fluid; therefore, when administered to the patient requiring water, it provides no water at all —it merely expands the extracellular fluid volume and ignores the patient's requirements for water for renal excretion, insensible loss, and metabolic needs of the body. Consequently, it should never be used for this purpose.

It should always be remembered that one should *never give water alone by a parenteral route.* If pure water not containing electrolytes were injected directly into the bloodstream, the red blood cells would absorb water, swell and burst.

ELECTROLYTE SOLUTIONS A wide variety of electrolyte solutions are available for parenteral administration. Some of the more common solutions are listed in Table 16-6 for quick reference. Included in the table are the following:

Electrolyte content
Trademarks (brand names)
Precautions for administration
Usual rate of administration

Administration of Potassium Solutions Potassium may be given in the form of commercially prepared electrolyte solutions, or a potassium salt may be added as a supplement to an intravenous fluid, such as 5 or 10 per cent dextrose in water.

The nurse should keep the following facts in mind when potassium-containing solutions are administered (see Table 16-6):

1. As a general rule, no more than 30 mEq. of potassium should be infused in 1 hour. (Some authorities say 20 mEq. per hour.)
2. Potassium solutions should never be allowed to run with the flow valve wide open or be given under pressure; high concentrations of potassium in the bloodstream can result in cardiac arrest.
3. Small ampules containing concentrated solutions of potassium salts for addition to I.V. fluids are meant to be mixed with at least 1 L. of solution. They should never be directly administered in concentrated form through the tubing or needle, due to the danger of cardiac arrest.
4. It is wise to limit the potassium concentration in 1 L. of fluid to 40 mEq., never more than 80 mEq., since an accidental rapid infusion rate is less dangerous when potassium content is moderate.
5. Potassium should be administered intravenously only after adequate urine flow has been established. The presence of oliguria or anuria is an indication to withhold potassium until initial hydrating or pump-priming solutions (such as 5% D/W or 0.45% saline) have demonstrated adequate renal function, since potassium is mainly excreted by way of the kidneys; when the kidneys are non-functional, a high potassium level builds up in the bloodstream. An exception to this rule may be the occasional administration of

Solution*	Tonicity	pH (approximate)	mEq./L. Na+	K+	Ca++	Mg++	NH4+	Cl−	Lactate	HCO3−	Acetate	Gluconate	HPO4−−	Brand Names	Reasons for Use	Comments
Sodium Chloride 0.45% *(One-half isotonic saline)*	Hypotonic	(4.5–7.0) 5.3 Abbott Lab. 5.5 Baxter Lab. 6.0 Cutter Lab.	77					77							Supply daily salt requirements Supply water for excretory purposes	Available commercially with varying concentrations of carbohydrates
Sodium Chloride 0.9%	Isotonic	(4.5–7.0) 5.7 Abbott Lab. 5.5 Baxter Lab. 5.0 Travenol Lab. (Viaflex) 6.1 Cutter Lab.	154					154							Replace Na^+ and Cl^- Expands extracellular fluid volume Correct mild metabolic alkalosis	Widely used as a routine electrolyte replacement solution even though it supplies only Na^+ and Cl^- (Many feel its routine use should be replaced by a solution that more closely resembles extracellular fluid, such as Lactated Ringer's) Does not supply free water for excretory purposes Cl^- is supplied in excess of normal plasma Cl^- level—excessive use of isotonic saline can cause Cl^- to replace part of the body HCO_3^- (metabolic acidosis) Sometimes erroneously referred to as "normal saline" or "physiologic saline" Available commercially with varying concentrations of carbohydrates Ordinarily given at a rate of 400-500 ml./hr.—may be given much faster in special instances (check with physician)

* K-containing solutions should be infused with caution and are contraindicated when these conditions are present: oliguria, potassium excess, renal disease, Addison's disease. (See section on K-solutions)

Table 16-6. *(Cont.)*

*Solution**	*Tonicity*	*pH (approximate)*	*mEq./L.*											*Brand Names*	*Reasons for Use*	*Comments*
			Na^+	*K^+*	*Ca^{++}*	*Mg^{++}*	*NH_4^+*	*Cl^-*	*Lactate*	*HCO_3^-*	*Acetate*	*Gluconate*	*HPO_4^{--}*			
Sodium Chloride 3%	Hypertonic	(4.5–7.0) 6.0 Cutter Lab. 5.0 Travenol Lab.	513					513							Rapid correction of severe low-salt syndrome	Contraindicated unless severe salt depletion is present
Sodium Chloride 5%	Hypertonic	(4.5–7.0) 5.6 Abbott Lab. 5.9 Cutter Lab. 5.0 Travenol Lab.	855					855								Use with caution in edematous patients Administer at a slow rate
Ringer's	Isotonic	(5–7.5) 5.8 Abbott Lab. 5.5 Baxter Lab. 6.0 Travenol Lab. (Viaflex) 5.9 Cutter Lab.	147	4	5			156							Replaces K^+ and Ca^{++} in addition to Na^+ and Cl^-	Contains an excess of Cl^- in relation to normal plasma Cl^- level Available commercially with carbohydrates
Lactated Ringer's (Hartmann's)	Isotonic	(6–7.5) 6.7 Abbott Lab. 6.5 Baxter Lab. 6.6 Cutter Lab.	130	4	3			109	28						Routine electrolyte maintenance solution Correct metabolic acidosis Replace fluid lost as bile, diarrhea, and in burns	Electrolyte concentration closely resembles extracellular fluid Same precautions as for any K-containing solution* (It is permissible to use Lactated Ringer's in burns since the amount of K^+ is so small as to be inconsequential) (May at times be administered cautiously in the presence of decreased urinary output) Available commercially with carbohydrates

[illegible]							[illegible] Cutter Lab.	[illegible] cellular fluid losses	[illegible] tion is identical to [illegible]c-tated Ringer's with the exception that it contains acetate instead of lactate as its HCO_3^- precursor Acetate is metabolized largely by muscle and other peripheral tissues rather than by the liver May be preferred to Lactated Ringer's in metabolic acidosis associated with liver dysfunction, hypothermia, circulatory insufficiency and extracorporeal circulation It requires less oxygen for metabolism than does Lactated Ringer's (particularly important in shock with its tissue hypoxia) Same precautions as for any K-containing solution* (May at times be administered cautiously in the presence of decreased urinary output) Available commercially with carbohydrate
Gastric (Cooke and Crowley)	Isotonic	(3.3–3.7)	63	17	70	150	Electrolyte No. 3 Cutter Lab. Travenol Lab. Isolyte G McGaw Lab.	Replace gastric fluid lost in vomiting and gastric suction	Should not be used as a routine maintenance solution pH of solution is acid, similar to that of gastric juice Contraindicated in hepatic insufficiency The ammonium ions are converted by the liver to urea and hydrogen ions, thereby replacing the H^+ deficit resulting from gastric juice loss

* K-containing solutions should be infused with caution and are contraindicated when these conditions are present: oliguria, potassium excess, renal disease, Addison's disease. (See section on K-solutions)

Table 16-6. *(Cont.)*

*Solution**	*Tonicity*	*pH (approximate)*	*mEq./L.*											*Brand Names*	*Reasons for Use*	*Comments*
			Na^+	*K^+*	*Ca^{++}*	*Mg^{++}*	*NH_4^+*	*Cl^-*	*Lactate*	*HCO_3^-*	*Acetate*	*Gluconate*	*HPO_4^{--}*			
																Same precautions as for any K-containing solution* Available commercially with carbohydrates Can be given at a rate up to 500 ml./hr. (check with physician)
Duodenal	Isotonic		138	12	5	3		108	50					Ionosol D-CM Abbott Lab.	Replace duodenal fluid loss Correct mild acidosis	Same precautions as for any K-containing solution* Available commercially with carbohydrates Rate should not exceed 660 ml./hr. (check with physician)
Duodenal (modified)	Hypotonic		79.5	36	4.5	3		63	60					Electrolyte No. 1 Cutter Lab. McGaw Lab. Travenol Lab.	Replace pancreatic and duodenal fluid losses Supply water for excretory needs Correct deficits of K^+, Ca^{++}, Mg^{++}, Na^+ and HCO_3^- Correct acidosis	Same precautions as for any K-containing solution (Note that the K^+ content is high)* Available commercially with carbohydrates
Sodium Lactate 1/6 M *(Alkalinizing Solution)*	Isotonic	(6–7.3) 6.9 Abbott Lab. 6.8 Cutter Lab. 6.5 Travenol Lab.	167						167						Correct severe metabolic acidosis	Contraindicated in liver disease, shock, and right-sided heart failure (lactate ions are improperly metabolized in these conditions) Contraindicated in alkalosis

								250-400 ml./hr. (ch[illegible] with physician)
Sodium Bicarbonate 1.4%	Isotonic		167			167	Correct severe metabolic acidosis	Contraindicated in metabolic and respiratory alkalosis
Sodium Bicarbonate 5% *(Alkalinizing Solutions)*	Hypertonic		595			595	Alkalinize urine (as in hemolytic reactions requiring rapid alkalinization of urine to reduce nephrotoxicity of blood pigments)	Contraindicated when hypocalcemia is present; alkalinization of plasma may produce signs of tetany Administer at a slow rate Administer with extreme caution to salt-retaining patients with cardiac, renal or liver damage (Severe acidosis in edematous patients should be treated with 5% bicarbonate solution in small volumes)
Ammonium Chloride 0.9% *(Acidifying Solution)*	Isotonic			168	168		Correct severe metabolic alkalosis in children	Contraindicated in disturbed hepatic function, renal failure or any condition with a high NH_4^+ level
Ammonium Chloride 2.14% *(Acidifying Solution)*	Hypertonic	5.0 Cutter Lab.		400	400		Correct severe metabolic alkalosis in adults	Contraindicated in disturbed hepatic function, renal failure or any condition with a high NH_4^+ level Excessive amounts of this solution can cause metabolic acidosis with: drowsiness hyperpnea nausea and vomiting confusion disorientation coma Give slowly—check with physician (rate should not exceed 380 ml./hr. in an adult)

* K-containing solutions should be infused with caution and are contraindicated when these conditions are present: oliguria, potassium excess, renal disease, Addison's disease. (See section on K-solutions)

Table 16-6. *(Cont.)*

Solution*	Tonicity	pH (approximate)	mEq./L. Na+	K+	Ca++	Mg++	NH_4^+	Cl−	Lactate	HCO_3^-	Acetate	Gluconate	HPO_4^{--}	Brand Names	Reasons for Use	Comments
Balanced electrolyte (Fox)	Isotonic		140	10	5	3		103			55			Isolyte E McGaw Lab. Polysal Cutter Lab.	Replaces gastrointestinal losses of: small intestinal juice, bile, diarrhea Burn treatment Postoperative fluid replacement Correct Na+ deficit	Electrolyte content similar to plasma except that it has twice as much K+ (K+ content is similar to that of intestinal juice) Same precautions as for any K-containing solution* Should not be given at a rate faster than 1 L. in 1½ hours (check with physician) Available commercially with carbohydrates
			140	10	5	3		103	8		47			Plasma-Lyte Travenol Lab.		
Butler (*Electrolyte No. 88*)	Hypotonic		57	25		5-6		49-50	25				13	Electrolyte No. 2 McGaw Lab. Travenol Lab. Ionosol B Abbott Lab.	Supply water Supply maintenance needs of Na+, Mg++, K+, and Cl− Replace fluid loss from the large intestine	Same precautions as for any K-containing solution* Available commercially with carbohydrate Should not be given at a rate faster than 500 ml./hr. in adults (check with physician)
Modified Butler (*Electrolyte No. 48*)	Hypotonic		25	20		3		22	23				3	Electrolyte No. 48 Baxter Lab. Cutter Lab. Ionosol MB Abbott Lab. Isolyte P McGaw Lab.	Supply water Used in pediatrics to treat dehydration of acidosis, diarrhea and burns	Same precautions as for any K-containing solution* Available commercially with carbohydrates Should not be given at a rate faster than 250 ml./hr. in adults

Solution												Polyonic M-56 Cutter Lab. Plasma-Lyte 56 Travenol Lab. Isolyte H McGaw Lab.	Supply electro-lytes for older children and adults	[illegible] tion* Available commercially with carbohydrates
Balanced Isotonic Solution	Isotonic	7.4 Abbott Lab. 6.2 Abbott Lab. 7.4 Cutter Lab. 7.4 Travenol Lab. 5.5 Travenol Lab.	140	5		3	98		27	23		Isolyte S McGaw Lab. Normosol-R Abbott Lab. Plasma-Lyte 148 Travenol Lab. Polyonic R 148 Cutter Lab.	Extracellular fluid replacement solution Recommended substitute for isotonic saline Correct mild acidosis	Same precautions as for any K-containing solution* Available commercially with carbohydrates Contains no calcium; therefore can be administered simultaneously with blood
Electrolyte No. 75 (Talbot)	Hypotonic		40	35			40	20			15	Electrolyte No. 75 Baxter Lab. Cutter Lab. Ionosol T Abbott Lab.	Supply water Supply maintenance electrolyte needs Correct K^+ deficit	Same precautions as for any K-containing solution* Contains more K^+ than most maintenance solutions Available commercially with carbohydrates
Maintenance electrolyte solution	Hypotonic		40	16	5	3	40	12	12			Polysal M Cutter Lab. Plasma-Lyte M Travenol Lab.	Supply water Supply maintenance electrolyte needs—contains Ca^{++} and Mg^{++} in addition to Na^+ and K^+	Same precautions as for any K-containing solution* Available commercially with carbohydrates

* K-containing solutions should be infused with caution and are contraindicated when these conditions are present: oliguria, potassium excess, renal disease, Addison's disease. (See section on K-solutions)

lactated Ringer's solution in the presence of oliguria; the potassium content of this solution is low and is probably not harmful unless anuria is present.

6. A solution containing sizable amounts of potassium (30 to 40 mEq./L.) is sometimes associated with pain in the vein it is entering; slowing the rate usually relieves this sensation. Because infiltration of a potassium solution into the subcutaneous tissues is painful, it is rarely administered by means of hypodermoclysis; when it is, the concentration should be no higher than 10 mEq./L. to avoid local pain.

Incompatible Combinations of Additives and Parenteral Fluids

The nurse is frequently required to add medications to parenteral fluids. There is a fast-growing number of medications and types of parenteral fluids on the market; thus, the number of possible combinations is astronomical. It is impossible, without help, for the nurse to know which medications can be safely mixed with certain intravenous fluids and such assistance must come from several sources:

pharmacist
physician
manufacturer's directions
publication of new admixture information

The pharmacist is best qualified to predict incompatibilities. Some hospitals have pharmacy-centralized intravenous additive programs, but, if there is no such program, the nurse must assume the responsibility for safely adding medications to infusion fluids, using the pharmacist as a resource person.

Some manufacturers of intravenous fluids have prepared charts noting the compatibility of various medications with their solutions; usually these charts show only physical incompatibilities, that is, soluble precipitates. Chemical and pharmacologic incompatibilities are more difficult to detect, because they do not always produce a visible change. Often manufacturers insert valuable information in their medication packages, which should be read thoroughly before adding the medication to an infusion fluid. When possible, it is best to add only one medication to each solution bottle, as the complex interaction between two additives may render the solution incompatible.

The intravenous administration of a solution containing insoluble matter may result in embolism or damage to the heart, liver, and kidneys. The formation of a precipitate when a medication is added to an intravenous fluid is an indication to discard the solution (unless directions accompanying the medication state otherwise). Solutions containing additives should be inspected for precipitate formation periodically during administration—some incompatibilities do not become apparent until the solution has been mixed for awhile. An administration set with a filter between the infusion tubing and the needle should be used when there is a danger of precipitate formation. (See Figure 16-20.)

The degree of solubility of an additive varies with the pH, as most incompatibilities are related to changes in pH. Solutions of a high pH seem to be incompatible with solutions of a low pH. (A chart listing the pH of certain drugs and parenteral solutions can help the nurse predict potential incompatibilities.)

When in doubt, the nurse responsible for adding medications to intravenous fluids should consult with the pharmacist, the physician, or both. To better prepare the nurse, the hospital should provide an effective in-service program on intravenous additives. Some hospitals have prepared charts listing specifically the medications that the nurse can mix with specific intravenous fluids.

Cutter Laboratories has compiled parenteral admixture information from the medical literature and other published material, Guide to Parenteral Admixtures, designed for use by any who are concerned with the preparation of admixtures. It consists of a number of compatibility charts; a separate page or section is devoted to each therapeutic agent and is arranged in alphabetical order within a loose-leaf binder. The compatibility of the agents with various parenteral fluids is indicated, and compatibilities of the title agent in combination with other drugs, in various fluids, is also given. Mixtures which show evidence of physical incompatibility are designated "X". If there is no evidence of physical incompatibility, the mixture is marked "C". The mixture is marked "₵" if there are conflicting reports on compatibility. The guide is kept current by supplements which furnish new admixture information.

SPECIAL EQUIPMENT FOR INFUSIONS

DROP SIZE REDUCTION When potent medications are added to intravenous solutions, extreme precautions must be taken to prevent too rapid administration.

Abbott Laboratories has developed the Microdrip for precision drop control, delivering approximately 60 drops for 1 ml. Baxter/Travenol Laboratories has developed an administration set adaptor (M-50 Minimeter) for reduction of drop size to 1/50 ml. (delivers approximately 50 drops/ml.). Cutter Laboratories has a set that delivers approximately 60 drops/ml. (Saftiset Sixty Set), and McGaw Laboratories also has a pediatric set that delivers approximately 60 drops/ml.

VOLUME CONTROL SETS There are several commercial sets designed to administer limited amounts of solution in precise volume, all of which are extremely useful in the infusion of potent medications, such as the vasopressors. They are also valuable in pediatric intravenous therapy.

Abbott Laboratories has designed a rigid plastic cylinder (Soluset) that is available in 100 ml. or 250 ml. capacities, and the maximum amount of solution that can be infused is limited

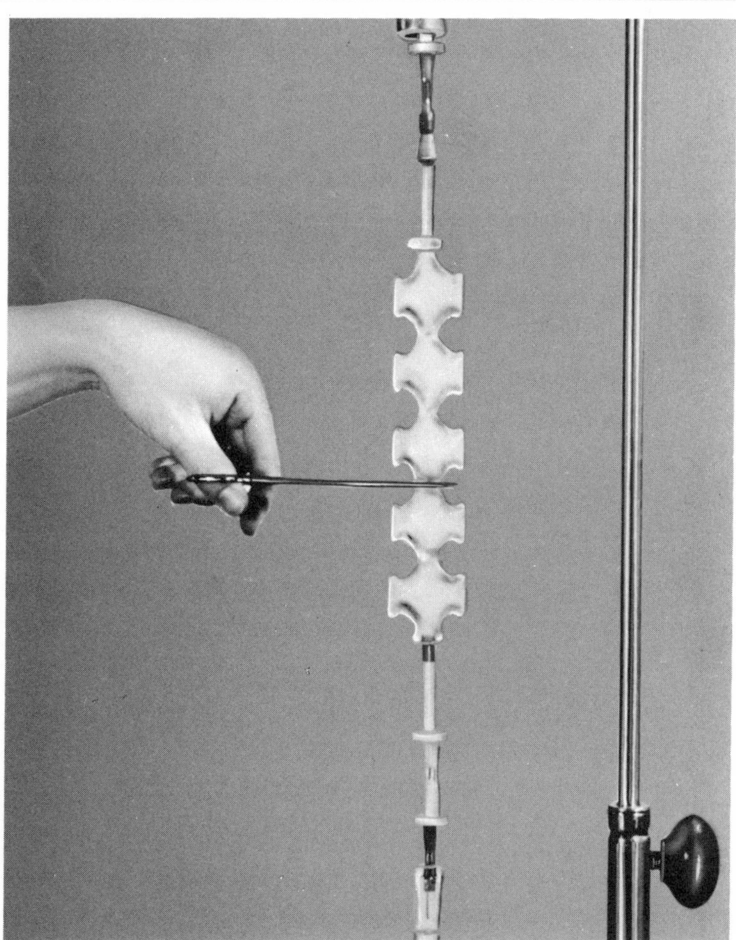

Fig. 16-9. Pedatrol Administration Set. (Baxter Laboratories, Morton Grove, Illinois)

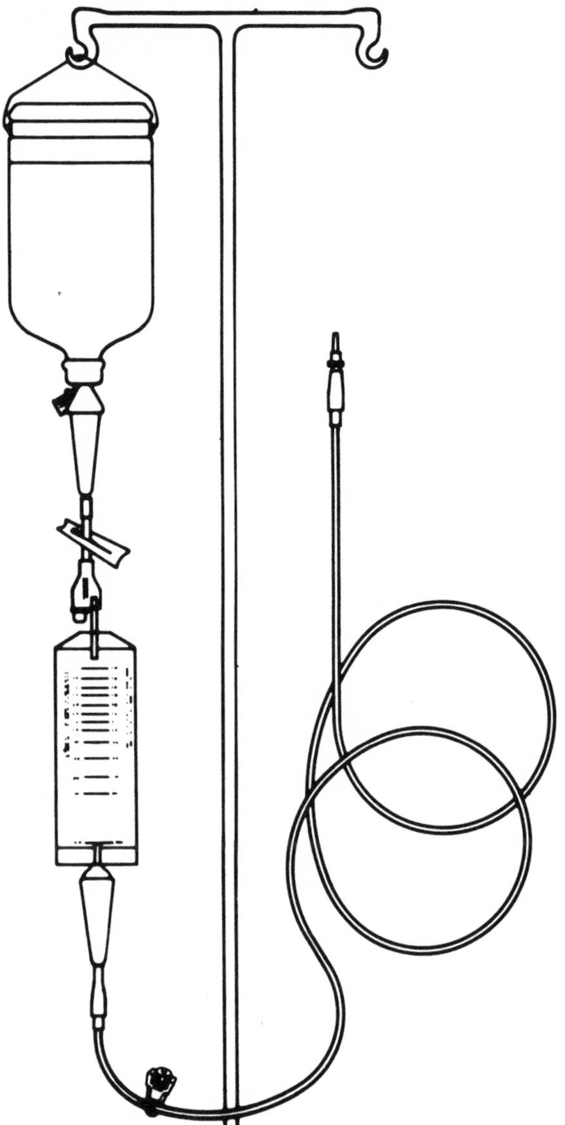

Fig. 16-10. Volu-Trole® Set. (Cutter Laboratories, Inc., Berkeley, California)

to the amount in the cylinder. Amounts larger than capacity may be given by refilling the chamber. The Soluset-100 is fitted with a Microdrip orifice, which provides approximately 60 drops/ml., whereas the Soluset-250 provides approximately 15 drops/ml.

Baxter/Travenol Laboratories has designed the pliable plastic Pedatrol set, divided into 5 aliquots of 10 ml. each. (See Figure 16-9.) By simply moving a hemostat's position on the set, the maximum amount of solution to be infused can be limited to 10, 20, 30, 40 or 50 ml.; when empty, the set can easily be refilled from the solution bottle above. Travenol Laboratories also has the In-Line Buretrol set, especially designed for use in pediatrics for metered intravenous administration of blood or solutions; it has a capacity of 150 ml., with markings at 1 ml. intervals.

McGaw Laboratories has developed the Metriset, a calibrated chamber that controls volume to 100 ml., wherein medications may be added directly into the set through a medication plug. Lastly, Cutter Laboratories has a pediatric measuring apparatus (Volu-Trole Set) consisting of a regular I.V. infusion set plus a flexible transparent plastic metering chamber graduated in 10 ml. divisions (approximately 60 drops/ml.). See Figure 16-10.)

BOTTLE ARRANGEMENTS A simple intravenous infusion involves a setup such as the one illustrated in Figure 16-11. However, to add more fluid or to change fluids while an infusion continues, a series hookup is used. (See Figure 16-12.) The two bottles are connected by plastic tubing, with the airvent closed in the primary bottle and the secondary bottle vented—the secondary bottle will empty first. If the specific gravity is higher in the secondary bottle, there will be no mixing of solutions; there will be mixing if the specific gravity is higher in the primary bottle.

A parallel hookup may be used to administer two solutions alternately or simultaneously. (See Figure 16-13.) This type of hookup is more dangerous than a series hookup, because if either of the bottles empties completely and its clamp closure is not complete, large quantities of air will leak in by way of the empty bottle and form air bubbles in the infusion tubing. The nurse must exercise great care when using a Y-type set; complete clamp closure should be made when there is still a little fluid in the bottle. Well meant intentions to administer every drop in the bottle are not warranted.

PLASTIC CONTAINERS Travenol Laboratories has a number of intravenous solutions available in plastic containers (Viaflex™). (See Figure 16-14.)

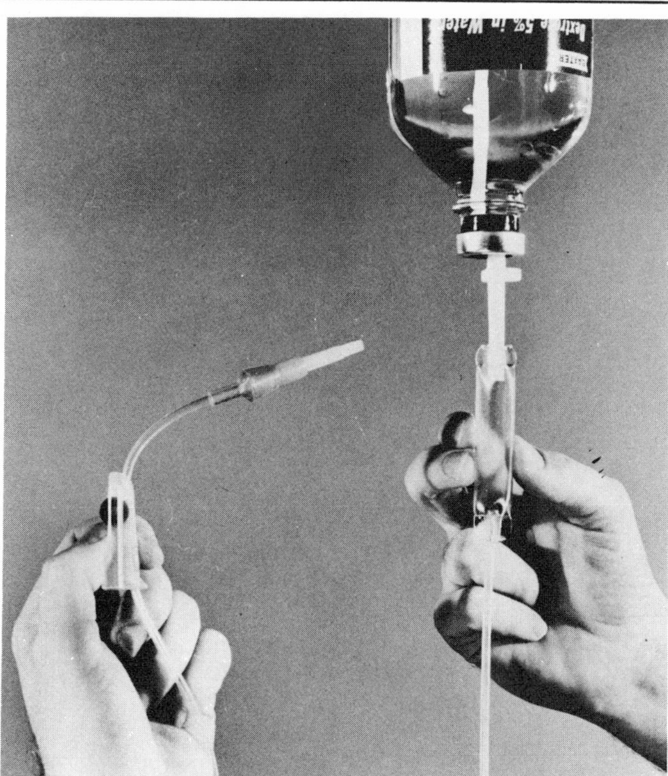

Fig. 16-11. Simple intravenous infusion set. (Baxter Laboratories, Morton Grove, Illinois)

These containers eliminate solution contamination by way of the air filter. One advantage of plastic bags is that they are more easily stored than glass bottles. Another is that infusion can be speeded up by applying external pressure to the sides of the bag. The nurse should be aware of the manufacturer's warning: "Do not use plastic container in series connections. Such use could result in air embolism due to residual air (approximately 15 ml.) being drawn from the primary container before administration of the fluid from the secondary container is completed."

DEVICES TO CONTROL FLOW RATE Disposable soft plastic tubing loses its shape when compressed and has the characteristic of totally collapsing when clamped. Standard intravenous administration sets lose about 52% of the initial flow rate in the first hour of use, meaning that the nurse must frequently adjust the clamp to maintain the desired rate of flow. Several devices are available to help the nurse maintain a more accurate flow rate with less difficulty.

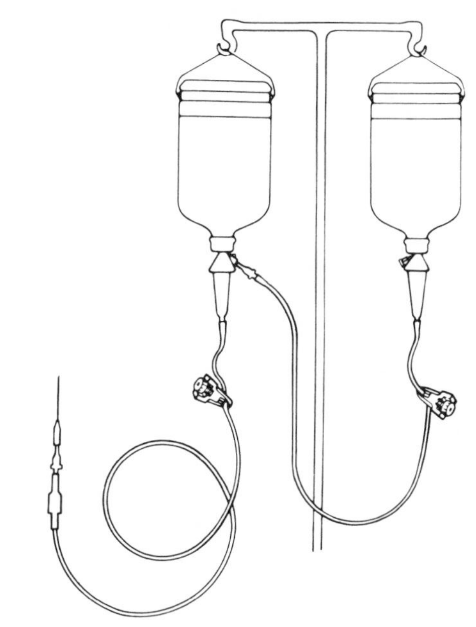

Fig. 16-12. I.V. Tandem Setup (Saftiset™ Tandem Set). (Cutter Laboratories, Inc., Berkeley, California)

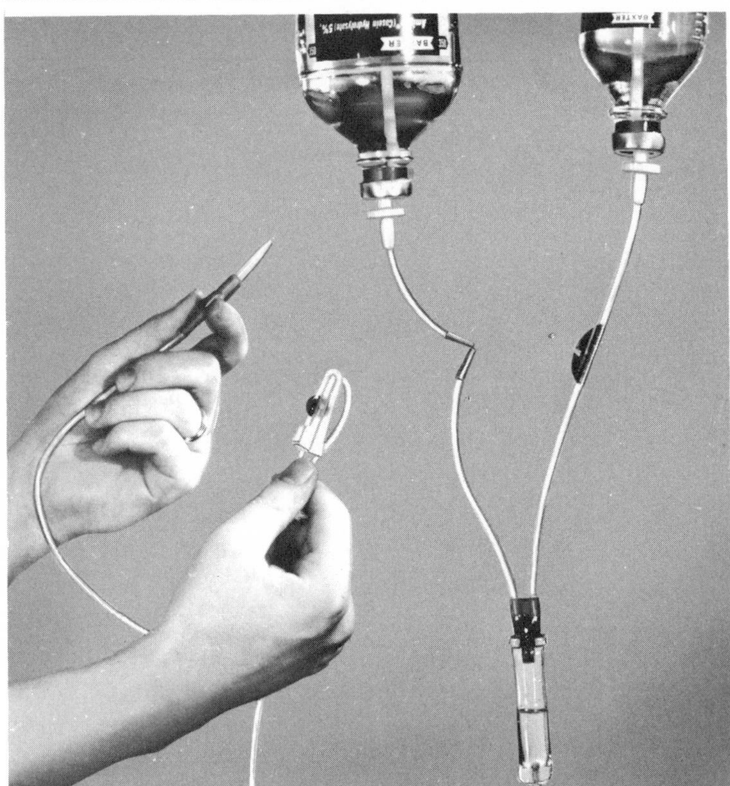

Fig. 16-13. Bottles connected in parallel (Y-type setup). (Baxter Laboratories, Morton Grove, Illinois)

One such device is the Accu-Flow Set; it has a silicone rubber section of tubing which can be carefully adjusted with a screw-type clamp. (See Figure 16-15.) Another device is the ARDL clamp, which has a tapered V-shaped groove along one surface; it provides greater dependability than clamps that squeeze the tubing between two flat surfaces. The Accu-Flow Set and the ARDL clamp are associated with only about a 10% decrease in flow rate in the first hour of infusion.

INFUSION PUMPS Infusion pumps can pump intravenous fluids at an exact predetermined rate, providing a constant flow rate, as opposed to the variable rate furnished by the gravity flow method. They are particularly helpful in pediatric and adult intensive care units.

One type of pump is the IVAC 500 infusion pump. (See Figure 16-16.) This apparatus can pump from 1 to 99 drops per minute; the desired flow rate is set by a dial on the front of the pump. Any change in the rate is automatically corrected

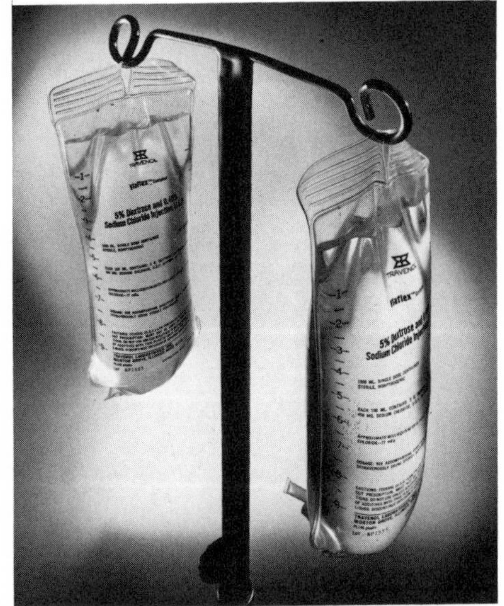

Fig. 16-14. Plastic parenteral fluid container—Viaflex™. (Travenol Laboratories, Inc., Morton Grove, Illinois)

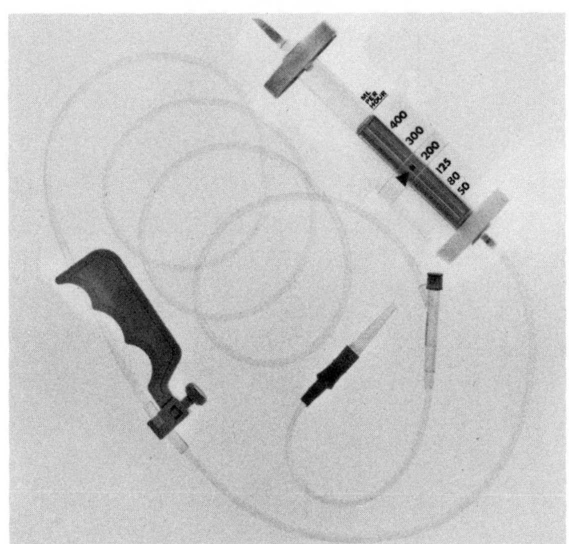

Fig. 16-15A. Complete view of Acca-Flow set. (United States Surgical Corporation, New York, New York)
Enclosed within the meter section is the drip chamber. Adjustment of the clamp will bring the ball in the meter section to the desired number. When the ball is within the confines of the number, the slide with the red arrow is placed opposite to indicate the rate of fluid flow as prescribed.

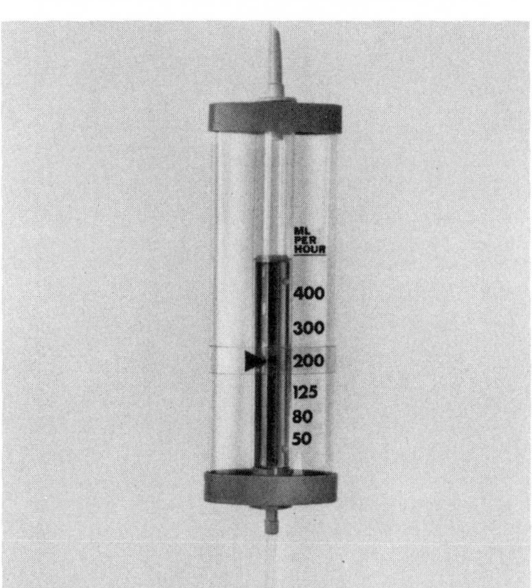

Fig. 16-15B. Closeup view of the drip chamber and meter. One can tell at a glance that this infusion is flowing at the original setting of 200 ml./hr. because the ball is visible directly through the red plastic marker. The meter enables the nurse to monitor the flow rate without counting drops and to quickly note a change from the desired rate.

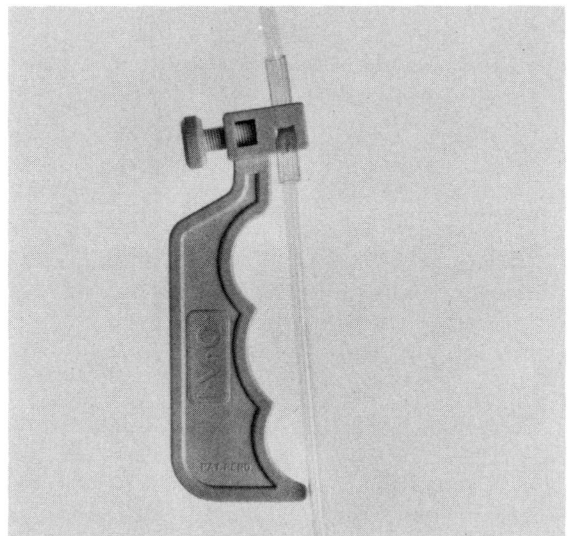

Fig. 16-15C. Multi-lumen construction of tubing at the clamping site (viewed here in cross-section) allows more accurate control of flow rate.

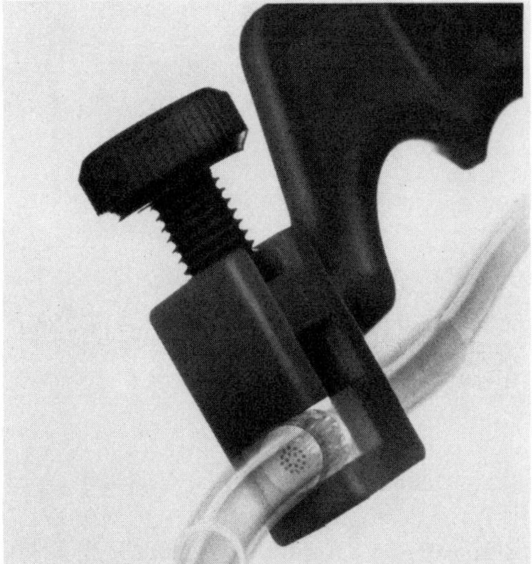

Fig. 16-15D. Screw clamp with hand grip insures easy adjustment of drip rate. Use of a segment of Silastic multi-lumen tubing at the clamp site eliminates the phenomenon of plastic "creep."

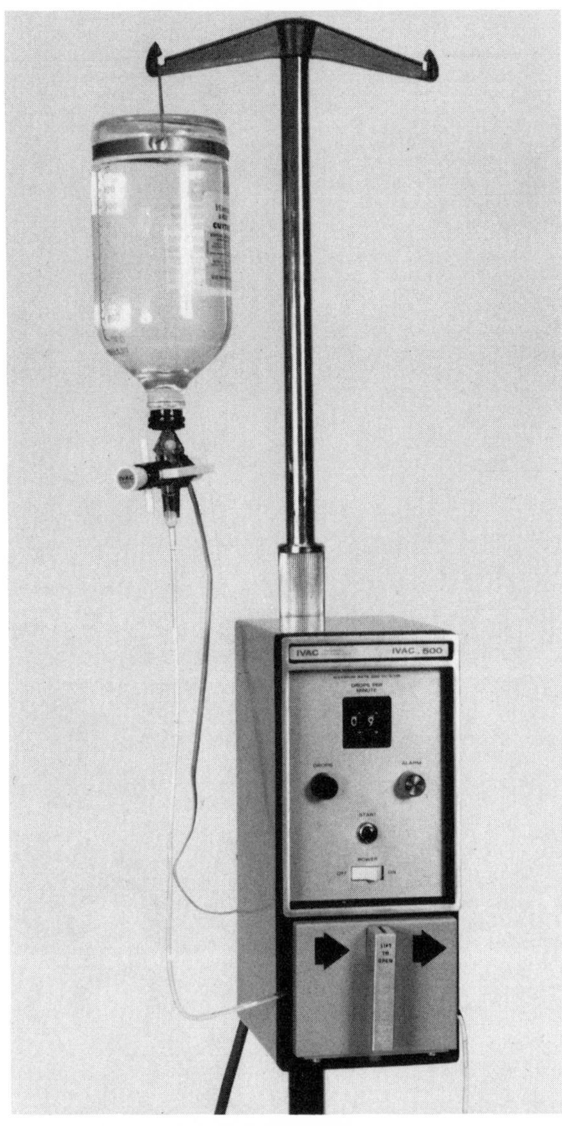

Fig. 16-16. IVAC 500 Infusion Pump. (IVAC Corporation, San Diego, California)

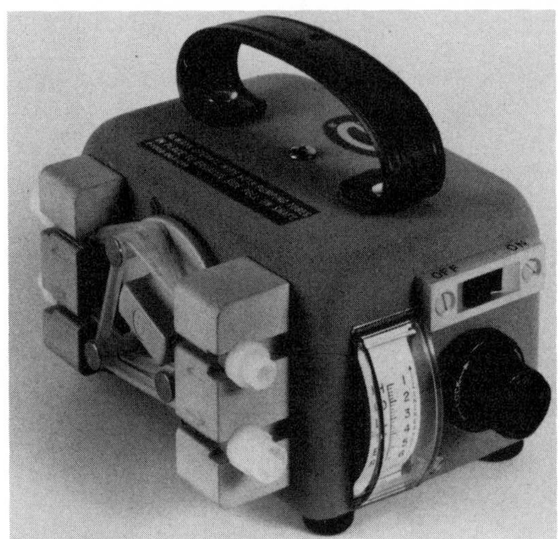

Fig. 16-17. Holter Roller Pump (Series 900). (Extracorporeal Medical Specialties, Inc., King of Prussia, Pennsylvania)

to maintain the prescribed flow regardless of back pressure changes, tubing diameter changes, tubing crimps or the solution level. The IVAC 500 cannot infuse air because its drop sensor will detect the last drop of fluid and automatically stop the solution flow. In this event, the pump will generate a visual and, if desired, an audible alert, and when connected, it will also initiate a call at the nurse's station.

Another type of infusion pump is the Holter Pump. (See Figure 16-17.) The new Holter Series 900 precision roller pumps are available in 8 basic models offering flow rates from .33 to 1300 ml. per hour. These pumps permit two separate fluids to be pumped simultaneously at varying rates (depending on the pumping chamber selection). The new Holter pumps are small and lightweight, thus enabling them to be easily moved or suspended from an I.V. stand by the strap. A new bottle of solution should be added, or the pump stopped, before the container runs dry, because air will be pumped if pumping is continued after the solution bottle is emptied.

COMPLICATIONS OF INTRAVENOUS FLUID ADMINISTRATION

Patients receiving parenteral fluids should be observed often to detect the early appearance of complications. The nurse should periodically check the rate of flow, the amount of solution in the bottle, the appearance of the injection site and the patient's general response to the infusion.

Complications sometimes occurring with intravenous infusions include:

Pyrogenic reactions
Local infiltration
Circulatory overload
Thrombophlebitis
Air embolism
Speed shock

PYROGENIC REACTIONS The presence of pyrogenic substances in either the infusion solution or the administration setup can induce a febrile reaction. (Pyrogens are foreign proteins capable of producing fever.) Such a reaction is characterized by:

An abrupt temperature elevation (from 100 to 106° F.) accompanied by severe chills (the reaction usually begins about 30 minutes after the start of the infusion)
Backache
Headache
General malaise
Nausea and vomiting
Vascular collapse with hypotension and cyanosis, which may occur when the reaction is severe

The severity of the reaction depends upon the amount of pyrogens infused, the rate of flow and the patient's susceptibility. Patients having fever or liver disease are more susceptible than others.

If these symptoms occur the nurse should stop the infusion at once, check the vital signs and notify the physician. The solution should be saved so that it can be cultured if necessary.

The wide use of commercially prepared solutions and administration sets has dramatically decreased the number of pyrogenic reactions. It must be remembered, however, that contaminants can enter the solution flask after the seal is broken. It is, therefore, a wise practice to indicate on the bottle the date and time that the seal was broken; electrolyte and dextrose solutions should be in use no longer than 24 hours—important to remember when patients are on slow "keep open" infusions. Administration sets should be changed at least every 24 hours, and any evidence of cloudiness or other particulate matter in a normally clear solution is an indication to discard it. Unless the nurse uses the most careful technique, contaminants can be introduced when medications are added to the infusion fluid. (See Figure 16-18.)

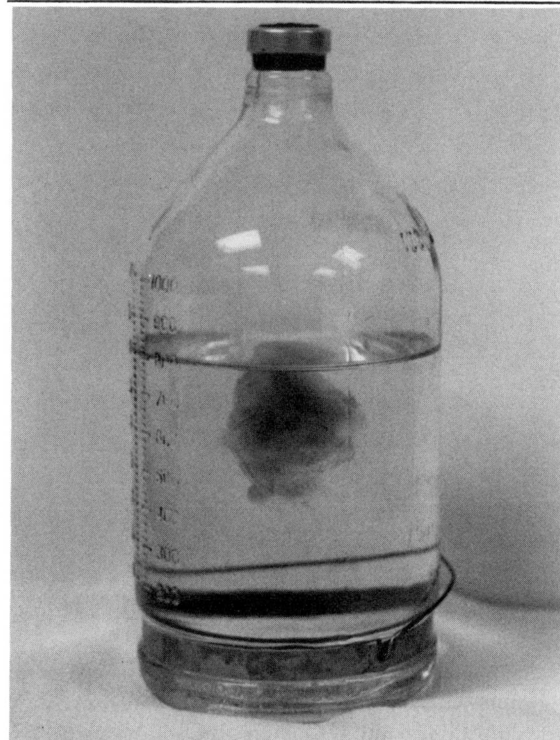

Fig. 16-18. Mold in this I.V. bottle indicates break in aseptic technique.

Because traffic generates airborne contamination, medications should be added in an isolated area. Some hospitals are equipped with Laminar Flow Clean Air Work Stations; these stations provide a filtered air screen to reduce contamination of intravenous fluids during handling. (See Figure 16-19.)

A final filter is another safety device to prevent the infusion of bacteria and particulate matter. (See Figure 16-20.) The filter is situated between the infusion tubing and the needle, allowing for final sterilization filtration immediately before the solution enters the bloodstream. It also prevents air from entering the circulatory system during mechanical infusion. (Changing the filter set every 24 hours prevents a potential buildup of material.)

LOCAL INFILTRATION The dislodging of a needle and the local infiltration of solution into

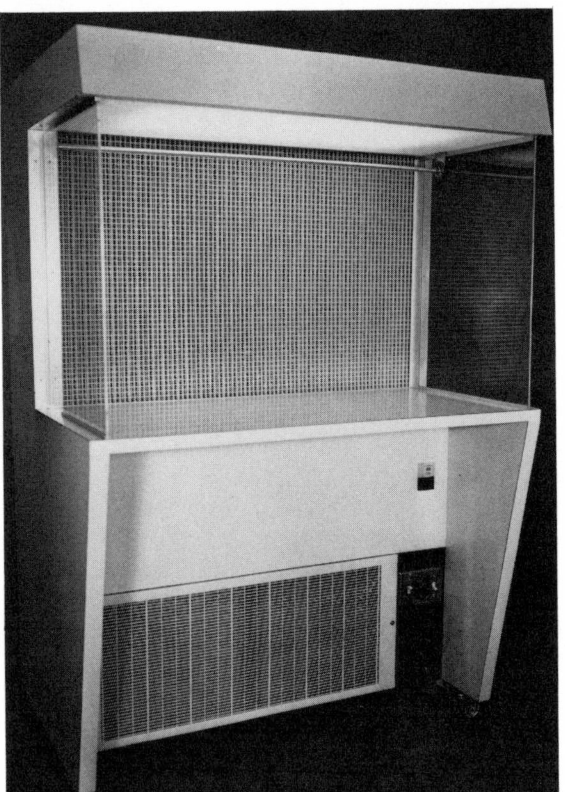

Fig. 16-19. Laminar Flow Clean Air Work Station. (Travenol Laboratories, Inc., Morton Grove, Illinois)

the subcutaneous tissues is not uncommon, especially when a small, thin-walled vein is used and the patient is active. Infiltration is characterized by:

- Edema at the site of injection
- Discomfort in the area of the injection (the degree of discomfort depends on the type of solution)
- Significant decrease in the rate of infusion, or a complete stop in the flow of the fluid
- Failure to get blood return into tubing when the bottle is lowered below the needle (this method is not always foolproof—sometimes the needle lumen is partially in the vein with its tip in the subcutaneous tissue)

Hypertonic carbohydrate solutions, potassium solutions, and solutions with a pH varying greatly from that of the body (such as protein hydrolysates, sixth molar sodium lactate, or ammonium chloride) often cause great pain if they infiltrate into the subcutaneous tissues. Tissue slough may result from the local irritation, especially when norepinephrine (Levophed) is the offending solution.

The infusion should be immediately discontinued when infiltration is apparent. When in doubt, an infiltration can be confirmed by applying a tourniquet to restrict venous flow proximal to the injection site; if the flow continues, regardless of the venous obstruction, the needle is obviously not in the vein.

CIRCULATORY OVERLOAD Overloading the circulatory system with excessive intravenous fluids may cause the following symptoms:

- Increased venous pressure
- Venous distention
- Increased blood pressure
- Coughing
- Shortness of breath, increased respiratory rate
- Pulmonary edema with severe dyspnea and cyanosis

The nurse should be particularly alert for this reaction in patients with cardiac decompensation. If the above symptoms occur, the infusion should be stopped and the physician notified immediately. If necessary, the patient can be raised to a sitting position to facilitate breathing.

THROMBOPHLEBITIS The condition associated with clot formation in an inflamed vein is known as thrombophlebitis. Although some degree of venous irritation accompanies all intravenous infusions, it is usually of significance only in infusions kept going in the same site for more than 12 hours. Thrombophlebitis at an infusion site may be manifested by:

- Pain along the course of the vein
- Redness and edema at the injection site
- If severe, systemic reactions to the infection (tachycardia, fever and general malaise)

Mechanical factors can produce thrombophle-

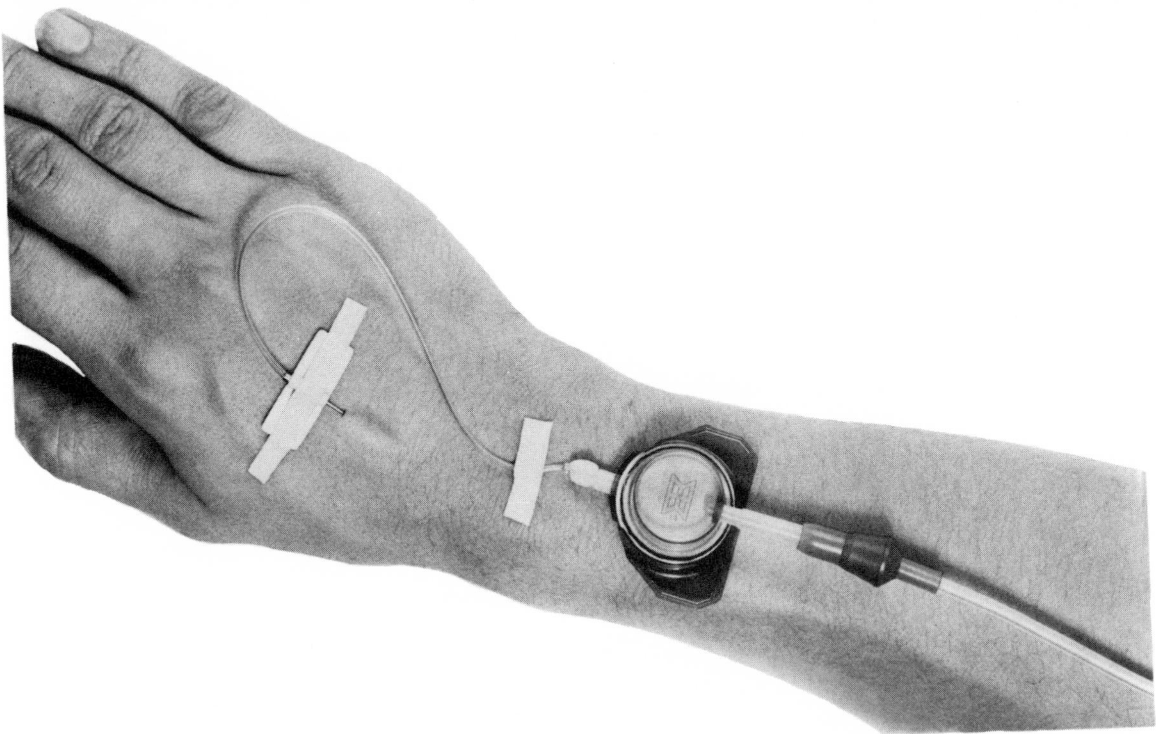

Fig. 16-20. Final Filter. (Travenol Laboratories, Inc., Morton Grove, Illinois)

bitis. Needle movement can cause venous irritation when the infusion site is near a joint; careless technique in venipuncture, or in removing an infusion needle, can seriously traumatize the vein.

Irritating solutions, such as alcohol, can be instrumental in causing thrombophlebitis. Hypertonic solutions are often associated with venous irritation; carbohydrate solutions in excess of 10 per cent almost always produce this reaction. Solutions with an alkaline or acid pH are more frequently associated with thrombophlebitis than are the solutions that approximate body pH.

Dextrose solutions are irritating to veins because of their low pH. (The U.S.P. specification for pH of dextrose solutions ranges between 3.5 and 6.5.) Five per cent dextrose in water has a pH ranging between 4.0 and 5.0, a low pH necessary to prevent caramelization of the dextrose during sterilization and to preserve the solution's stability during storage. Studies have shown a significant decrease in thrombophlebitis when buffered dextrose solutions have been used. For example, Abbott Laboratories provides a sodium bicarbonate 1% additive solution (Neut) to increase the pH of intravenous solutions, the addition of which will raise the pH to a less irritating level. This small amount of basic solution will not alter the patient's plasma pH. However, increasing the pH of solutions containing additives can produce incompatibility problems, since some additives are only stable at a low pH.

Once thrombophlebitis is detected, the infusion is stopped. Consideration should be given at this time to obtaining a change in the order for the infusion; otherwise, more veins may be lost. The infusion may be started in another site to allow the traumatized vein to heal. Usually, cold compresses are applied to the thrombophlebitic site, after which warm moist compresses can be employed to relieve discomfort and promote healing.

AIR EMBOLISM The danger of air embolism is present in all intravenous infusions, even though it usually occurs when blood is given under pressure. Small amounts of air are not always harmful, yet as little as 10 ml. may be fatal in some patients.

The nurse should take these measures to prevent the occurrence of air embolism:

1. Inspect the disposable tubing for cracks or defects.
2. The needle and any other attachments in the setup should be tightly fitted to the infusion tubing to prevent the entrance of air.
3. Discontinue an infusion before the bottle and tubing are completely emptied; otherwise, air from the bottle will enter the bloodstream if there is a negative pressure in the vein receiving the infusion. (If the vein has a positive pressure, the fluid will stay at this level; normally venous pressure is 4 to 11 cm. above the level of the heart.)
4. Kerr has pointed out that the extremity receiving the infusion should not be elevated above the level of the heart since this results in venous collapse and negative venous pressure. Negative pressure in the vein receiving the infusion draws in air if there are any defects in the apparatus or if the solution flask is emptied.
5. The clamp used to regulate the fluid flow rate should be kept at a low level—preferably no higher than the level of the heart, certainly no higher than 4 to 11 cm. above the heart. If the flow regulating clamp is placed above this height, a negative pressure will develop in the tubing below. The negative pressure can be great enough to draw in sizable amounts of air if there are any defects in the apparatus.
6. Permitting the infusion tubing to drop below the level of the extremity may help prevent air from entering the vein if the infusion flask empties unobserved. There is nothing wrong with enlisting the patient's help in observing the infusion bottle and notifying the nurse when the infusion is about to run out. A tape can be placed on the side of the infusion flask showing the level at which the patient should buzz the nurse.
7. The first bottle to empty in a Y-type set (parallel hookup) should be completely clamped off; otherwise, air will be drawn into the vein from the empty bottle.
8. Instructions for use of blood pumping apparatus should be carefully followed when blood or, indeed, any fluid is given under pressure. (See section on blood administration.)
9. Some types of electric infusion pumps will pump air into the vein if the infusion bottle is allowed to empty. (See section on electric infusion pumps.)

The presence of an air embolism is manifested by sudden vascular collapse, with the following symptoms:

Cyanosis
Hypotension
Weak rapid pulse
Venous pressure rise
Loss of consciousness

The occurrence of these symptoms in the patient receiving an infusion should lead one to suspect air embolism.

If an air embolism occurs, administration tubing should be promptly clamped. Some physicians place the patient on his left side with his head down, on the theory that this allows the air to rise into the right atrium and away from the pulmonary outflow tract.

SPEED SHOCK Too rapid administration of solutions containing drugs may induce a systemic reaction called *speed shock*. The bloodstream is flooded with the drug, and toxic concentrations are supplied to organs such as the heart and brain, which have a rich blood supply; syncope and shock may occur. Symptoms, of course, vary with the offending drug. The nurse should check the flow rate often and reduce it if untoward symptoms develop.

ADMINISTRATION OF BLOOD, PLASMA AND DEXTRAN

Blood

Whole blood can be preserved with a solution of sodium citrate, citric acid, and glucose. Sodium citrate acts as an anticoagulant by combining with ionized calcium and thus interrupting the clotting mechanism, whereas citric acid and glucose prolong the viability of red blood cells. Blood preserved with acid-citrate-dextrose (A.C.D.) solution can be kept safe for use up to 21 days after collection from the donor, if stored at 4°C. (39°F.). Whole blood can also be preserved with citrate phosphate dextrose solution (C.P.D.) for up to 21 days. Blood preserved in C.P.D. anticoagulant has a higher pH while containing less acid than A.C.D. blood; it therefore imposes less acid load. This is particularly important if a large volume of blood is infused.

BLOOD TRANSFUSION REACTIONS Whole blood transfusions are indicated in the presence of a significantly decreased blood volume. Blood replacement therapy is often lifesaving, but, without careful attention to its hazards, it may also be lethal. Because the nurse shares a large responsibility in assuring safe blood administration, she should be familiar with complications associated with its use.

Stored Blood and Potassium Excess Continual destruction of red blood cells occurs when blood is stored; at the end of 21 days only 70 to 80 per cent of the original number of cells remain. The longer the blood ages, the higher its plasma potassium level becomes. One day old blood has a plasma potassium content of approximately 7 mEq./L.; blood stored for 21 days has a plasma potassium content of approximately 23 mEq./L. Not only is potassium released from the destroyed red blood cells, but there is also a transfer of potassium from the intact cells into the surrounding plasma.

Aged blood should not be given to patients with oliguria or anuria, since there is great danger of causing potassium excess. Potassium excess may be recognized by the following symptoms:

- Gastrointestinal hyperactivity (nausea, intestinal colic and diarrhea)
- Vague muscular weakness, first in the extremities, later extending to the trunk
- Paresthesia of hands, feet, tongue and face
- Flaccid paralysis (involving respiratory muscles last)
- Apprehension
- Slowed pulse rate (may also be irregular)
- Cardiac arrest and death when plasma potassium level reaches 10 to 15 mEq./L. (due to marked dilation and flaccidity of the heart)

According to LeVeen, the high incidence of cardiac arrest during surgery is correlated with the rapid infusion of large quantities of aged blood.

Citrated Blood and Calcium Deficit Calcium deficit can be caused by the rapid administration of large volumes of citrated blood. It should be recalled that A.C.D. solution contains citrate in excess of that needed to combine with the calcium in the blood collected. The binding of blood calcium will be more serious if a partial flask of blood is withdrawn from the donor. If citrate ions (furnished by sodium citrate) are infused too rapidly, the liver is unable to remove them and they combine with ionized calcium in the bloodstream. The reduced level of circulating calcium ions may cause these signs of neuromuscular irritability:

- Tingling of the fingers and the circumoral region
- Muscular cramps
- Hyperactive muscular reflexes
- Carpopedal attitude of hands
- Convulsions
- Laryngeal stridor
- Cardiac arrest

Calcium deficit due to excessive administration of citrated blood is more prone to occur in patients with liver damage, and blood should be given slowly to such patients to eliminate this hazard.

Circulatory Overload Discussed earlier in the chapter as a possible complication of all intravenous infusions, circulatory overload is particularly likely to occur in massive blood replacement for hypovolemia or when blood is given to a patient with normal blood volume. In addition to inducing pulmonary edema, the increased blood volume may cause hemorrhage into the lungs and the gastrointestinal tract.

To guard against the occurrence of circulatory overload, many physicians monitor venous pressure during the rapid replacement of large volumes of blood. (The procedure is discussed in the last section of this chapter.) Aged patients and patients with cardiac damage should be closely observed for circulatory overload even when small volumes of blood are given; venous pressure monitoring is frequently used to protect such patients from overload.

Administration of packed red blood cells, obtained by centrifuging whole blood and drawing off approximately 200 to 225 ml. of plasma, is sometimes necessary when a patient with congestive heart failure or fluid volume excess requires blood. Packed cells are administered in a minimal amount of fluid and are thus less prone to overload the circulatory system, but because of the increased density, they are more difficult to infuse than whole blood.

Allergic Reactions Prospective donors with known food and drug allergies are rejected in order to decrease the incidence of allergic reactions following blood transfusions. Blood from a donor with hypersensitivities may cause itching, erythema, urticaria, chills, wheezing, bronchospasm and angioneurotic edema; severe allergic reaction may produce anaphylactic shock. Appearance of any of these symptoms is an indication to immediately stop the transfusion. Antihistamines, such as diphenhydramine (Benadryl) or tripelennamine (Pyribenzamine), usually relieve mild symptoms, but severe reactions require treatment with an injection of 0.5 ml. of 1:1000 solution of epinephrine, or with adrenal steroids.

Serum Homologous Hepatitis Associated with blood transfusion is the risk of transmitting serum hepatitis, and, therefore, persons known to have had hepatitis are not allowed to give blood. Nonetheless, not all patients with hepatitis have had the condition diagnosed; thus, the danger always exists. There is no way to completely eliminate this risk, but recent advancements have been made and researchers have found an agent (Australian antigen) that is linked with serum hepatitis. More importantly, tests have been devised to detect the agent and allow blood banks and hospitals to screen blood for serum hepatitis. Unfortunately, the accuracy of the tests is estimated at only about 25%.

The incidence of Australian antigen in voluntary donors is about 1:11,000. Statistics indicate that paid donors cause up to 5 times as many cases of serum hepatitis as unpaid donors. (Drug addicts often sell blood to raise money for more drugs, with serum hepatitis fast spreading among them, because most use unsterile equipment for intravenous injections.) It is regrettable that in many cities, as much as half the blood comes from commercial sources.

The incubation period for serum hepatitis is from 6 weeks to 6 months; symptoms include malaise, anorexia, vomiting, abdominal discomfort, enlarged liver with tenderness, diarrhea, headache, fever and jaundice. Serum hepatitis is particularly serious in the elderly and in patients already debilitated by serious illness or injury.

Hypothermia Cold solutions are quickly warmed as they mix with circulating blood during usual administration rates. Rapid massive replacement of cold blood has caused cardiac arrest, and one study in a New York hospital showed a significant decrease in cardiac arrest (from 58.3% to 6.8%) when cold blood was warmed to body temperature during rapid massive infusion (6 pints or more per hour). When it is deemed necessary to warm blood, a heat exchange coil may be used. (See Figure 16-21.) The blood is warmed by immersing the long coiled tubing in a warm water bath and allowing the blood to flow through the coil. The adult coil warms approximately 150 ml./minute. (A single pediatric coil is available and warms approximately 50 ml./minute.)

Pyrogenic Reactions A pyrogenic reaction has been described earlier in the chapter as a possible complication of all intravenous infusions. Substances capable of producing a pyrogenic reaction during blood transfusion include foreign material in the administration setup, denatured proteins, bacterial polysaccharides, leuko-agglutinins and platelet-agglutinins. Such a reaction is sometimes confused with an incompatible

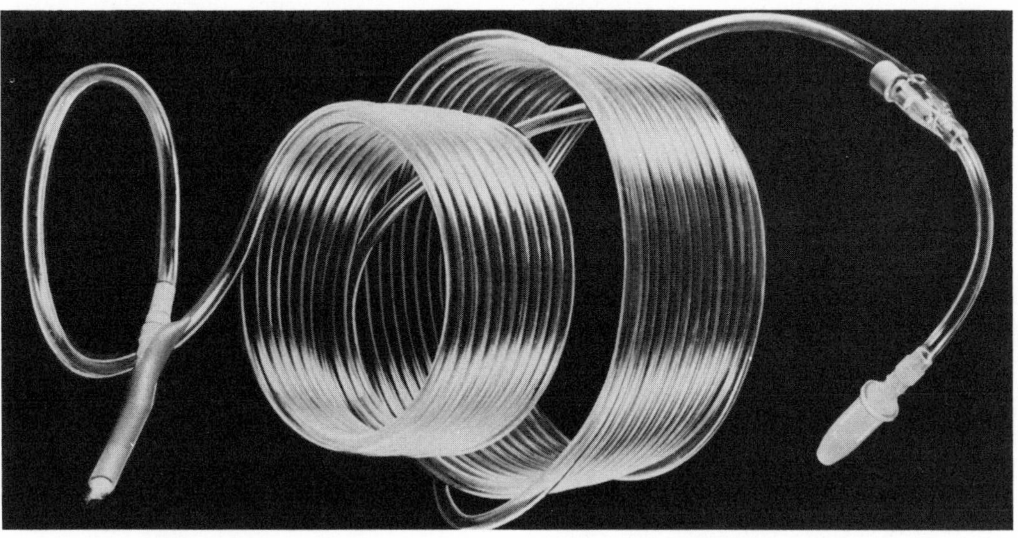

Fig. 16-21. Heat exchange coil to warm blood. (Cutter Laboratories, Berkeley, California)

blood reaction, and so it should be noted that a pyrogenic reaction tends to occur toward the end of a transfusion or even after it is completed. The most predominant symptoms are fever and chills; back pain, characteristic of incompatible blood reaction, is often absent. The onset of malarial chills can also be confused with a pyrogenic reaction but this, of course, is more of a problem in tropical and semitropical climates.

Bacterial Contamination Blood should be inspected before use for signs of bacterial growth, such as discoloration or gas bubbles; if these are present the blood should be discarded. If blood used for transfusion is grossly contaminated, the recipient usually develops symptoms of shock. Treatment may consist of vasopressors, steroids and antibiotics.

Incompatible Blood Reaction The most dreaded reaction to blood transfusion is that caused by incompatible blood, most often caused by the careless administration of the wrong blood. It can also be caused by blood accidentally hemolyzed from improper handling. Some hemolytic reactions result from inadequate crossmatching. A transfusion of incompatible blood causes hemolysis of the red blood cells with the liberation of hemoglobin into the plasma. Symptoms of a hemolytic reaction may occur within the first 10 to 15 minutes of the transfusion and may include:

- Lumbar and flank pain (flank pain caused by hemoglobin precipitation in the renal tubules)
- Feeling of coldness
- Feeling of fullness in the head
- Feeling of constriction in the chest
- Urge to defecate or urinate
- Fever and severe shaking chills (hemolytic reaction may cause a considerable degree of fever and general toxicity; these effects, in the absence of renal shutdown, are rarely fatal)
- Later hemoglobinuria and acute renal tubular necrosis may occur
- The only signs of serious transfusion reaction in an anesthetized or otherwise unconscious patient may be increasing tachycardia, shock and bleeding

Because an acute hemolytic reaction becomes evident during transfusion of the first 20 to 100 ml. of blood, it is highly desirable that the patient be carefully observed during this part of the infusion. If the transfusion is stopped early, acute renal tubular necrosis and death rarely occur; if more than several hundred ml. are infused, renal shutdown and death are common. Renal shutdown is due to blockage of the tubules with hemoglobin and to the powerful vasoconstriction caused by toxic substances released from the hemolyzed blood.

The blood transfusion should be discontinued immediately when a hemolytic reaction is evident. The blood bottle and set should be refrigerated so that further compatibility tests may be made. All urine should be saved and observed for discoloration; urine is sent to the laboratory for evaluation of hemoglobin content. The onset of a hemolytic reaction may be delayed when factors of less moment than the ABO system are involved. For example, a patient who has received multiple transfusions in the past may have become sensitized to Rh or to the minor factors, and his hemolytic reaction might have a delayed onset.

Hemolytic reactions are more prone to occur in patients who have had past transfusions and tend to be proportionate to the number of such transfusions, regardless of when given.

Treatment of an incompatible blood reaction usually consists of rapid administration of dilute fluids to promote diuresis. Alkaline fluids, such as sixth molar sodium lactate, increase the solubility of hemoglobin and aid in its excretion. An osmotic diuretic (usually mannitol) may be given intravenously to promote fluid excretion by the tubules and to overcome renal vasoconstriction; further treatment is dependent upon the amount of renal damage present. It is impossible to overstress the need to check and recheck all labels for both donor and patient, as errors in labeling still constitute a frequent cause of reaction.

SAFE BLOOD ADMINISTRATION To help assure that blood transfusions be as safe as possible, the nurse should keep the following points in mind:

1. Be aware of the complications associated with blood administration; keep their descriptions in mind while observing the patient.
2. *Give the right blood to the right patient.*
   A. Read the labels identifying the blood and check them carefully with the patient's full name, obtained from the wrist identification band. The bed card should not be relied on solely to identify the patient; these cards are often not up to date.
   B. The patient should be called by name and his response observed; this practice in itself is not foolproof because some patients respond to any name!
   C. Location of the patient should not be relied upon as the sole means of identification; patients are moved frequently in most hospitals.
   D. Particular precautions are necessary when the patient has a common name; many errors have been made by not checking further than the last name and first initial. This is not to imply that two patients with the same uncommon name cannot be confused; it *has* happened.
3. Blood sent to nursing divisions should be started within 30 minutes, because rapid deterioration of red blood cells occurs after blood has been exposed to room temperature for more than two hours. Ward refrigeration is inadequate for storing blood because it is not controlled and has no alarm to signal fluctuation of temperature. (Accidental freezing of blood renders it unsuitable for use.)
4. The patient's temperature should be taken before the transfusion to serve as a baseline for later temperature comparisons. An elevated temperature during a transfusion may indicate either a pyrogenic or an incompatible blood reaction, and for this reason the temperature should be checked hourly during the blood administration and for several hours afterwards.
5. The blood should be inspected before use for discoloration or gas bubbles; if present, the blood is probably contaminated and must be discarded.
6. Blood should always be given through

a filter to remove the particulate matter formed during storage. Care should be taken to keep the filter unclogged.

7. Do not start whole blood with 5 per cent dextrose in water, or hook whole blood in series or in parallel with it. Even though 5 per cent dextrose in water is an isotonic solution, it contains no electrolytes and can cause hemolysis of red blood cells when allowed to mix with blood. (This reaction does not occur when 5 per cent dextrose in water is given into the bloodstream, because it is rapidly diluted.) Isotonic saline is quite compatible with blood and is usually used to start blood.
8. Do not use a calcium-containing solution to start citrated blood or hook it in series or parallel with citrated blood, as calcium ions may cause the blood to clot and clog the infusion apparatus.
9. If it is necessary to warm blood before administration, a heat exchange coil can be used, as described earlier. Hot water should never be used to heat blood because excess heat destroys red blood cells.
10. The first 50 ml. of blood should be delivered slowly over a 30-minute period. The patient should be continually observed during the first 15 minutes and frequently thereafter, and if no adverse reactions occur, the rate may be increased as ordered.
11. Unless the patient has severe hypovolemia, blood transfusions should be given no faster than 500 ml. every 30 minutes. The presence of factors such as cardiac, renal, or liver damage may necessitate much slower rates. A patient with normal blood volume should receive blood at a slow rate to prevent circulatory overload.
12. Blood under pressure must be administered with great caution. Glass blood containers must be vented and hence contain air, and so when blood is given under pressure, it is vital that the fluid level in the bottle be closely watched so that air is not accidentally pumped into the vein. Figure 16-22 shows a pump set used with a glass container for rapid administration of blood. The bulb is compressed to pump in blood; when released, the desired drip rate is easily reestablished. This type of pump set is also available for use with plastic blood containers, none of which contain air—eliminating the danger of air embolism. In this case, blood can be given under pressure by a blood pump administration set or by applying a pressure sleeve to the filled container. (See Figure 16-23.) Air, forced into the sleeve by means of a pressure bulb, exerts force on the flexible blood container and increases the flow rate.

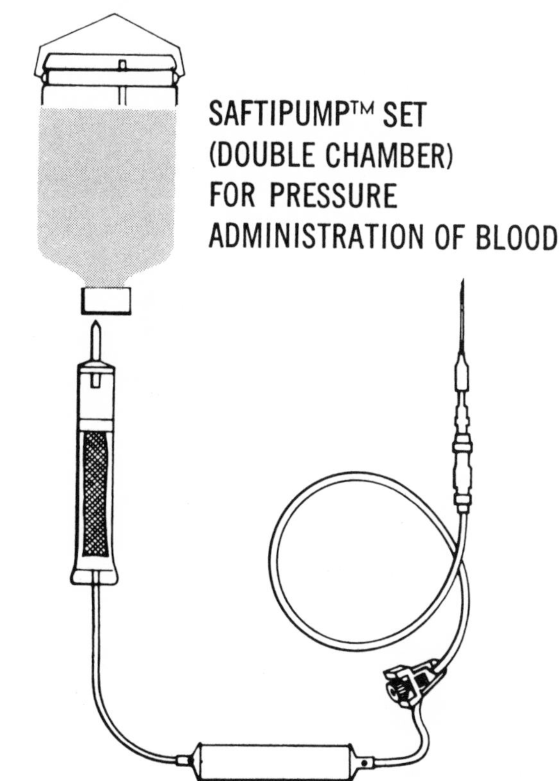

Fig. 16-22. Saftipump™ Set (double chamber) for pressure administration of blood. (Cutter Laboratories, Inc., Berkeley, California)

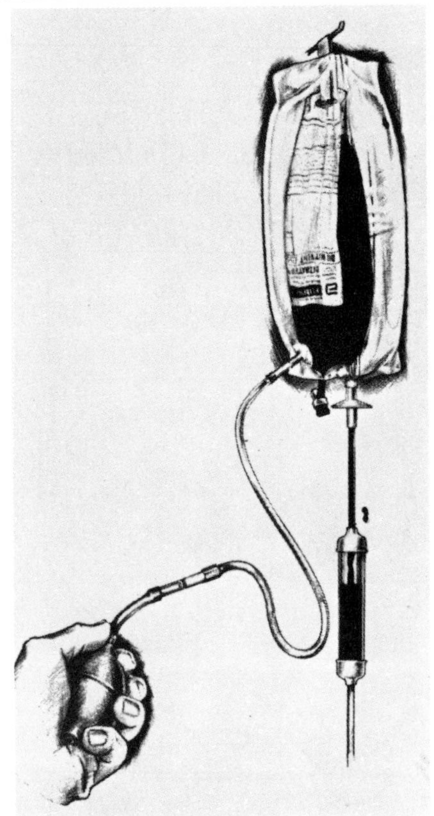

Fig. 16-23. Plastic blood bag with pressure cuff. (Abbott Laboratories: The Use of Blood, p. 60. North Chicago, Illinois, 1965)

Plasma

Plasma is the liquid component left after blood has been centrifuged and the red blood cells removed. It is prepared commercially and dispensed as liquid, frozen, or dried plasma.

Storage of plasma presents less of a problem than blood storage; therefore, it is more readily available than blood. For this reason plasma is often used in emergency situations to restore blood volume until whole blood can be obtained. Plasma is indicated for the replacement of volume when there is little or no deficit of red blood cells, as in severe burns or crushing injuries.

There is less chance of transmitting hepatitis when single donor plasma is used, and consequently, the use of pooled plasma (derived from the blood of many donors) is to be discouraged because of the increased risk of viral contamination. It was thought that storage of plasma at 30 to 32°C. for six months or more would inactivate the hepatitis virus, but cases of hepatitis have been reported with the use of plasma so stored.

Serum albumin is the chief protein of plasma. A 5 per cent solution can be used in the emergency treatment of hypovolemic shock; a 25 per cent solution can be used to treat the hypoproteinemia of nephrotic and cirrhotic edema. There is no hepatitis hazard associated with the use of albumin.

Dextran

Dextran is a polymer of glucose having a large molecular weight. It is often used for emergency treatment of hypovolemic shock.

When infused into the bloodstream, the large dextran molecules increase intravascular osmotic pressure and draw in interstitial fluid to restore blood volume. When blood loss is not severe, dextran may serve as the total replacement fluid. If blood loss is severe, dextran should be followed by whole blood when available.

Dextran does not require special storage. Because it is prepared synthetically rather than from blood, there is no danger of serum homologous hepatitis.

Dextran 70* has a molecular weight close to that of serum albumin—about 70,000. Dextran 70 6% is available in isotonic saline or in non-electrolyte solutions (such as 5% D/W or 10% invert sugar in water). The latter is used for patients requiring a low sodium intake. Dextran is for intravenous use only, and the usual dose is 500 ml. More than this amount can be given but is not recommended, since dextran is not broken down rapidly and will expand the intravascular space for some time. By so doing, it limits the rapidity of red blood cell replacement.

Dextran may act as an allergen and occasionally causes reactions of varying degrees of severity. Symptoms of a severe allergic reaction may include:

* Gentran 75—Travenol Laboratories
Macrodex—Pharmacia Laboratories

Generalized urticaria	Nausea and vomiting
Chest tightness	Dyspnea
Wheezing	Hypotension

The patient should be observed closely for anaphylaxis during the first 30 minutes of the infusion. (Allergic symptoms have been known to appear after the administration of as little as 10 ml. of dextran.) If any of these symptoms appear, the infusion should be stopped immediately; Adrenalin may be necessary to control a severe reaction. In mild reactions withdrawal of the dextran will usually suffice to relieve the symptoms.

Particular caution is necessary when dextran is administered to patients with heart disease or renal disease, because of the danger of congestive heart failure and pulmonary edema. Careful monitoring of venous pressure during rapid dextran administration is sometimes indicated to guard against circulatory overload. (A precipitous rise in venous pressure is an indication to stop the infusion immediately.) If venous pressure is not monitored, the infusion must be given more slowly and the patient observed carefully for signs of circulatory overload. The physician should indicate the desired flow rate.

A transient increase in bleeding time is sometimes seen several hours following the administration of dextran (particularly if more than 1,000 ml. has been given). For this reason, patients should be observed for any bleeding tendencies. Dextran should be used with caution in patients with thrombocytopenia and severe bleeding disorders.

A dextran of lower molecular weight—about 40,000—has been developed; it is referred to as dextran 40*. Ten per cent dextran 40 is available in 5% D/W and in 0.9% sodium chloride. Like dextran 70, it expands the plasma volume and is used in the treatment of shock; however, because of its smaller molecular weight, it has a shorter action period and is more readily excreted.

Studies have shown that capillary blood flow is often decreased or stopped in shock, probably due to blockage of these small vessels with red blood cells. Dextran 40 enhances blood flow, particularly in the small vessels, by increasing blood volume, decreasing blood viscosity, and by reducing the aggregation of red blood cells in the capillaries.

Blood samples for typing, cross-matching, and other tests should be obtained before the dextran infusion is started (dextran can interfere with the accuracy of some laboratory tests).

Poorly hydrated patients receiving dextran are in danger of becoming more dehydrated. (Recall that dextran acts by pulling water from the extravascular space.) Other parenteral fluids should be administered as necessary to prevent extravascular dehydration and to maintain an adequate urinary output.

VENOUS PRESSURE MEASUREMENT DURING INFUSIONS

Venous pressure is sometimes measured frequently during rapid intravenous fluid replacement in hypovolemic patients to warn of impending circulatory overload. It is the best single sign for determining the adequacy of fluid replacement. The nurse may be called upon to measure and record venous pressure, and therefore should have an understanding of the basic principles involved.

Venous pressure can be measured in peripheral veins (as in the arm) or in cannulated central veins in either the inferior or superior caval systems. Central venous pressure measurement is the more accurate of the two, but the procedure is more complicated. Peripheral venous pressure reflects central pressure fairly well if the limb in which it is measured is not acutely compressed between the manometer and the heart. When accuracy is of the utmost importance, venous pressure should be measured in a central vein.

When venous blood return into the right atrium is in physiologic balance with blood flow from the right atrium, venous pressure is 4 to 11 cm. of water (40 to 110 mm. of water). More important than the absolute values are the upward or downward trends it takes; these are

* Gentran 40—Travenol Laboratories
LMD 10%—Abbott Laboratories
Rheomacrodex—Pharmacia Laboratories

determined by taking frequent readings. A decreased blood volume causes a decreased venous blood return into the right atrium and thus a decreased venous pressure, whereas an increased blood volume causes an increased venous blood return and thus an elevated venous pressure.

In an individual with normal cardiac function, the following is true:

A normal venous pressure indicates an adequate circulating blood volume

A decreased venous pressure indicates an inadequate circulating blood volume and the need to increase fluid flow rate

An increased venous pressure indicates an excessive circulating blood volume and the need to decrease fluid flow rate

In an individual with cardiac disease and acute failure, increased venous pressure is present because there is an inadequate blood flow out of the right atrium, due to the ineffective pumping action of the heart. Venous pressure measurement is particularly helpful in guiding the treatment of patients with cardiac damage and blood volume changes, such as in the postoperative management of open-heart surgical patients.

Equipment used to measure venous pressure during intravenous fluid administration is simple. A glass water manometer may be used in conjunction with a three-way stopcock to connect to the needle or catheter and to the infusion setup. Commercial sets have been devised to further simplify the procedure of venous pressure measurement.

The position of the patient is important when venous pressure is measured. The patient should be flat in bed, because this is the position of greatest stability of circulatory dynamics. The zero mark on the manometer should be at the level of the patient's right mid-atrium (approximately the midaxillary line).

When measuring venous pressure, the stopcock is first turned to allow fluid to flow through to the patient. Next, the stopcock is turned to allow fluid to enter the manometer. Finally, the stopcock is turned so that fluid goes from the manometer to the patient. The fluid in the manometer will fluctuate with respirations when it reaches the level of venous pressure.

17 Fluid Balance in the Surgical Patient

THE BODY'S RESPONSE TO SURGICAL TRAUMA

Although a surgical procedure may be lifesaving, the body responds to it as trauma. Postoperative responses bear a direct relationship to nursing care.

Endocrine Response (Stress Reaction)

PERIOD OF FLUID RETENTION AND CATABOLISM The stress reaction described by Selye, representing a response to surgical trauma, is present for the first 2 to 5 days. The intensity of changes depends on the severity and duration of the trauma.

A scale of 10 has been proposed to grade the severity of trauma. An appendectomy or a simple herniorrhaphy is rated low on the scale, around 1 or 2, whereas severe trauma, such as deep burns or pelvic evisceration, rates high on the scale. In the middle of the scale are abdominal surgical procedures such as subtotal gastrectomy or colectomy. Postoperative apprehension and pain enhance the stress reaction, and extreme preoperative apprehension can initiate the stress reaction *before* surgery.

The endocrine responses may be briefly outlined as follows:

1. Increased ACTH (adrenocorticotropic hormone) secretion from the anterior pituitary
2. Increased mineralocorticoid and glucocorticoid secretion from the adrenal cortex (in response to stimulation by ACTH)
   A. Mineralocorticoids (desoxycorticosterone [DOCA] and aldosterone) cause:
      a. Na^+ retention
      b. Cl^- retention
      c. K^+ excretion
   B. Glucocorticoids (mainly hydrocortisone) cause:
      a. Na^+ retention
      b. Cl^- retention
      c. K^+ excretion
      d. Catabolism
         (1) protein breakdown
         (2) gluconeogenesis and elevated blood sugar
      e. Fat mobilization
      f. Drop in eosinophil count
3. Increased ADH (antidiuretic hormone) secretion from posterior pituitary, causing decreased urinary output
4. Vasopressor substances (epinephrine and norepinephrine) secreted from the adrenal medulla to help maintain blood pressure, a response stimulated by fear, pain, hypoxia and hemorrhage

The body's response to stress appears purposeful. For example, sodium retention, chloride retention, potassium loss and increased ADH secretion help to maintain blood volume. Sodium and chloride retention cause water retention; cellular potassium loss releases cellular water into the extracellular space, and ADH secretion causes decreased fluid excretion by way of the kidneys. Glucocorticoids cause protein breakdown, make amino acids available for healing at the site of trauma, and cause conversion of protein and fat to glucose (gluconeogenesis), creating a ready supply of glucose for use during the stress period. (The elevated blood sugar may be mistaken for diabetes mellitus.)

Normally, a decreased protein intake causes a drop in urinary nitrogen excretion. (Approximately 1 Gm. of nitrogen is contained in 6.25 Gm. of protein.) The early postoperative patient, however, loses more urinary nitrogen than normal even though his protein intake is low or absent; because body nitrogen losses exceed intake, the patient is said to be in negative nitrogen balance. Many authorities feel it is useless to try to attain positive nitrogen balance until the period of catabolism has passed.

Laboratory findings during the stress period include reduced eosinophil count and elevated level of serum 17-hydroxycorticosteroid hormones; both indicate increased adrenal activity.

The changes described above are *normal* responses to trauma and do not require corrective measures; in fact, "correction" can be harmful. For example, a high water intake may erroneously be thought necessary to increase the low urinary output of the first few postoperative days. If fluids are forced, the output remains low due to the water-retaining effects of increased ADH secretion and sodium retention; the extra water is retained by the kidneys, and symptoms of water excess may appear. The changes evoked by stress must be understood so that their effects are not misinterpreted. Although aware of the effects of stress, the physician should, nevertheless, institute a careful investigation if the output seems unduly low, particularly if it is prolonged.

PERIODS OF DIURESIS AND ANABOLISM

After the second to fifth postoperative days, adrenal activity is decreased and a mild water and sodium diuresis occurs. The body also begins to retain potassium. Following an uncomplicated abdominal operation, it is not uncommon for a normal adult male to lose from 4 to 9 lbs. during the first postoperative days.

Anabolism, the building up of body protein, usually begins by the seventh to the tenth postoperative day. At this time the urinary nitrogen losses are decreased even though the patient is consuming protein foods. Thus, the renal excretion of nitrogen no longer exceeds the nitrogen intake from protein foods, and the patient begins to gain weight, provided oral intake is adequate.

Tissue Injury

The operative site is edematous for the first few days after surgery. The fluid closely resembles plasma; its volume is roughly proportionate to the amount of tissue trauma. While the amount of fluid lost in edema is not in itself significant, it may enhance the extracellular fluid volume deficit created by peritonitis, hemorrhage, or other complications. The edema fluid is reabsorbed and excreted during the diuretic phase of the stress reaction.

Immobilization

Despite the emphasis on early ambulation, postoperative patients are much less physically active than normal. Immobilization favors increased renal nitrogen and calcium excretion and negative nitrogen balance, with muscle atrophy occurring from disuse. However, except for weight loss and temporary weakness, immobilization for a few days does not significantly affect metabolism.

Starvation Effect

Most patients eat inadequately, or not at all, during the first few postoperative days; thus, a starvation effect is induced. Accompanying starvation is a daily weight loss of about one-half lb., reflecting a decrease in lean and fatty tissue mass. Renal nitrogen excretion is increased as a result of lean tissue catabolism.

The weight loss following surgery is generally constant as revealed by accurate weighing procedures and recording the findings on a weight chart. A weight gain, in the face of starvation, indicates fluid retention. Usually the patient will regain his normal weight in 2 or 3 months if preoperative nutrition was good, operative trauma was of only moderate severity, and there was prompt return of gastrointestinal function.

PREVENTION OF POSTOPERATIVE COMPLICATIONS BY CAREFUL PREOPERATIVE PREPARATION

Nutrition

A patient in good nutritional condition preoperatively withstands postoperative negative nitrogen balance and early starvation without serious effects. On the other hand, the nutritionally depleted patient goes to surgery under a serious handicap—a poor tolerance for operative stress. Increased susceptibility to infection results from a diminished ability to form antibodies, and from the superficial atrophy in the mucous membrane linings of the respiratory and gastrointestinal tracts that often accompanies malnutrition. Hypoproteinemia follows prolonged negative nitrogen balance and increases susceptibility to shock from hemorrhage. The body gives top priority for nutrients to the incision site, and good wound healing is seen in some nutritionally depleted patients; in others, wounds fail to heal. Diminished supplies of protein and vitamin C retard wound healing.

When surgery is elective, the patient with a real or potential fluid balance problem is hospitalized early for preoperative evaluation and buildup. Weisberg advocates baseline electrolyte studies for all infants, adults over 50, and any patient subjected to an exploratory laparotomy or gastrointestinal surgery. During this time the patient is given a well-balanced diet to provide the body with substances to make its own repairs and to help the patient weather the impending surgical trauma. Specific oral or parenteral medications may be deemed necessary after evaluation of clinical and laboratory findings.

A primary nursing responsibility in the preoperative period is getting the patient to eat—sometimes difficult, especially when the patient's illness is such that his appetite is diminshed. Fear and depression, common before surgery, may also deter the patient's desire to eat. (For nursing measures to promote eating see Chapter 14.) The benefits of activity are sometimes overlooked in the preoperative period; activity stimulates appetite and sleep, as well as general well-being.

Another important nursing responsibility is reporting inadequate oral intake, as when all efforts fail to promote eating. Nasogastric tube or parenteral feedings may then have to be given. (For nursing responsibilities in administering tube feedings see Chapter 14.) Anorexia accompanies malnutrition; correction of malnutrition with tube feedings often restores the patient's appetite. (For nursing responsibilities in parenteral nutrition see Chapter 16.)

Emotional Response

Emotional stimuli may produce changes in electrolyte metabolism, which are mediated through the hypothalamus and anterior pituitary gland with the adrenal cortex as the target organ. The patient's attitudes toward surgery may thus significantly affect his postoperative course. Some fear of surgery is natural; undue fear and apprehension, however, may initiate the adrenocortical stress reaction. Discomfort due to venipuncture or to insertion of a gastric tube, as part of the preoperative preparation, may contribute to the stress reaction.

Most nurses can recall more than one postponement of surgery because the patient was not emotionally ready for the experience.

The nurse has an ideal opportunity to observe the patient's behavior and to detect signs of apprehension or severe depression that may be missed by the surgeon. Patients display fear in different ways: some refuse to discuss the oncoming surgical event; others can talk of nothing else. (Significant behavior observations should be discussed with the physician.)

No nursing function is more important than providing emotional support for the surgical patient. The most effective support comes from persons who have a sincere interest in the patient's welfare and a respect for his feelings. Thoughtful explanations before new procedures and experiences do much to relieve fear. Inspiring confidence by performing all nursing functions with skill and confidence is also a form of emotional support. Willingness to listen when the patient feels like talking helps; many patients find it easier to verbalize fears to an understanding nurse than to a relative or close friend. This is understandable when one considers the patient's desire to spare his loved ones additional worry. (Some patients regard fear of surgery as a weakness and prefer to hide such fears from those close to them.)

Body Weight

All surgical patients should have an admission weight recorded on the chart. The preoperative body weight serves as a baseline for comparison with subsequent body weight measurements. Obtaining the weight of an ambulatory patient presents no problem; the patient confined to bed can be weighed on a bed scale. (For procedures in weighing the patient see Chapter 12.)

Intake-Output

Patients requiring preoperative electrolyte studies are placed on the nursing intake-output measurement list. An accurate record of fluids gained and lost from the body is of great importance in detecting inadequate intake and abnormalities in renal function and fluid balance. (For nursing responsibilities in measurement of fluid intake and output see Chapter 12.)

Medications

STEROIDS Some physicians routinely ask all surgical patients if they have recently taken cortisone or any other steroid preparation. When a patient is on steroid therapy there is less need for adrenal secretion and the glands tend to atrophy from disuse; after withdrawal of steroid therapy, the adrenals gradually resume their function. However, if steroids are suddenly withdrawn and the patient is subjected to massive trauma, such as a major surgical procedure, the atrophied adrenal glands may be unable to respond to the stress signal; adrenocortical failure may follow cessation of adrenocortical substitution therapy. Symptoms include hypotension, nausea and vomiting, thready pulse, subnormal temperature early with later hyperpyrexia, hallucinations, confusion, stupor or coma. The reaction usually occurs in the first 24 hours.

Preoperative patients who have received steroid therapy should have their adrenal function checked by the ACTH infusion test. If this discloses decreased adrenocortical responsiveness, steroids must be given to cover the operative and postoperative periods.

Today, due to medical specialization, one patient may have two or three physicians prescribing medications at the same time. The fact that the patient may recently have received steroids is often overlooked, and, in fact, many patients do not know what medicines they have taken; if this is the case, the nurse can ask for a description of the medication and why it was given. Conditions for which steroid therapy is often used should be kept in mind (for example, rheumatoid arthritis, asthma, dermatitis, and ulcerative colitis). When in doubt, the physician should check with those who prescribed medications for the patient.

DRUG ALLERGIES OR IDIOSYNCRASIES The physician or the nurse should always ask the prospective surgical patient if he knows of any drug allergies, sensitivities, or idiosyncracies he may have. If the patient does not understand the question, typical symptoms of sensitivity, such as urticaria, asthma and the like, can be mentioned. One can also ask the patient if a physician has ever cautioned him to avoid a specific medication because of an unusual reaction to it. In questioning the newly admitted patient, the nurse will do well to remember that he is often upset and may have difficulty remembering.

Some patients assume that their physician remembers any drug allergies from office interviews prior to hospital admission, and unless specifically asked, they may not volunteer information. Allergies must be discovered before the patient is sedated or anesthetized; it is too late to ask when he is unconscious or semi-reactive after surgery, since most medications are ordered in the immediate postoperative period. Failure to ascertain the presence of allergies may be disastrous. The most dreaded allergic reaction is anaphylactic shock; other less dangerous reactions include skin eruptions and asthma.

Idiosyncratic reactions to drugs deserve consideration. For example, a narcotic may cause more depression in one patient than in another of equal weight and age. A dose creating the desired effect in one patient may overwhelm the patient who is unusually reactive to the drug. The aged are particularly sensitive to narcotics and should be given much smaller doses than younger adults; this is particularly important in aged surgical patients.

Pulmonary Ventilation

Inadequate pulmonary ventilation is common after surgery and can lead to respiratory acidosis (primary carbonic acid excess) or atelectasis. During the preoperative period, the nurse should teach the patient how to deep-breathe and cough postoperatively, explaining that these activities are excellent preventives against lung complications. Once the patient is properly motivated and knows what is expected of him, the nurse will have greater success in carrying through the common postoperative order to "have the patient cough and deep-breathe every hour."

Intermittent positive pressure treatments are sometimes used preoperatively and postoperatively to improve pulmonary ventilation in patients with chronic pulmonary conditions, such as emphysema. If other deep breathing devices are to be successfully used postoperatively, the patient should be allowed to practice their use *preoperatively.*

Chronic Illnesses

Certain chronic illnesses greatly increase the hazard of postoperative water and electrolyte imbalances. Such illnesses include:

Diabetes mellitus
Addison's disease
Renal disorders
Cardiac disorders
Hepatic disorders
Thyroid disorders
Pulmonary disorders

The presence of any of the above conditions requires careful preoperative preparation so that postoperative disturbances can be kept at a minimum.

The physician does a careful history and physical examination before surgery to detect pre-existing illness. However, the patient may forget an important item and mention it later to the nurse, in which case, the information should be brought immediately to the physician's attention. The nurse should also be alert for symptoms of chronic illness.

Special Considerations in the Aged

Conscientious preoperative preparation often means the difference between success or failure of surgery in the aged, since the decreased body homeostatic adaptability of these patients predisposes to difficulty when they are exposed to stress.

These facts apply to the aged:

1. Malnutrition is more common in the aged than in younger adults.
2. Thirst is not as accurate a gauge of fluid needs as it is in younger adults. Sodium excess occurs with relative frequency in the aged because the thirst stimulus is often not intact and water intake is inadequate. In fact, many aged patients fail to recognize thirst when they are confused, whereas elderly patients who are alert and have access to water are not apt to develop sodium excess. Conditions causing water loss, such as fever and hyperpnea, contribute to a rise in plasma sodium. Clinical signs include dry, sticky mucous membranes and excitement. The nurse should offer the patient adequate water, and when in doubt, the intake and output should be recorded. (A urinary volume that greatly exceeds oral intake is a signal to increase fluid intake.)
3. The aged patient will develop sodium deficit faster than younger adults; thus the nurse should be particularly alert for sodium deficit when the patient is losing body fluids containing sodium. This is particularly apt to occur when there is a free intake of water—either orally or parenterally. Sometimes the elderly patient may drink too much water; thirst satisfaction may require excessive water.
4. Moderate fluid volume deficit and decreased circulating blood volume are not uncommon in the aged *before* operation.
5. The plasma pH tends to remain fixed on the low side of normal, largely due to decreased pulmonary and renal function.
6. Decreased pulmonary function is common in the aged. It has been demonstrated that vital capacity is reduced with an increased residual volume, as rigidity of the chest wall interferes with normal pulmonary excursions. Since diminished respiratory

function interferes with carbon dioxide elimination, many aged patients are in a state of impending respiratory acidosis. Because of this decline in pulmonary function, the nurse must help the aged patient achieve maximal ventilation. This can be accomplished by keeping the respiratory tract free of excessive secretions, providing maximal allowed activity, turning the bedfast patient from side to side at regular intervals and avoiding restrictive clothing or tight chest restraints.

7. Because renal response to pH disturbances is not as efficient in the aged, imbalances occur faster. There is a tendency toward metabolic acidosis as a result of decreased renal function.
8. Changes in pH are less well tolerated in the aged. Anemia, with its decreased hemoglobin, depletes one of the major buffer systems; emphysema is not uncommon in the aged and disrupts pH control.
9. The volume and acidity of gastric juice decreases gradually with age. Hypochlorhydria or achlorhydria is present in about one-third of patients over 60. The aged patient with decreased gastric acidity may not develop metabolic alkalosis with vomiting or gastric suction; the primary disturbance in such a patient may be sodium deficit or potassium deficit.
10. Hypoxia is not well tolerated in the aged; for this reason local or spinal anesthetics are preferable to inhalation anesthetics.
11. Hypotension is poorly tolerated by the aged, and unless corrected quickly, is frequently complicated by renal damage, stroke, or myocardial infarct. (Shock becomes irreversible earlier than in younger patients.)

Preoperative dietary management is particularly important; optimal nutrition helps the aged patient withstand the electrolyte deficits and pH changes occurring after surgery. Electrolyte solutions may be given intravenously prior to surgery to supplement dietary intake; deficits of potassium and sodium especially should be corrected.

Small, frequent blood transfusions are sometimes used to restore blood volume and to correct anemia. Ambulation and activity improve appetite and sleep. An accurate account should be kept of the patient's urinary output. In addition, renal function tests and an ECG may be indicated. And finally, a conservative dose of preoperative medication is used to help avoid respiratory depression and hypoxia.

Immediate Preoperative Preparation

ENEMAS A cleansing enema may be ordered either the night before or on the morning of abdominal or rectal surgery. Occasionally one still sees an order for "tap water enemas until returned clear"; fortunately, it is seen less and less. As many as five to ten enemas may be needed before the solution is "returned clear"; large amounts of sodium and potassium are lost with the enema return, thus depleting the patient of valuable electrolytes when he can ill afford to lose them. Most surgeons feel that one cleansing enema, properly given, suffices.

WITHHOLDING FLUIDS A few years ago one commonly saw the order "nothing by mouth after midnight" for all surgical patients, whether the patient was scheduled for surgery at 7:00 a.m. or 12:00 noon. Recently emphasis has been placed on allowing fluids up to six hours before surgery. The goal, of course, is to allow the patient to take needed fluids as long as possible and still prevent the complications resulting from a full stomach during anesthesia.

VITAL SIGNS All vital signs should be checked before the preoperative medication is given. An elevated temperature should be reported immediately; postponement of surgery may be necessary until the source of the fever is disclosed. An unusually rapid pulse and respiratory rate may indicate undue apprehension and should be reported.

A more accurate appraisal of the patient's blood pressure may be obtained by checking it both the evening before and the morning of surgery, and after sedative medication has been given. Postoperative blood pressure findings must be compared with the patient's usual blood pressure if they are to be evaluated correctly. For example, some patients normally have a systolic pressure of 90; unless this reading is established as the patient's norm, it may be inaccurately interpreted as a symptom of early shock.

POSTOPERATIVE GAINS AND LOSSES OF WATER, ELECTROLYTES AND OTHER NUTRIENTS

Need for Intake-Output Measurement

Surgery often brings into play abnormal routes of fluid loss, such as gastric or intestinal suction, vomiting, or drainage from an ileostomy or colostomy. Failure to measure the amounts and kinds of fluids lost makes adequate replacement therapy almost impossible, and without an accurate account of gains and losses, the early discovery of water and electrolyte imbalances is unlikely. It behooves the nurse, then, to automatically place postoperative patients on the intake-output list and to make a conscientious effort to keep the intake-output record accurate.

The 8-hour and 24-hour totals are significant in assessing fluid balance in general; it is equally important to know the types and amounts of fluids making up the total. For example, to state that a patient has lost a total of 3,000 ml. of fluid in 24 hours is not as revealing as an itemized analysis of the loss:

1,000 ml. urine
800 ml. gastric suction
200 ml. bile from T-tube drainage
1,000 ml. estimated perspiration

The aim of fluid replacement therapy is to restore to the body the quantities of water and electrolytes lost. Special parenteral fluids are available to replace losses of gastric juice, intestinal juice, bile, and others.

(Chapter 12 tabulates the electrolyte content of most of the body fluids of concern in postoperative care plus imbalances to be expected with large losses of each fluid. The reader is encouraged to review this section because of its importance for the formulation of intelligent postoperative care.)

Urinary Output

In health, the daily urinary output is roughly equal to the volume of liquids taken into the body. However, during postoperative stress reaction the urine volume may tend to be low regardless of the amount of fluids taken in. Following a major surgical procedure, the 24-hour urine output may be only 600 to 700 ml. for the first few postoperative days. Therefore, unless the stress reaction's influence on urinary output is understood, the low volume and high specific gravity may be confused with fluid volume deficit. As mentioned earlier, attempts to increase urine volume by forcing fluids fail, and forced fluids are retained by the body and may cause several complications, among which are: (1) water excess (sodium deficit), if the extra fluids were primarily 5 per cent glucose in water; (2) pulmonary edema; (3) increased edema at the operative site. In intestinal surgery the increased edema may be sufficient to cause partial or complete obstruction.

Fluid Intake

The usual daily fluid intake during the stress reaction should be about 1,500 to 2,000 ml., varying with the patient's need for replacement.

PARENTERAL FLUIDS Nausea, gastrointestinal surgery and gastrointestinal suction contraindicate oral fluids. A parenteral route, almost always the intravenous, is then relied on to furnish the body with needed substances.

As little as 100 Gm. of carbohydrate given daily can reduce protein breakdown (catabolism) by as much as one-half. This amount is contained in 2 L. of 5 per cent glucose solution or 1 L. of a 10 per cent glucose solution.

Five per cent glucose in water or in hypotonic (quarter strength isotonic) saline is often given intravenously during the first few postoperative days; the physician may choose saline in instances in which sodium has been lost incident to the surgical procedure, and in which there is no indication of sodium retention.

After adequate renal function has been established, potassium is given daily to prevent potassium deficit, if the patient is not yet eating. Forty mEq. per day suffices unless large volumes of gastrointestinal fluids, rich in potassium, are being lost by vomiting, suction, or fistulas. (Nursing responsibilities in administering potassium solutions are discussed in Chapter 16.) As a general rule, a solution containing 40 mEq./L. of potassium may be given at a rate of 500 ml. per hour to normal adults; this is equivalent to 20 mEq. of potassium (suitably diluted) per hour. In older patients, it is best to give potassium solutions at a slower rate, preferably no faster than 20 to 30 mEq. over a three to four hour period.

After the fluid retention of stress has subsided, a larger amount of fluid is given. If oral intake is still prohibited, an attempt must be made to supply body needs solely with parenteral fluids. Magnesium replacement may be necessary when parenteral fluid administration is prolonged. Magnesium deficit is not as rare as was once thought; prolonged administration of magnesium-free fluids dilutes the plasma magnesium level and may produce symptoms of deficit, particularly when magnesium loss has resulted from gastric suction. Parenteral vitamin preparations of the B complex group and vitamin C should be given daily when parenteral therapy is necessary for more than 2 days.

Amino acid preparations (protein hydrolysates), or intact protein preparations such as Sustagen, are beneficial after the catabolic phase has passed and the body is again able to build tissues. Many authorities feel it is useless to give amino acids during the catabolic phase, because the body is unable to use them and they are excreted in the urine. Others believe they are helpful in decreasing the extent of the negative nitrogen balance. The increased solute load of amino acid preparations can be harmful in the aged patient whose kidneys are already overtaxed.

Parenteral solutions containing alcohol may be used postoperatively to supply calories and reduce pain. (Nursing responsibilities in the administration of carbohydrate solutions, electrolyte solutions, alcohol and protein hydrolysates are discussed in Chapter 16.)

ORAL INTAKE Many physicians prefer that patients undergoing gastrointestinal suction receive nothing by mouth; others allow "ice chips sparingly" to relieve thirst. The term "sparingly" is open to interpretation by the staff, and more ice chips may be given than was intended by the physician, because of a thirsty patient's constant plea for more ice.

Drinking plain water causes a movement of electrolytes into the stomach to make the solution isotonic; before the water and electrolytes can be absorbed they are removed by the suction apparatus. This process can deplete the body of valuable electrolytes, primarily sodium, chloride and potassium. Profound states of metabolic alkalosis or of sodium deficit have been caused by the unwise practice of giving plain water to a patient undergoing gastric suction. *If ice chips are to be given, they should be made from isotonic saline or a balanced electrolyte solution indicated by the physician*—Lytren, for example.

When oral feedings are allowed, the nurse should encourage the patient to eat those foods most likely to replace his probable deficits. For example, a patient with an ileostomy should receive high potassium foods; a patient with a cholecystectomy and bile drainage should receive high sodium foods. Contraindications to high potassium intake (such as renal disease) and to high sodium intake (such as cardiac disease) should, of course, be considered. The patient should be returned to a full diet as early as possible, because good nutrition decreases both the duration and the complications of convalescence.

POSTOPERATIVE PROBLEMS IN WATER AND ELECTROLYTE BALANCE

Water Excess

Water excess (sodium deficit) is also referred to as water intoxication or hyponatremia, an imbalance most likely to occur in the first 1 or 2 postoperative days, while the water retention effect of stress is still present. Excessive administration of water-yielding fluids, such as 5 per cent glucose in water, predisposes to this condition. Symptoms of water excess (sodium deficit) include:

1. Behavior changes
   A. Inattentiveness
   B. Confusion
   C. Hallucinations
   D. Shouting and delirium
   E. Drowsiness
2. Acute weight gain
3. Overbreathing
4. Normal or elevated blood pressure
5. Skin color normal, or pinker than usual
6. Neuromuscular changes
   A. Cramping of exercised muscles
   B. Isolated muscle twitching
   C. Weakness
   D. Headache
   E. Blurred vision
   F. Incoordination
   G. Elevated intracranial pressure may occur with hypertension, bradycardia, decreased respiration, projectile vomiting and papilledema
   H. Convulsions
   I. Hemiplegia

The nurse should suspect water excess (sodium deficit) when several of these symptoms occur in the early postoperative period. Behavior changes are usually noticed first. The aged and the very young are particularly susceptible to this imbalance.

Prevention of body fluid disturbances demands the study of daily accurate body weight measurements; a sudden weight gain in the early postoperative period is an indication to decrease fluid intake. Fluid intake during the water-retention of stress should not exceed body fluid losses; a reasonable 24-hour intake for most patients is about 1,500 to 2,000 ml. Here again, much depends upon how accurately the nurse performs body weight and intake-output measurements.

Mild water excess can be corrected by prohibiting further water intake; however, serious illness or death may supervene if the condition is allowed to go untreated.

Respiratory Acidosis

Normally carbon dioxide is given off by the lungs during exhalation. Respiratory acidosis (primary carbonic acid excess) occurs when the lungs retain carbon dioxide, because of decreased respiration depth or blockage of oxygen-carbon dioxide exchange at the alveolar level. Breathing excessive amounts of carbon dioxide will also produce this imbalance. The surgical patient may develop respiratory acidosis for one or several reasons:

1. Depression of respiration by anesthesia
2. Blockage of oxygen-carbon dioxide exchange in the lungs due to atelectasis, pneumonia, or bronchial obstruction
3. Depression of respiration with too frequent or too large doses of narcotics
4. Shallow respiration due to abdominal distention and crowding of the diaphragm
5. Excessive breathing of carbon dioxide during anesthesia
6. Shallow respiration due to pain in the operative site or large cumbersome dressings

A threat to postoperative ventilation is posed by surgical procedures involving the diaphragm, such as hiatus hernia repair. Also, patients having thoracic or high abdominal incisions are particularly prone to develop ventilatory problems. For example, vital capacity is decreased by 40% of normal on the day after subtotal gastrectomy. However, this loss of reserve still allows for adequate oxygen and carbon dioxide exchange if preoperative ventilation was normal. In addition to causing respiratory acidosis, decreased ventilation interferes with the correction of metabolic acidosis. (Recall that the lungs attempt to compensate for metabolic acidosis by eliminating more carbon dioxide.)

Indiscriminate use of oxygen in the postoperative period increases the chance of overlooking respiratory acidosis. Cyanosis is usually the chief criterion for detecting inadequate ventilation;

oxygen therapy may prevent cyanosis and keep the skin color pink even though respiratory acidosis is progressing. When oxygen is necessary, it is usually given by nasal catheter rather than by tent. (Some physicians feel that an oxygen tent predisposes to respiratory disorders, since excessive amounts of carbon dioxide can be inhaled in a tent from which carbon dioxide is not adequately absorbed.)

The nurse can help prevent respiratory acidosis by encouraging the patient to cough and breathe deeply at regular intervals, unless contraindicated by the type of surgery. Even when coughing is to be avoided in neurological or eye surgery the patient can be encouraged to breathe deeply. Administration of narcotics requires good nursing judgment, with enough medication given to make coughing tolerable, yet not enough to produce shallow respiration. The timely use of analgesics enables the patient to expand his thoracic cavity with less discomfort during deep-breathing treatments. It is best to position the patient in high Fowler's to allow for better gas distribution throughout the lungs. The sitting position allows for greater lung expansion because gravity pulls the abdominal organs away from the diaphragm. The nurse should splint the patient's incision while he coughs; this causes him to be less fearful and less apt to splint himself by muscular contraction, which limits ventilation. Of course, the patient should be taught how to splint his own incision when assistance is not available.

Turning the patient at regular intervals helps prevent pneumonia and atelectasis and thus discourages respiratory acidosis. Early ambulation probably helps avoid this complication by increasing the patient's breathing efforts.

Some physicians order IPPB (intermittent positive pressure breathing) treatments to improve pulmonary ventilation; others may prefer the use of blow bottles or devices such as the Dale-Schwartz rebreathing tube or the Adler rebreather.

The nurse should remember that seemingly small doses of barbiturates or narcotics may produce respiratory depression and acidosis in the aged patient. If the ordered dose appears inadequate, or produces adverse effects, the nurse should report her observations to the physician and seek new orders. Conscientious physicians welcome such nursing observations; they realize that what may be a therapeutic dose in one patient may be ineffective or harmful to another. Observations made by the nurse take on added weight because she spends more time with the patient than does the physician.

Gastric Dilatation

Gastric dilatation can occur within the first few postoperative days; before peristalsis returns, liters of fluid can be trapped in the stomach. The extracellular fluid volume may be significantly decreased and these symptoms of shock may develop:

Dyspnea
Cyanosis
Rapid thready pulse
Cold extremities

Additional symptoms include regurgitation of blood-tinged fluid, effortless vomiting, and epigastric discomfort. Symptoms of metabolic alkalosis (primary base bicarbonate excess) may result from the pooling of stomach secretions in the massively distended viscus.

Treatment includes gastric suction, water and electrolyte replacement therapy, and, in some instances, blood transfusion. Gastric dilatation can often be prevented by instituting gastrointestinal suction until peristalsis returns.

Ileus

Peristalsis is inhibited for two to four days after intra-abdominal manipulation, and for this reason, patients with abdominal surgery usually receive nothing by mouth until bowel sounds indicate the return of peristalsis. Gastric intubation is often employed early in the postoperative period to prevent the bowel from becoming greatly distended with swallowed air and gastrointestinal fluids.

If paralytic ileus persists longer than normal, the patient must be maintained on intravenous fluids and gastric suction until peristalsis returns. Factors that may prolong the expected period of ileus postoperatively include bacterial and chemical peritonitis, excessive handling of the intestines during surgery, advanced age or actual mechanical obstruction.

Large amounts of water and electrolytes may be sequestered into the bowel. The amount of fluid "lost" in this manner is not revealed by body weight change. Clinical signs of fluid volume deficit, decreased urinary volume and increased urinary specific gravity help indicate the amount of fluid trapped in the bowel. (See the discussion of bowel obstruction in Chapter 19.)

Use of Plain Water as Irrigating Fluid for Suction Tubes

Plain water should never be used to irrigate suction tubes because it depletes the body of valuable electrolytes. The mechanism is the same as that operating when plain water is drunk while gastrointestinal suction is being used. (See Chapter 14 for a discussion of this subject.) Isotonic solution of sodium chloride largely eliminates the hazard and should be used unless the physician requests a specific fluid, such as an oral electrolyte mixture.

Imbalances Associated With Specific Body Fluid Losses

Metabolic alkalosis is most commonly seen in surgical patients as a result of the loss of large amounts of gastric secretions, either through vomiting or gastric suction. It is closely associated with potassium deficit, produced by the excessive loss of potassium-rich intestinal secretions or by prolonged parenteral therapy without potassium replacement. Potassium deficit is enhanced by the stress reaction in the early postoperative period.

Metabolic acidosis (primary base bicarbonate deficit) follows excessive loss of alkaline intestinal secretions, bile and pancreatic juice.

(The reader is referred to Chapter 12 for a more thorough discussion of imbalances prone to occur with specific body fluid losses.)

Hemorrhage and Shock

Severe hemorrhage and hypovolemic shock are dreaded complications of surgery. The nurse should be alert for, and report, symptoms of hemorrhage and hypovolemic shock such as:

- Rapid pulse with decreased volume
- Apprehension
- Restlessness
- Rise, then rapid fall in blood pressure
- Visual evidence of bleeding at the site of operation or elsewhere
- Pallor
- Cold extremities
- Thirst
- Loss of consciousness

Prompt correction of the cause of hemorrhage and replacement of fluids are mandatory to prevent irreversible shock. Blood is the fluid of first choice, but dextran, plasma or electrolyte solutions may be used until blood is available. (Sometimes vasopressors are used to maintain adequate blood pressure.) Elevating the legs releases about 500 ml. of blood and thus partially relieves the effect of hypovolemia on the vital organs; some feel it is more effective to place the patient in Trendelenburg's position (entire body tilted head down on an inclined plane). Studies have indicated that the Trendelenburg position may do more harm than good because it impairs cardiac filling; it may also embarrass pulmonary ventilation by allowing the abdominal contents to crowd the lungs.

The period of hypotension must be kept at a minimum because it results in decreased blood flow and damage to vital organs, primarily the brain, the heart and the kidneys. The brain is extremely sensitive to anoxia. Irreversible brain damage occurs when the blood supply is occluded for three minutes; neurons, once destroyed, cannot be replaced. Hypotension in a patient with arteriosclerosis is particularly dangerous because of the high incidence of thrombosis, resulting in either cerebral vascular accident or myocardial infarct. Acute renal insufficiency may follow prolonged hypotension, particularly in the aged.

Acute Renal Insufficiency

Acute renal insufficiency often complicates surgery. Usually it is secondary to reduction of renal blood flow (as in shock) or to a hemolytic blood transfusion reaction. The aged patient has a higher incidence of acute renal insufficiency.

In acute renal insufficiency the urinary output is greatly decreased and may be less than 100 ml. in 24 hours. Metabolic acidosis, less frequently sodium deficit, may be present, and the specific gravity is fixed at a low level.

Only enough fluids should be given to replace insensible losses and abnormal losses from suction tubes or fistulas. Extremely accurate intake-output records and body weight measurements are mandatory. Alkaline solutions, such as sodium lactate or sodium bicarbonate, or Butler-type solutions can be given to correct the acidosis. The plasma potassium level rises if anuria persists; peritoneal dialysis helps meet this problem. (Nursing responsibilities in peritoneal dialysis are discussed in Chapter 20.)

Spontaneous diuresis occurs within 1 to 2 weeks in many patients with acute renal insufficiency, provided appropriate treatment has been given; yet months may pass before renal function returns to normal.

The nurse can help prevent acute renal insufficiency by being alert to, and reporting, *early* symptoms of shock; prompt correction of shock prevents a pronounced reduction in renal blood flow. (Nursing responsibilities in preventing hemolytic blood transfusion reactions are discussed in Chapter 16.)

18 Fluid Balance in the Badly Burned Patient

INTRODUCTION

Burns cause a series of major water and electrolyte changes. The purpose of this chapter is to explore these changes and their implications for nursing care. A background discussion of physiologic changes accompanying burns precedes the discussion of treatment and nursing care.

EVALUATION OF BURN SEVERITY

The severity of water and electrolyte changes is largely dependent on the *burn depth* and the *percentage of body surface* involved.

Burn Depth

Burns are classified as first, second, or third degree, according to the depth of skin damage. Factors considered in determining burn depth include:

Amount of sensation remaining (pinprick test may be done to denote the degree of sensation)
Appearance of the burned surface
Nature of burning agent plus length of exposure to it
(See Table 18-1.)

In a first-degree burn, vasodilation is the only important change, whereas a second-degree burn is characterized by damaged capillaries and the appearance of blebs containing fluid.

Third-degree burns result in thrombosed capillaries and the formation of an eschar (dead tissue), and each per cent of a third-degree burn is about twice as severe as each per cent of a second-degree burn.

Percentage of Surface Involved

The "rule of nines" is commonly used to estimate the severity of burns in adults. It divides the body surface into areas of 9 per cent or its multiples:

Head	= 9%
Each arm	= 9%
Each leg	= 18%
Front of torso	= 18%
Back of torso	= 18%
Genitalia	= 1%

Unless used cautiously, this method can result in dangerously high estimates. A more detailed breakdown is beneficial, since it contributes to a complete understanding of percentage of surface involved. (See Figure 18-1.)

After the percentage of second-degree and third-degree burns is estimated, the therapeutic approach is planned. Burns may be classified as critical, moderate, or minor.

Age as a Factor in Burn Severity

The mortality rate in burns increases with age. To illustrate the effect of advanced age on burn mortality, compare these statistics: a burn covering 15 to 24 per cent of the body surface carries a mortality of 6 per cent in persons from 15 to 44 years old, whereas an equal burn in persons 65 years and older carries an 80 per cent mortality. Even minor burns present a serious threat to the aged, since they frequently have pre-existent cardiovascular-renal damage and cannot respond to stress as well as their younger counterparts. In general, healthy persons under 40 years of age have about a 50-50 chance for survival from a 50 per cent second-degree or third-degree burn.

Table 18-1. Diagnosis of Burn Depth*

	Degree	Nature of Burn	Symptoms	Appearance	Course
Epidermal Burn	First	Sunburn	Tingling	Reddened; blanches with pressure	Complete recovery within a week
		Low-intensity flash	Hyperesthesia	Minimal or no edema	Peeling
			Painful		
			Soothed by cooling		
Intradermal Burn	Second	Scalds	Painful	Blistered, mottled red base, broken epidermis, weeping surface	Recovery in 2 to 3 weeks
		Flash flame	Hypesthesia		Some scarring and depigmentation
			Sensitive to cold air	Edema	Infection may convert to third degree
Subdermal Burn	Third	Fire	Painless	Dry; pale white or charred	Eschar sloughs
			Symptoms of shock	Broken skin with fat exposed	Grafting necessary
			Hematuria and hemolysis of blood likely	Edema	Scarring and loss of contour and function

* From Sako, Y.: Emergency management of the acutely burned patient. Hospital Medicine, p. 7, Wallace Laboratories, New York, October, 1964.

WATER AND ELECTROLYTE CHANGES IN BURNS

Loss of Body Fluids in Burns

Body fluids are lost in severe burns as:

- Plasma leaves the intravascular space and becomes trapped as edema fluid
- Plasma and interstitial fluid are lost as exudate
- Water vapor is lost from the denuded burn site
- Blood leaks from the damaged capillaries

PLASMA-TO-INTERSTITIAL FLUID SHIFT Intravascular water, electrolytes and protein are lost through damaged capillaries at the burn site. Clinically, the shift results in edema; the magnitude of this shift depends upon the burn depth and the percentage of surface area involved. Consider a specific example: an adult with a body surface of 1.75 $m.^2$ has about 10.5 L. of extracellular fluid. If he sustains a 50 per cent burn, the volume of edema fluid formed during the first day or two would approximate 5.25 L., a quantity exceeding the total plasma volume of the patient. Obviously all of the edema fluid is not derived from plasma; some of it comes from the body cells and some from administered fluids.

Proportionately greater amounts of water and electrolytes than of protein are lost from the plasma. (Protein molecules are larger and thus fewer escape through the damaged capillaries.) As a result, the circulating plasma protein be-

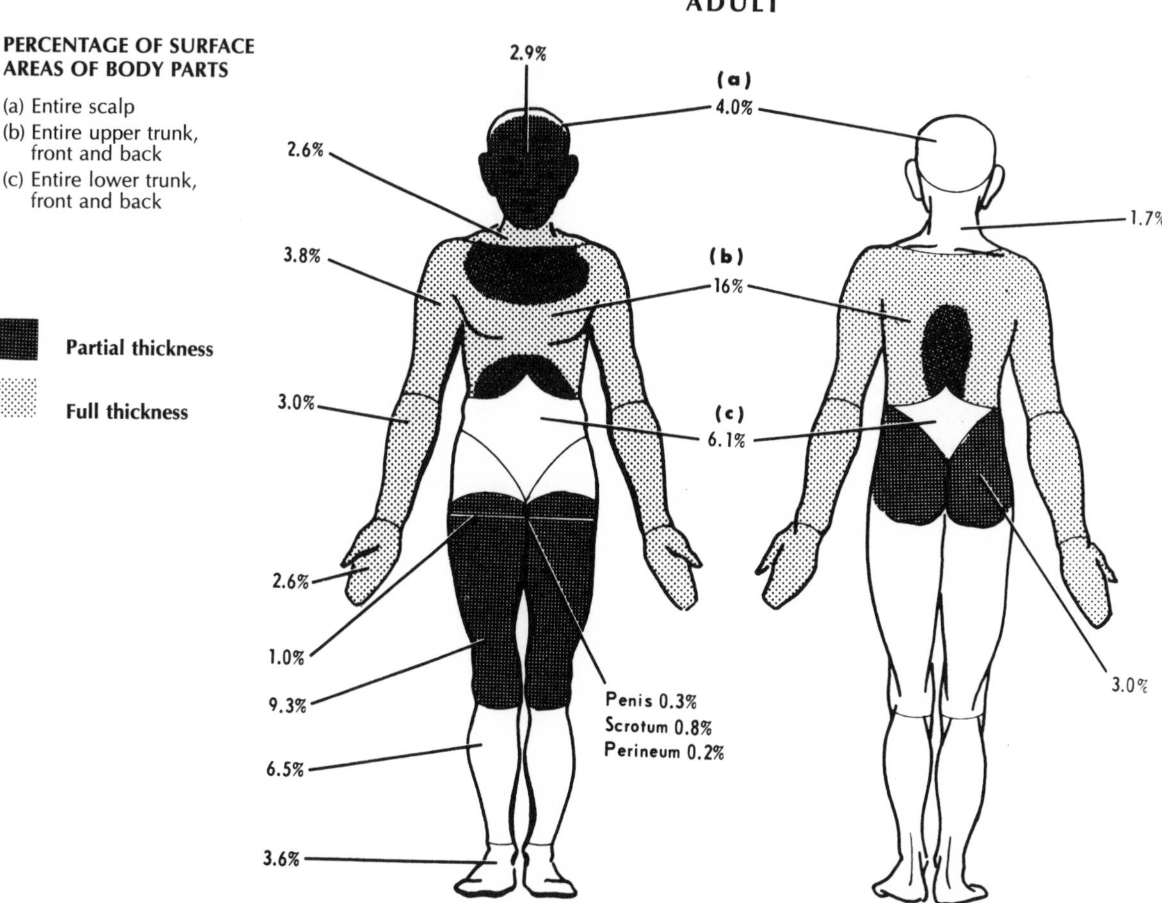

Fig. 18-1. Surface diagram constructed from Meeh's data. Persons aged eight or up, except for the very obese. (Moyer, C.: Treatment of large burns. Arch. Surg., *90*:856. June 1965)

comes more concentrated; the increased osmotic pressure draws fluid from undamaged tissues in all parts of the body, and generalized tissue dehydration results. It is sometimes difficult to visualize the presence of severe dehydration in a patient so obviously edematous; one must remember that the edema represents trapped fluids unavailable for body use.

BURN EXUDATE A protein-rich fluid is lost through the leakage of approximately equal parts of plasma and interstitial fluid from the burned surface. Visible fluid loss by way of the surface is mostly limited to second-degree burns, and the amount of fluid lost in this manner is proportional to the percentage of second-degree burns; such losses do not increase appreciably in burns involving 50 per cent or more of the body. Burn exudate has approximately two-thirds as much protein as plasma.

WATER VAPOR AND HEAT LOSS The intact skin serves as a barrier against the loss of water and heat. When skin is destroyed by a burn, increased water and heat loss result, and the larger the burned surface, the greater the loss of water vapor and heat. Burned infants are particularly vulnerable to heat loss.

The average water vapor loss from a major burn wound is thought to be from 2.5 to 4.0 L.

per day. Maintenance of an environment saturated with water vapor decreases the transcutaneous water loss; for example, wounds covered with 0.5 per cent silver nitrate dressings and dry covers lose only half the amount of water vapor lost through exposed wounds. Patients treated by exposure often shiver and complain of feeling cold; external heat sources should be provided for comfort. Radiational heat loss is significantly decreased when the temperature of the room is maintained at 30 to 32° C. A heavy dressing or a bed cradle will decrease convective heat loss.

Other Effects Fever contributes to fluid loss by increasing the metabolic rate, and infection is also dreaded; the presence of the latter may cause the rectal temperature to rise to 104-107° F. and extend the burn depth.

Vomiting is frequently observed in severely burned patients; it may be a sign of circulatory collapse, acute gastric dilatation, or paralytic ileus.

WATER AND ELECTROLYTE CHANGES IN MAJOR BURN PHASES

The nurse should be aware of the water and electrolyte changes occurring in burns so that she can recognize significant changes in the patient. Observations are more meaningful when one has at least some idea what to look for. An outline of expected water and electrolyte changes is presented in Table 18-2. The reader is referred to earlier chapters for detailed descriptions of these imbalances. Planned nursing observations are discussed in Chapter 12.

Physiologic Basis for Treatment and Nursing Care During the Fluid Accumulation Phase

The adequacy of early burn treatment largely depends upon the physician's and the nurse's understanding of physiologic derangements caused by

Table 18-2. Water and Electrolyte Changes in Different Burn Phases

Phase	*Water and Electrolyte Changes*	*Comments*
Fluid Accumulation Phase (Shock Phase)	Plasma-to-Interstitial Fluid Shift (edema at burn site)	Plasma leaks out through the damaged capillaries at the burn site—edema forms
First 48 hours	Generalized Dehydration	Undamaged tissues give up fluids to help increase plasma volume—part of it leaks through the damaged capillaries and helps form edema
	Contraction of Blood Volume	Loss of plasma causes a decreased circulatory volume
	Decreased Urinary Output	Secondary to: Decreased renal blood flow Increased secretion of ADH (antidiuretic hormone) Sodium and water retention caused by stress (increased adrenocortical activity) Severe burns may cause hemolysis of red blood cells; the ruptured cells release Hb. and it is excreted by the kidneys (hemoglobinuria can cause severe renal damage)
	Potassium Excess	Massive cellular trauma causes the release of K^+ into the extracellular fluid (recall that most of the body's K^+ is located *inside* the cells; only small amounts are tolerated in plasma)
	Sodium Deficit	Large amounts of Na^+ are lost in the trapped edema fluid and in the exudate (recall that Na^+ is the chief extracellular ion and large amounts are lost when extracellular fluid is lost)

Table 18-2. Water and Electrolyte Changes in Different Burn Phases—(Continued)

Phase	*Water and Electrolyte Changes*	*Comments*
		Research work done under the direction of C. A. Moyer indicates sodium deficit in unburned tissues is closely linked with burn shock (partial correction of Na^+ deficit relieved burn shock symptoms in some patients even though a substantially decreased blood volume persisted)
	Metabolic Acidosis (base bicarbonate deficit)	Develops within a few hours due to: Accumulation of fixed acids released from injured tissues; Ineffective tissue perfusion
	Calcium Deficit	May occur after 12-24 hours in extensively burned patients—may be particularly marked in infants and children (presumably due to saponification of fat in the burned subcutaneous adipose tissue)
	Hemoconcentration (elevated hematocrit)	Relatively greater loss of liquid blood components in relation to blood cell loss
Fluid Remobilization Phase	Interstitial Fluid-to-Plasma Shift	Edema fluid shifts back into the intravascular compartments
(Stage of Diuresis) Starts 48 hours post-burn	Hemodilution (hematocrit decreased)	The blood cell concentration is diluted as fluid enters the vascular compartment and, in addition, at this time a decrease in the number of cells becomes evident (destruction of red blood cells at the burn site causes anemia—as much as 10% of the total number of RBCs may be destroyed)
	Increased Urinary Output	Fluid shift into the intravascular compartment increases renal blood flow and causes increased urine formation
	Sodium Deficit	Sodium is lost with water when diuresis occurs
	Potassium Deficit (may occasionally occur in this phase)	Beginning about the fourth or fifth post-burn day, K^+ shifts from the extracellular fluid into the cells
	Metabolic Acidosis	
Convalescent Phase	Calcium Deficit	Since calcium may be immobilized at the burn site in the slough and early granulation phase of burns, symptoms of calcium deficit may occur (recall that for some unknown reason calcium rushes to damaged tissues)
	Potassium Deficit	Extracellular K^+ moves into the cells, leaving a deficit of K^+ in the extracellular fluid
	Negative Nitrogen Balance (present for several weeks following burns)	Secondary to: Stress reaction; Immobilization; Inadequate protein intake; Protein losses in exudate; Direct destruction of protein at the burn site
	Sodium Deficit	

burns, the organization of equipment, and the ability to act quickly and skillfully.

Need for Early Treatment

The shift of fluid from plasma to the interstitial space is rapid and well underway by the end of the first hour. The maximal speed of edema formation is reached by the end of the first 8 to 10 hours; the shift continues until the 36th to 48th hour. (By this time, the capillaries have healed sufficiently to prevent further fluid loss.) The decreased plasma volume can lead to hypovolemic shock and renal depression (due to decreased renal blood flow) unless quickly corrected by fluid replacement therapy. Oliguria or anuria are particularly threatening during this phase because of the excessive amounts of potassium flooding the extracellular fluid. (Remember that potassium is mainly excreted in urine; decreased urinary output causes a dangerous excess to build up in the bloodstream.) The sodium deficit requires prompt attention, as does the acidosis so frequently present.

Initial Patient Evaluation

Ideally a burn team made up of physicians and nurses skilled in the care of burn patients is on hand to treat burn emergencies. Unfortunately, the number of specialized burn units in the United States is inadequate and most burned patients must be cared for in general hospitals. When at all possible, patients should be transferred to a burn center for treatment. (Fortunately, burned patients withstand travel fairly well.)

Some hospital emergency rooms are staffed with at least one house physician. Unfortunately, however, *many* emergency rooms are staffed only with R.N.s and "on-call" physicians. While the nurse in this situation cannot initiate therapy without medical orders, she can obtain valuable information to expedite treatment when the physician arrives. Pertinent questions include:

1. When did the burn occur?
   (The degree of fluid shift is related to the length of time the burn has been present.)
2. What was the nature of the burning agent?
   (Notice in Table 18-1 that burns are classified in relation to burning agents frequently associated with them.)
3. What was the length of exposure to the burning agent?
   (Questions 2 and 3 are intended to help the physician establish the burn depth—appearance of the burns on admission is often misleading.)
4. Were any medications given prior to hospital admission?
   (Sometimes narcotics are given at the scene of the accident; it is important to avoid repeating drugs too soon, especially if respiratory tract burns or shock are present.)
5. Was the burn sustained in an enclosed area where heat and fumes were inhaled?
   (This question is highly significant in establishing the likelihood of respiratory burns.)
6. Are there any pre-existent illnesses, such as cardiac or renal damage or diabetes, that will require therapy in addition to burn treatment?
   (Failure to ascertain the presence of such illnesses is not uncommon in the initial rush.)
7. What is the normal pre-burn weight?
   (The pre-burn weight is a baseline for comparison for later weight changes; the weight is also instrumental in determining drug doses.)
8. Is pain present? If so, how severe?
   (It should be remembered that severe pain can cause a drop in blood pressure and further complicate the patient's condition.)
9. Is the patient known to have any drug allergies?
10. What is the status of tetanus immunization?
    (All patients with severe burns should receive prophylaxis against tetanus.)
11. Are there any associated injuries requiring treatment?
    (For example: head injuries or fractures)

While asking these questions, the nurse can be busy with other activities, such as readying fluid equipment, removing loose clothing not stuck to the burns, and removing constrictive jewelry before edema becomes severe. The unit that is to receive the patient after initial treatment should be notified so that every necessary preparation can be made and all initial patient evaluation can be prepared.

The physician will usually request that blood be drawn for determination of electrolytes, hemoglobin, hematocrit, glucose and urea nitrogen; arterial blood may be drawn for determination of pH, pCO_2 and pO_2.

Observing for Burn Shock

The nurse should be particularly alert for symptoms of burn shock:

Extreme thirst (due to generalized cellular dehydration)

Increasing restlessness
(persistent slight to moderate restlessness may be due to apprehension and discomfort produced by the burn rather than to inadequate fluid resuscitation)

Sudden high pulse rate
(heart beats faster to compensate for decreased blood volume)

Respiratory rate is often increased, but the character of breathing should be normal unless there are complicating factors

Blood pressure, when measurable, is either normal or low
(the body may be too extensively burned to permit application of a blood pressure cuff)
(the supine burned patient can often tolerate a large fluid volume deficit with little or no change in blood pressure; however, upon sitting or standing, hypotension and even syncope may occur—thus, the badly burned patient should be left supine for at least the first 48 to 72 hours)

Cool pale skin in unburned areas
(indicative of cutaneous vasoconstriction—a compensatory mechanism that helps preserve normal blood flow)

Oliguria
(due to decreased renal blood flow and to increased levels of ADH and aldosterone)

Delirium or coma
(presumably these symptoms are due to inadequate cerebral blood flow and are serious signs)

Seizures sometimes occur
(may be the result of cerebral ischemia)

Fortunately, burn shock is slow in onset and can be prevented or corrected by the intravenous administration of fluids in sufficient volume to maintain an adequate urinary output.

Initial Urine Observations

An indwelling urinary catheter is usually inserted when burns involve 20 per cent or more of the body surface; the catheter should be connected to a device for hourly measurement of the urine flow. If the patient voids before the catheter is inserted, the urine should be measured and saved. It should be observed for discoloration due to blood; if present, the patient probably has severe third-degree burns. Hemolysis of red blood cells at the burn site (due to trauma) causes the release of hemoglobin and consequently, hemoglobinuria.

Initial Observations of Respiratory Tract

The nurse should observe the patient closely for symptoms of respiratory burns. These include:

Singed nasal hair
Hoarseness
Red painful throat
Dry cough
Moist rales and dyspnea
Stridor
Bronchospasm with prolonged wheezing

Such symptoms should be reported promptly. Burns about the face and neck can cause edema and pressure around the trachea; difficulty in breathing should, of course, be reported immediately.

Initial Wound Care

Dirt, debris or loose skin should be removed by the physician with sterile instruments. Many physicians favor scrubbing the burned area with soap and water or with antiseptics, whereas others feel this is unnecessary trauma in new major burn cases, unless the wound is known to be contaminated by dirt or polluted water. In any event, all wounds should be cultured. As a rule, general anesthesia for debridement should be avoided during the shock phase of burns; adequate analgesia can usually be achieved by small intravenous doses of narcotics. (Fluid resuscitation should be underway before analgesics are administered.)

Intravenous Fluids

Intravenous fluids are life-saving in the treatment of moderate and severe burns; burns involving 15% or more of the body surface (less in infants and the aged) usually require intravenous fluid therapy. Simple venipuncture may be performed in the adult if the burn wounds are less than 20% and if a large vein is available under unburned skin; burns of more than 20% of the body surface (10% in children) usually require a venous cutdown for parenteral fluid administration. The cutdown should be performed over unburned skin to minimize the chance of infection.

The aim of early fluid therapy is to give the least amount of fluids necessary to maintain the desired urinary output and keep the patient relatively free of burn shock symptoms.

Physicians are of varied opinions about the kinds of intravenous fluids used in burn treatment. Among those used initially are:

- Lactated Ringer's solution
- Isotonic saline
- Plasma and plasma substitutes
- Dextran
- Blood
- 5% dextrose in water or saline
- Alkalinizing solutions (1/6 M sodium lactate and 1.2% sodium bicarbonate)
- Hypertonic lactated saline

Lactated Ringer's solution is used to supply sodium and to help correct metabolic acidosis; one liter of this solution contains 130 mEq. of sodium and 28 mEq. of lactate, a bicarbonate precursor.

Isotonic saline (0.9% sodium chloride) can also be used to supply sodium, as one liter of isotonic saline contains 154 mEq. of sodium and 154 mEq. of chloride. It has the disadvantage of supplying an excessive amount of chloride ions which contribute to the acidosis rather than correcting it.

The use of plasma and plasma substitutes is advocated by some physicians, who reason that plasma or other colloids must be given to replace the plasma leaked through injured capillaries into the burn site. Artz and Moncrief regard clinical dextran (average molecular weight 75,000) in saline as an excellent plasma volume expander that has been extensively used in the treatment of burns with "very rewarding benefits." They point out that most clinicians prefer plasma as a colloid solution because of its protein content. Plasma contains sodium (sometimes as much as 200 mEq./L.) and thus helps correct sodium deficit. However, it should be remembered that the use of plasma is associated with the risk of serum hepatitis. (See Chapter 16.) Some physicians feel that plasma and other colloids are unnecessary in burn therapy.

A few physicians still advocate the use of blood in early burn resuscitation; however, many feel that blood is contraindicated initially because the patient already suffers from hemoconcentration. Blood administration is associated with risks of hepatitis and transfusion reaction. (See Chapter 16.) In addition, blood is difficult to obtain and is expensive.

A non-electrolyte solution, usually 5% dextrose in water, may be used to replace the normal insensible water loss and the increased transcutaneous water vapor loss. In addition, alkalinizing fluids, such as 1/6 M sodium lactate and 1.2% sodium bicarbonate are sometimes used to correct the metabolic acidosis associated with burns.

The use of a hypertonic lactated solution for fluid resuscitation in burned patients is advocated

Table 18-3. Formulas for Use of Intravenous Fluids in Burn Therapy

Formula	*Adults*	*Children*
	Brooke formula (Burns > 50% counted as 50%)	
	First 24 Hours	
a) Colloids (plasma, dextran or blood)	0.5 ml./kg./1% burn	Same as adults
b) Lactated Ringer's solution	1.5 ml./kg./1% burn	Same as adults
c) Electrolyte-free solution (5% D/W)	2000 ml.	According to age
	Second 24 Hours	
	Give: one-half the amount of a & b and all of c	
	Massachusetts General Hospital formula	
	First 24 Hours	
a) Plasma	125 ml. per 1% burn	90 ml./1% burn × BSA (m^2)
b) Saline	15 ml. per 1% burn	10 ml./1% burn × BSA (m^2)
c) 5% dextrose in water	2000 ml.	According to calculated normal fluid needed for age and body surface area
	Second 24 Hours	
	Give: one-half of a & b and all of c	

by Monafo.* (See patient care study.) One liter of this solution contains: 250 mEq. of sodium, 100 mEq. of lactate, and 150 mEq. of chloride. Hypertonic lactated saline (HLS) supplies sodium in a minimal fluid load; the HLS solution is given rapidly enough to maintain a urinary output of 30 ml. per hour in adults and proportionately less in children. Because the solution is hypertonic, moderate but transient blood hyperosmolarity results. The plasma sodium level is generally between 145 and 160 mEq./L. when HLS is used in contrast to the less than normal 135 mEq./L. usually maintained when isotonic or hypotonic sodium solutions are used. It may be necessary to administer an electrolyte-free solution if the hypernatremia becomes severe.

Whenever intravenous fluids are given there is a danger of giving too much or not enough; both hazards are always present in burn therapy. To serve as a guide for the amount to be given early to burned patients, several formulas have been devised. (See Table 18-3.)

The nurse must be alert for symptoms of inadequate or excessive fluid administration. Inadequate fluid therapy in burned patients is indicated by:

Decreased urinary output (see Table 18-4)
Thirst
Collapsed veins
Restlessness and disorientation
Poor skin turgor
Hypotension and increased pulse rate

Circulatory overload is indicated by:

Venous distention
Shortness of breath

* Monafo, Wm.: Treatment of Burns–Principles and Practices, St. Louis, Warren H. Green, Inc., 1971.

Moist rales
Increased blood pressure
Increased venous pressure
(as measured on manometer)

Central venous pressure measurement may be necessary at times to monitor the effects of intravenous fluid replacement therapy, particularly in infants, the aged, and patients with cardiac and renal disease; it is generally indicated when the burned surface is greater than 50 or 60%. The margin for therapeutic error is small when the patient has deep extensive burns. Frequent checks of venous pressure allow more aggressive fluid replacement therapy without the risk of circulatory overload. Normal venous pressure is from 4 to 11 cm. of water, and a level of 15 to 20 cm. represents a significant elevation. When venous pressure becomes elevated above a point designated by the physician, the fluid infusion rate is curtailed.

If possible, the patient should be weighed daily, for at least the first week, to get an indication of the amount of fluid retention present. Sudden weight gains indicate fluid retention; loss of weight accompanies the stage of diuresis and indicates loss of edema fluid. An in-bed scale may be used if the patient is immobilized. (See Chapter 12.)

Oral Electrolyte Solutions

Oral salt solution therapy is effective in combating burn shock. It may be the sole source of fluids for the patient with minor burns and may be used in conjunction with intravenous fluids in more seriously burned patients. (Early, only potassium-free solutions should be used.) Oral electrolyte solutions should not, of course, be administered if the gastrointestinal tract is not functional. (Recall that paralytic ileus and gastric dilatation may be complications of severe burns.) Some physicians prefer that the severely burned patient be given nothing by mouth for the first day or two.

Thirst is an early symptom following burns. The patient permitted unlimited quantities of plain water is in danger of developing water intoxication (sodium deficit) because of simple dilution. It is characterized clinically by:

Headache
Depression
Apprehension
Tremors
Muscle twitching
Blurring of vision
Vomiting
Diarrhea
Disorientation
Excessive salivation
Mania
Generalized convulsions

The nurse must explain to the seriously burned patient that plain water should be taken only in limited amounts, if at all. (It is usually not allowed until the second or third postburn day.) The demand for oral liquids should be met with the oral electrolyte solution prescribed by the physician; the exact contents and proportions desired vary among physicians. A commonly used solution consists of 1 teaspoon of sodium chloride and 3 teaspoons of sodium bicarbonate in 1 L. of chilled water. Occasionally isotonic saline or sixth molar sodium lactate is used.

The solution should be carefully prepared; errors between teaspoons and tablespoons can be serious. Oral electrolyte solutions have a definite taste and some patients find them difficult to accept. However, the patient with intense thirst usually welcomes any type of oral liquid. Measures which help to make the solution more palatable include chilling it, making ice chips from it, flavoring it with lemon, or disguising it in juices (when allowed). Orange juice and other potassium-containing fluids (see Table 14-4, Chapter 14) should be withheld until renal function is established and the physician approves their use. They are usually allowed by the third or fourth day. (Potassium is contraindicated in the first 2 days after burns because of the likelihood of potassium excess; see Table 18-2.)

Oral electrolyte solutions are not given in the presence of:

1. Acute gastric dilatation

2. Frequent vomiting
3. Peripheral vascular collapse
4. Mental confusion (there is danger of aspirating fluid into the lungs)

Observations of Urinary Output as a Basis for Therapy

Urinary output is the best single index of the adequacy of fluid replacement therapy; the nurse should take measures to assure its accurate measurement.

The output may be measured every one-half hour or hour as a guide to fluid replacement therapy. One commercial device available for measurement of small volumes of urine is the Davol Uri-Meter, described in Chapter 12. Any clear cylinder with small calibrations may be used. When dealing with small volumes any error can be significant.

Absent or decreased urinary output can be due to:

Inadequate fluid replacement
Gastric dilatation
Renal failure

Remember that a clogged catheter may falsely indicate oliguria.

If the urinary output has been inadequate for 3 hours or more, a test can be performed to differentiate between the oliguria of inadequate fluid therapy and that of renal failure. One can carry out this test by infusing a solution composed of 5 per cent dextrose in 0.2 per cent sodium chloride or in 0.33 per cent sodium chloride over a period of 40 to 60 minutes. If the oliguria is due to inadequate fluid therapy, the urinary volume will increase; if it is due to renal failure, the output will remain small. Fortunately, renal failure in burns is uncommon.

Haste may cause a clogged catheter to be overlooked; to prevent this, the catheter should be irrigated at regular intervals with a carefully measured amount of solution. The volume of irrigating solution used should be noted; if less than this amount is withdrawn, the deficit should be noted and subtracted from the hourly urine volume. Conversely, if more fluid is withdrawn than was put in, the excess should be added to the hourly urine volume. Obviously, failure to record an irrigation correctly could lead to a false high or low urinary volume.

Table 18-4. Desired Urinary Output

Age Group	*Desired Urine Flow (ml./hr.)*
Adult:	
Male	30-50
Female	25-45
Child:	
1-10	10-25
1 or under	5-10

Weisberg, H.: Water, Electrolyte and Acid-Base Balance, ed. 2, p. 386. Baltimore, Williams & Wilkins Co., 1962.

Gastric dilatation is not uncommon in burned patients. When it is present, fluids taken orally become trapped in the distended stomach. Thus, even though oral fluids are swallowed, they are not available for body use and urine formation. Gastric distention can be detected by effortless vomiting, nausea, epigastric distress and grunting respiration. If vomiting occurs, a Levine tube is inserted to prevent aspiration of the vomitus. Additional parenteral fluids are needed to make up for the fluid lost in gastric suction; a gastric replacement solution is preferred. The severe stress imposed by a serious burn may produce a Curling's ulcer in the stomach with resultant hematemesis.

The physician usually indicates the desired urinary volume plus the variations in either direction to be reported. (See Table 18-4 for desired hourly urine volumes.)

The desired urinary volume should be realistic and approach the minimum, not the maximum. Attempts to increase fluid input sufficiently to cause large urine volumes in the aged or the very young are dangerous; the kidneys will not excrete excessive fluids because of the body's reaction to stress (increased retention of sodium and water, plus increased secretion of the antidiuretic hormone).

Specific gravity tests are performed on urine, wherein a low reading indicates adequate hydration, and a high reading indicates inadequate hydration. (See Chapter 12.)

An accurate intake-output record is a necessity.

Treatment of Respiratory Tract Burns

Respiratory burns can cause dyspnea, stridor, and copious mucous secretions. Burns about the face and neck may produce sufficient edema to embarrass respiration. In these instances, an airway must be established, and if possible, an endotracheal tube is inserted; if not, a tracheostomy is performed. Massive involvement of respiratory tissue is nearly always fatal, even when tracheostomy is performed.

Fluid should be suctioned frequently from the respiratory tract to prevent its accumulation. In addition, humidifiers are used to loosen secretions, and oxygen should be administered to decrease anoxia. Use of respiratory support, such as positive pressure apparatus, may be necessary. Prophylactic antibiotics are given to prevent infection of the lungs and consequent increased edema. Some physicians prescribe corticosteroids, endotracheally or systemically, to decrease the pulmonary inflammatory reaction. Lastly, parenteral fluids are administered cautiously to avoid overloading the circulatory system and causing pulmonary edema. (The desired urinary volume is slightly less when respiratory tract burns are present.)

Topical Antibacterial Agents

A number of agents may be applied locally to burn wounds to prevent or control infection. Among those in use are:

Mafenide acetate (Sulfamylon) 10% cream
0.5% aqueous silver nitrate solution
Other silver preparations
Gentamicin sulfate (Garamycin) 0.1% cream

While these local agents are often effective in controlling infection, they may, in varying degree, alter body electrolyte levels or cause other undesirable effects.

MAFENIDE Mafenide acetate (Sulfamylon) is a white, water-soluble cream that can diffuse through avascular burn tissue to help control infection. It is smeared on open burns with a gloved hand, or a sterile tongue blade, once or twice daily. The cream can be left on the wound uncovered or a light fine mesh gauze dressing can be used; dry cream and exudate must be removed before more cream is applied. Because it is water soluble, it can be washed off by tub bathing, shower, or bed bath. The antibacterial spectrum of mafenide includes the Clostridia and a variety of other gram-negative and gram-positive organisms commonly found in major burn wounds. It is widely used because it is clinically effective and simple to use. However, the use of mafenide is associated with certain problems:

(1) metabolic acidosis
Mafenide is absorbed into the burn wound and is apparently eliminated principally in the urine. The drug is a potent carbonic anhydrase inhibitor; the tendency to metabolic acidosis is apparently due to carbonic anhydrase inhibition at the renal tubular level. Absorption of the drug causes urinary bicarbonate excretion to increase and the urine pH to become alkaline, which results in a plasma base bicarbonate deficit (metabolic acidosis). Most patients tolerate mild acidosis fairly well; however, at times, the acidosis requires treatment with bicarbonate solutions or discontinuing the use of mafenide.

(2) hyperventilation
The respiratory system becomes the only functional method for maintaining body pH in the normal range because the renal buffering mechanism is impaired. Hyperventilation is a compensatory action to lighten the pCO_2 and raise the plasma pH. (Usually the acidosis is only partially compensated for by the respiratory system.) Hyperventilation is particularly evident in patients with burns of 50% or more of the body surface. After absorption, mafenide is metabolized into an acid, placing further demands on the lungs to maintain a normal pH. As a re-

sult, respiratory compensation may overshoot and cause a high arterial pH and a low pCO_2 (respiratory alkalosis).

(3) pain on application
Application of the cream causes most patients to complain of stinging, especially in the first few weeks. (The use of analgesics is sometimes necessary.)

(4) allergic reaction
This is mild in most cases but may occasionally require that the drug be discontinued.

AQUEOUS SILVER NITRATE SOLUTION (0.5%) The application of an aqueous 0.5% silver nitrate solution to burns is a frequent means of combatting infection. It is a potent antibacterial agent against organisms that regularly colonize burn wounds. Silver nitrate is inexpensive, readily available, and non-allergenic. Unlike creams and ointments, silver nitrate can be applied over new skin grafts; the result is uninterrupted wound bacteriostasis and a high rate of graft take. The silver nitrate dressings are at least one inch thick, are held in place with stockinette, and are wet every two hours with warmed 0.5% silver nitrate solution. Dry sheets and a cotton blanket are used to cover the patient; the covers minimize convection currents and the rate of heat loss. Patients are usually comfortable with these dressings until the eschar is removed. However, despite the many advantages of silver nitrate, its use is associated with certain problems:

(1) leaching of electrolytes (Na, Cl, K, Ca, and Mg) and vitamins from the burn wound
This is due to the hypotonicity of the silver nitrate solution as well as to the ion-binding potential of the silver ion. 0.5% silver nitrate contains only 29.4 mEq./L. of $AgNO_3$, and the solute composition of the solution is much different from that of body fluids. *The patient's plasma electrolyte levels must be monitored closely so that adequate replacement therapy can be instituted; children should be monitored especially closely. Patients treated with topical 0.5% silver nitrate dressings should routinely receive supplementation of sodium chloride, potassium, calcium, and water soluble vitamins, especially vitamin C.*

(2) staining
The staining property of silver nitrate is esthetically objectionable to the patient and to the staff. Silver nitrate stains everything it touches brown or black; however, this is not an insurmountable problem if certain procedures are followed. (See patient care study.)

(3) dressings must be re-wet every two hours with warmed silver nitrate solution
Failure to keep the dressings wet results in an increased concentration of silver nitrate at the wound site (due to evaporation of water from the dressings). Concentrations of silver nitrate greater than 1 or 2% are caustic and damage tissue.

The bacteriostatic and bactericidal properties of silver have resulted in the use of colloidal silver and various silver salts to inhibit bacterial growth on burn wounds; among other salts being used are silver lactate, silver sulfadiazine, and silver acetate.

GENTAMICIN Gentamicin sulfate (Garamycin) may be applied topically and used systemically to treat burns. It is effective against a wide range of gram-negative and gram-positive organisms. Application of the cream is not associated with pain. The drug is not appreciably absorbed from the burn wound. Garamycin is primarily eliminated by the kidneys; it should be used systemically with caution on patients with impaired renal function. Nephrotoxicity or ototoxicity may occasionally be manifested when Garamycin is used systemically, particularly when renal function is impaired.

Control of Pain

The amount of pain present varies with the depth of the burn, the extent of surface area involved, and the patient's pain threshold. Third-degree burns are painless because the nerve endings are destroyed; however, pain is experienced around the periphery of third-degree burns where first-degree and second-degree burns are present.

Burned patients complaining of severe pain may be given small doses of meperidine or morphine through the intravenous cannula put in place for fluid administration. The subcutaneous or intramuscular route should never be used to administer narcotics to a burned patient with circulatory collapse. Peripheral tissue perfusion is erratic when shock is present; thus, absorption of the drug may not occur or may be delayed. Failure to achieve the desired effect may prompt repeated doses by the same route. When peripheral circulation is improved after fluid resuscitation, there may be a rapid absorption and cumulative overdosage of the narcotic resulting in respiratory depression. Consequently, the administration of 100 mg. or more of meperidine to an inadequately resuscitated patient in or near burn shock can be lethal.

An 18-year-old boy received superficial intradermal burns over 80% of his body in a flash fire and explosion at a motel that occurred at 8:00 a.m. He was initially alert and oriented when seen by a local physician who prescribed no treatment. He was taken 25 miles by automobile to his family physician; by this time 4 hours had elapsed since his accident. He was given 100 mg. of meperidine subcutaneously (but no intravenous fluids) and placed in an ambulance for transfer to St. John's Mercy Hospital—a distance of 75 miles. When he arrived, 8 hours after the accident, he was comatose and cyanotic, with infrequent, gasping shallow respirations. An endotracheal tube could not be inserted because of facial and cervical edema. Although tracheostomy and cannula phlebotomy were performed immediately, spontaneous breathing never resumed and the pupils remained fixed and dilated. There was persistent oliguria until his death in coma, 20 hours later. (*Comment: this patient had a potentially curable lesion; most of his burns were intradermal and shallow. Delayed resuscitation, together with an ill-advised dose of narcotic, led to his untimely and unnecessary death.*)*

It is important not to confuse the restlessness of burn shock with pain. A patient thrashing about in bed, without complaints of pain, may well be in burn shock. In this case, a narcotic is contraindicated; the physician usually orders an increased rate of parenteral fluid administration.

Adynamic Ileus with Gastric Dilatation

This is common during the first day or two in patients with burns of 50% or more of the body surface. Usual symptoms include nausea, effortless vomiting, hiccoughing, and abdominal distention. Oral intake should be withheld if vomiting is present, as the danger of tracheal aspiration of vomitus is great. The emesis should be measured and observed for blood. A nasogastric tube may be inserted if symptoms persist; rarely is it necessary to leave the tube in longer than 24 hours. (Nasogastric tubes irritate the esophagus and stomach and may contribute to ulceration.)

The appearance of abdominal distention after the first few days postburn may indicate the presence of invasive wound sepsis, since ileus commonly occurs with this condition. Ileus may also be associated with gastroduodenal perforation. Stools should be routinely observed for blood since ulcers of the gastrointestinal tract are not uncommon in burned patients.

Physiologic Basis for Treatment and Nursing Care During the Fluid Remobilization Phase

Remobilization of edema fluid represents an interstitial fluid-to-plasma shift which begins on the second or third day after the patient has been burned. Its usual duration is from 24 to 72 hours.

Observing Urinary Output

Reabsorption of edema fluid takes place about the second to fifth postburn day. The blood volume is greatly increased and large amounts of urine are excreted. The nurse should be alert for increasing urine volume and report its presence to the physician.

If the expected diuresis does not occur, the possibility of renal damage must be considered.

* Monafo, Wm.: Treatment of Burns–Principles and Practices, pp. 54-55. St. Louis, Warren H. Green, Inc., 1971.

Observing for Pulmonary Edema

Fatal pulmonary edema may occur because the renocardiovascular system is not capable of handling the volume of water and electrolytes shifting from the interstitial fluid into the plasma. (Recall that the volume of edema fluid in a burn may equal the total normal plasma volume.)

The nurse should be alert for signs of circulatory overload and pulmonary edema:

Venous distention
Shortness of breath
Moist rales
Cyanosis
Coughing of frothy fluid

Parenteral Fluid Therapy

Once the fluid remobilization phase is reached, parenteral fluids should be sharply curtailed or discontinued; infusion of large volumes of fluids could easily cause circulatory overload with pulmonary edema. Oral fluids and food may supply adequate fluid and nutrition during this phase if tolerated; if not, moderate quantities of intravenous fluids may be necessary to meet daily needs. If possible, a high protein and high caloric diet is started by the second or third day.

Physiologic Basis for Treatment and Nursing Care During the Convalescent Period

NUTRITION Good nutrition is of first importance for burned patients, all of whom have great nutritional needs, several times those of the healthy person. Frequent oral feedings of foods or commercial mixtures high in protein, calories and vitamins should be started as soon as possible. Vitamin preparations containing at least members of the B complex and vitamin C should be administered. If the patient refuses oral feedings, tube feedings may be employed. Gastrostomy feedings are often safer because the danger of aspiration pneumonitis, associated with nasogastric tube feedings, is eliminated. The nurse should examine the abdomen for bowel sounds before the nasogastric tube feeding is instilled and during the first few hours thereafter; recall that gastric atony and dilatation are common after major burns. Instillation of the tube feeding into a distended atonic stomach results in regurgitation of the gastric contents and possible tracheal aspiration. (Nursing responsibilities in administration of tube feedings are discussed in Chapter 12.) The nurse should be alert for gastric bleeding or other indications of a Curling's ulcer. Because the patient often has a poor appetite and psychologic depression, the nurse must take every opportunity to make food appealing to him.

Oral electrolyte supplements may also be given, depending upon the electrolytes needed. Serum electrolytes should be determined daily.

While providing the patient with optimal nutrition pays rich dividends, failure to meet his nutritional needs may lead to what Blocker terms "burn decompensation." This state is characterized by chronic weight loss, decreased resistance to infection, anorexia, failure of skin grafts to take, cachexia and death.

Parenteral hyperalimentation may be necessary when the burned patient is unable to consume an adequate diet. (Parenteral hyperalimentation is described in Chapter 16.)

AMBULATION Early ambulation, even in severely burned patients, improves appetite, helps to prevent contractures, helps correct negative nitrogen balance and sustains the patient's morale. Patients treated by the *closed* method (dressings) are more mobile than those treated by the *open* method (exposure).

OBSERVING FOR SPECIFIC ELECTROLYTE IMBALANCES The convalescent phase is often complicated by inadequate electrolyte intake from the diet; if supplemental replacements are not given, the patient may insidiously develop deficits of potassium, sodium and calcium. The nurse should be alert for symptoms of these imbalances. (A thorough description of each is offered in Chapter 9. Observations to be made by the nurse are discussed in Chapter 12.) Plasma electrolyte levels should be checked on a regular basis.

Obviously, some of the major nursing problems have been omitted in the preceding discussion of burns, not because they are unimportant but because space does not allow.

PATIENT CARE STUDY*

Mrs. S., a 49-year-old obese woman, was burned while attempting to ignite a barbecue grill with a flammable liquid. Her nylon clothing ignited and melted. The flames were extinguished by rolling in a sewage ditch. Four hours after injury she was transferred to the burn unit from a nearby general hospital; burns covered approximately 50% of her body and appeared to be mostly intradermal.

An ankle cut down was immediately performed to provide a line for administration of fluids, analgesics, and antibiotics. An indwelling urinary catheter was inserted and attached to a calibrated receptacle (Uri-meter). During the first 48 hours postburn, seven L. of hypertonic lactated saline (HLS)** were given intravenously, to prevent burn shock. Oral intake during this period amounted to 6,385 ml. Prior to admission, two liters of 5% dextrose in lactated Ringer's solution and 250 ml. of Plasmanate were administered intravenously.

Urine flow was maintained at 30 to 50 ml. per hour by adjusting the rate of flow of the HLS solution. (To insure adequate renal perfusion and to avoid overhydration, with resultant pulmonary edema, a urine flow closely approximating these levels must be maintained.)

Vital functions, including urine flow, were recorded hourly for the first 24 hours (Figure 18-2). During the second day, the urine flow was recorded hourly, and the other vital functions every two hours. Blood pressure readings were not done because all extremities were burned. During the first 48 hours, small doses (10 to 15 mg.) of meperidine (Demerol) were given intravenously every 4 to 6 hours as needed for pain.

* This section was prepared by Marjorie Wright, R.N., Burn Unit Supervisor, St. John's Mercy Medical Center, St. Louis, Missouri.

** One liter of HLS contains 250 mEq. of sodium, 100 mEq. of lactate, and 150 mEq. of chloride.

The pre-burn weight was 186 pounds; during treatment for burn shock, the weight increased to 201 pounds. By the 43rd postburn day, the weight had stabilized at 158 pounds, where it remained until discharge.

On admission the wounds were cleansed with sterile saline, and all loose epidermis was removed. Dressings soaked with 0.5% silver nitrate solution were applied. (An important nursing function consisted of soaking the dressings every two hours with warmed 0.5% silver nitrate solution.) Forty-eight hours after injury, necrotic, odoriferous, purpuric patches appeared in the burn wound, and the necrosis spread rapidly. Cultures disclosed E. coli, Enterobacter, Proteus, and Pseudomonas aeruginosa—organisms obviously innoculated into the wounds when the patient rolled in the sewage ditch. Cultures of the sewage water subsequently grew the same flora. The necessary excision of all the infected eschars resulted in conversion of the wounds to subdermal injuries; small areas of the wound were debrided and dressed sequentially to reduce fluid loss, shivering, patient discomfort, and contamination of the less colonized wound areas. A Circoelectric bed was utilized at this point to facilitate care. Local application of silver nitrate dressings was continuous. In addition, porcine xenografts (animal skin) were used as temporary biological dressings to reduce fluid loss and to help clean the wounds; they were changed at 24 to 48 hour intervals.

By 60 hours postburn, Mrs. S. was eating and drinking well and urine flow was adequate; the intravenous and urinary catheters were removed. The patient was gotten out of bed to walk and to sit in a chair with her legs elevated.

Spot checks of the urine had been done Q.I.D. because of a family history of diabetes mellitus. On the 6th postburn day, glycosuria (4^+ on Clinitest) and hyperglycemia (355 mg.%) were noted. This represented latent diabetes unmasked by the burn trauma, and so a 2,500 calorie diabetic diet and regular insulin by the sliding scale were instituted.

On the 14th postburn day, mafenide (Sulfamylon) was applied to the heavily colonized thigh wounds. (Unlike silver nitrate, Sulfamylon is absorbed through the burn wound into the underlying tissues to control invasive sepsis.) During the septic period, Mrs. S. became delirious. (Mental aberration is not uncommon when serious sepsis is present.)

By the 16th postburn day, her mental status had deteriorated to the point where adequate nutrition could not be achieved by regular foods alone. Therefore, a liquid basic nutritional supplement, high in glucose, was given hourly, in small amounts, by mouth; during the next 48 hours she received 3,330 ml. of this substance (Vivonex, Eaton Laboratories). Urinary spot checks were now done every four hours. After two days on the supplement, Mrs. S. became unresponsive. The urine tests showed a high glucose content (4^+) and no acetone. A dramatic diuresis of 5 L. of urine in a 24-hour period occurred. Mrs. S. went into deep coma; her skin and mucous membranes were obviously dry, and her eyes were sunken. The diagnosis of nonketotic hyperosmotic coma was verified by immediate determination of the blood sugar (900 mg.%) and the serum osmolality (415 mOsm/L.). Other serum determinations at this time showed: sodium 162 mEq./L., potassium 2.8 mEq./L., and BUN 56 mg.%. To quickly compute the osmolality, the following formula may be used:

$$2(Na^+ + K^+) + \frac{BUN}{3} + \frac{Glucose}{18}.$$

The supplemental feedings were discontinued and 4 L. of 5% dextrose in water were administered intravenously in a four-hour period, and eighty units of regular insulin were given; within four hours, Mrs. S. was no longer in deep coma. She was awake and alert the following day. Her appetite improved and a 2,000 calorie diabetic diet was instituted. By the 34th postburn day, all urinary spot checks were negative.

Sulfamylon therapy to the thigh wounds was discontinued on the 19th postburn day when the invasive sepsis was controlled. Split thickness grafting was begun on the 28th postburn day; because of numerous systemic problems, skin grafting was performed using local infiltration anesthesia for the donor sites, an approach that avoided delay in permanent wound closure. Seven grafting procedures were done in all, and by the 43rd postburn day her wounds were nearly epithelialized. After all autografting was completed, the patient was transferred from the Circoelectric bed to a regular bed. Daily tub baths were begun to facilitate physical therapy and for patient comfort. Finally, by the 48th postburn day, Mrs. S. was walking with the use of a walker.

A stool specimen on the 29th postburn day showed occult blood (3^+). Thus, an antacid was administered for what was presumed to be a Curling's ulcer. However, no overt signs of bleeding occurred, and three repeat stool specimens eight days later were negative.

Three and a half liters of sedimented erythrocytes were administered to correct anemia between the 12th and 41st postburn days. (The blood transfusion requirements of severely burned patients are often this great.) Etiology of burn anemia is not fully understood but is likely due to a combination of factors: infection, poor nutrition, external blood loss, and lack of secretion of erythropoietin (a hormone).

With the progression of permanent wound closure, Mrs. S. was more comfortable, interested in her convalescence, and anxious to return to her home. She was discharged with healed wounds on the 54th postburn day. Approximately one month after discharge she developed viral hepatitis, which was likely contracted from the numerous blood transfusions. Fortunately, the hepatitis caused no serious immediate complication.

A burned patient, with or without complications, presents a formidable challenge to the ability of physicians and nurses. The rewards of a successfully treated patient are proportional to the magnitude of the clinical problems encountered. Other members of the burn team who directly contributed to Mrs. S.'s recovery include the dietitian, physical therapist, occupational therapist, and social worker. The family was included in the patient care regime as much as possible.

COMMENT An aqueous 0.5% silver nitrate solution is generally recognized as a highly efficient method of achieving bacteriostasis on burn wounds and has been used extensively in this unit for the past five years. The acceptance and

DATE 6-1-71 ICU DAY ADM. - BURN DAY

DIET	B	L	S
	NPO	LIQ	LIQ
APPETITE	—	G	G
WEIGHT	186 lbs		

SPECIAL PROC., MONITOR, L.P. DEFIBRILLATION, PACEMAKER, OXYGEN, BONE MARROW ASP.

X-RAY

OTHER DEBRIDEMENT + CULTURES PHOTOGRAPHS - $AgNO_3$ DRESSINGS BLOODWORK

Temperature scale: 105°, 104°, 103°, 102°, 101°, 100°, 99°, 98°, 97°

	DAY SHIFT								EVENING SHIFT								NIGHT SHIFT							
	7	8	9	10	11	12	1	2	3	4	5	6	7	8	9	10	11	12	1	2	3	4	5	6
PULSE	102	120	112	120	120	120	120	120	112	116	148	140	124	130		136	120	124	100	110	122	96	100	120
RESPIRATION	20	24	24	28	24	24	16	20	24	28	28	28	24	26		24	28	26	32	30	32	24	22	24
BLOOD PRESSURE																								

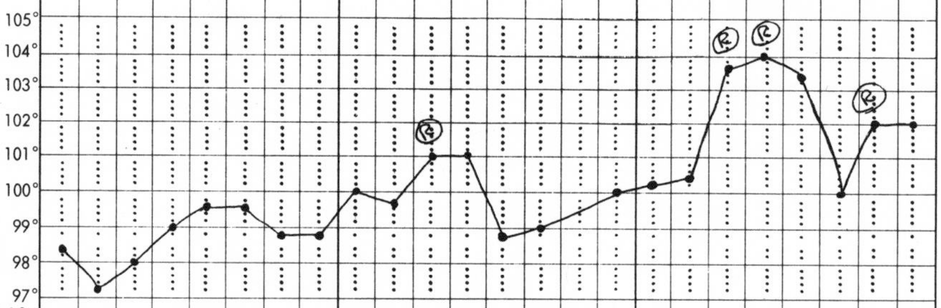

MEDICATIONS

MEDICATIONS	7	8	9	10	11	12	1	2	3	4	5	6	7	8	9	10	11	12	1	2	3	4	5	6
PRIOR TO ADM. DEMEROL 100 mg (M)	(5 HRS P.T.A.)																							
THORAZINE 25 mg (M)	(4 HRS P.T.A.)																							
HYPERTET 250 mg (M)		/																						
TETANUS TOXOID 0.5 cc (M)		/																						
DEMEROL 10 mg (V)			/													/30								
DEMEROL 15 mg (V)												/												
A.S.A. 20 grs (R) SUPPOSITORY																				/30				

FLUID INTAKE IN cc PER HOUR	7	8	9	10	11	12	1	2	3	4	5	6	7	8	9	10	11	12	1	2	3	4	5	6
PER O S			N.P.O.									200	200	200	200	200								
OTHER PER SHIFT												1000 cc								1680 cc				

IV P.T.A. c̄ #20 MEDICUT = 250 cc 5% PLASMA + 2000 cc D5LR

IV (PER HOUR)	7	8	9	10	11	12	1	2	3	4	5	6	7	8	9	10	11	12	1	2	3	4	5	6
ADM. = CUTDOWN #1 HLS-B 1000 cc	1000																							
#2 HLS-B 1000 cc c̄ 1 mil. U. Aq. PENICILLIN				500	D.C.'D.																			
#3 HLS-A 1000 cc c̄ 1 mil. U. Aq. PENICILLIN					1000																			
#4 HLS-A 1000 cc c̄ 0.5 Gm STAPHCILLIN							300		700															
HLS-B (500 cc of #2 LEFT)											500													
#5 HLS-B 1000 cc c̄ 0.5 Gm STAPHCILLIN														1000										
#6 HLS-B 1000 cc c̄ 1 mil. U. Aq. PENICILLIN																		1000						
#7 HLS-B 1000 cc c̄ 0.5 Gm STAPHCILLIN																							250	
PER SHIFT	(V) = 2800 cc + P.T.A.								2200 cc								1250 cc							
INTAKE 24 HOUR SUMMARY	(V) = 6250 cc																							

OUTPUT IN cc PER HOUR	7	8	9	10	11	12	1	2	3	4	5	6	7	8	9	10	11	12	1	2	3	4	5	6
VOIDED					*					*					**					*				
CATHETER	50	31	[4	6	4]	50	35	20	[5	12]	40	30	50	[70	85]	30	30	35	[13	12]	60	50	60	40
EMESIS 500 cc P.T.A.																								
OTHER SPECIFIC GRAVITY											1.015									1.023				
PER SHIFT	200 cc								322 cc								300 cc							
OUTPUT 24 HOUR SUMMARY	822 cc																							
STOOLS	X3 - SEMI LIQUID LIGHT BROWN								X1 - SOFT													NO		

ST. JOHN'S MERCY MEDICAL CENTER / ST. LOUIS, MISSOURI

ACUTELY ILL PATIENT RECORD

* I.V. INFUSION TOO SLOW

** I.V. INFUSION TOO FAST

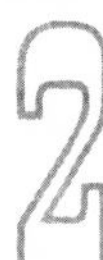

FORM 533

Fig. 18-2. Acutely ill patient record. (St. John's Mercy Medical Center, St. Louis, Missouri)

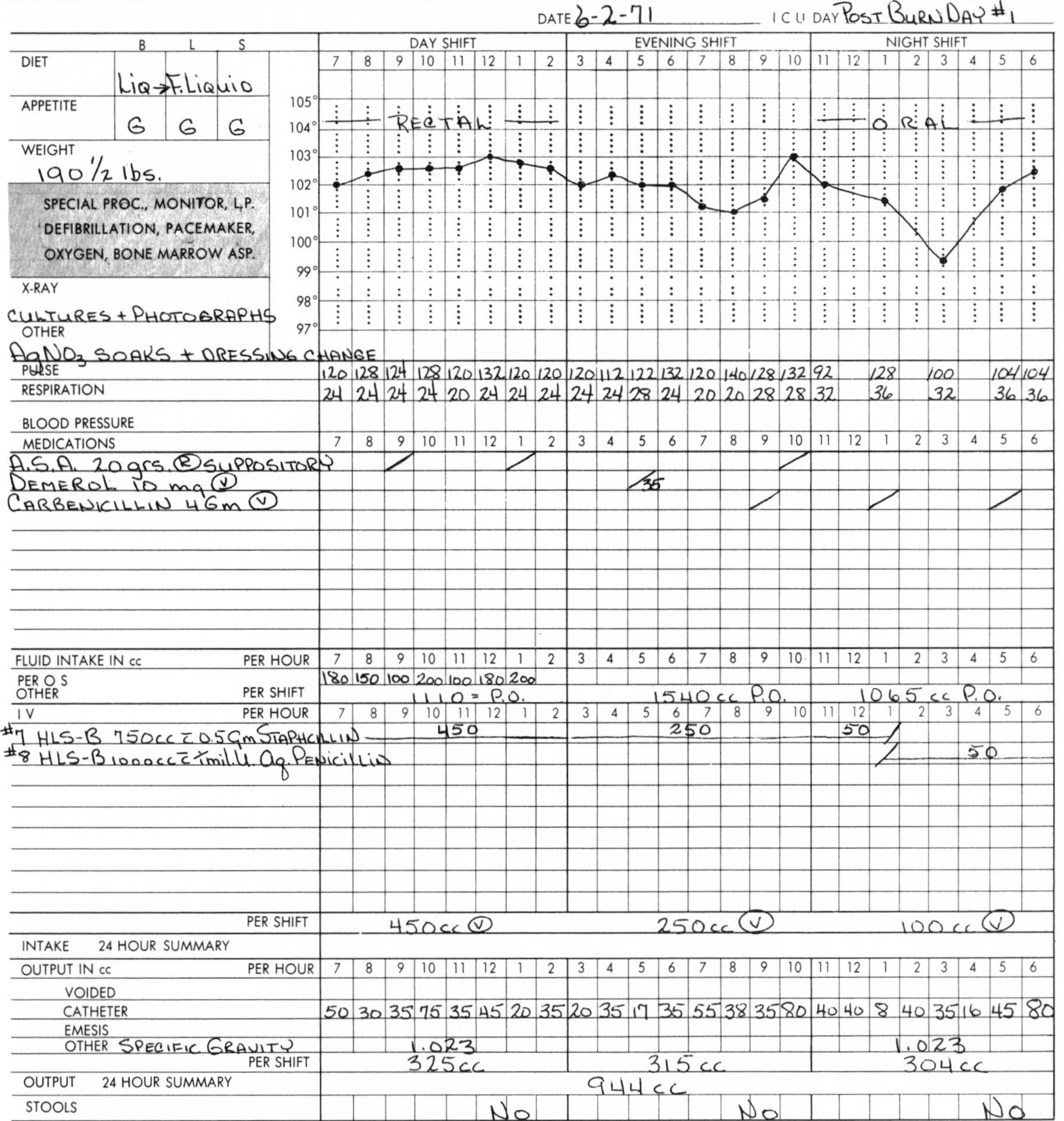

DATE 6-2-71 ICU DAY Post Burn Day #1

	B	L	S
DIET	Liq → F. Liquid		
APPETITE	G	G	G

WEIGHT 190 1/2 lbs.

SPECIAL PROC., MONITOR, L.P. DEFIBRILLATION, PACEMAKER, OXYGEN, BONE MARROW ASP.

X-RAY: Cultures + Photographs

OTHER: $AgNO_3$ soaks + dressing change

	DAY SHIFT								EVENING SHIFT								NIGHT SHIFT							
	7	8	9	10	11	12	1	2	3	4	5	6	7	8	9	10	11	12	1	2	3	4	5	6
PULSE	120	128	124	128	120	132	120	120	120	112	122	132	120	140	128	132	92		128		100		104	104
RESPIRATION	24	24	24	24	20	24	24	24	24	24	28	24	20	20	28	28	32		36		32		36	36
BLOOD PRESSURE																								

MEDICATIONS	7	8	9	10	11	12	1	2	3	4	5	6	7	8	9	10	11	12	1	2	3	4	5	6
A.S.A. 20 grs. Ⓡ suppository			/				/									/								
Demerol 10 mg Ⓥ											/35													
Carbenicillin 4 Gm Ⓥ															/				/				/	

FLUID INTAKE IN cc PER HOUR	7	8	9	10	11	12	1	2	3	4	5	6	7	8	9	10	11	12	1	2	3	4	5	6
PER O S	180	150	100	200	100	180	200																	
OTHER PER SHIFT	1110 = P.O.								1540 cc P.O.								1065 cc P.O.							

I V PER HOUR	7	8	9	10	11	12	1	2	3	4	5	6	7	8	9	10	11	12	1	2	3	4	5	6
#7 HLS-B 750cc c̄ 0.5 Gm Staphcillin				450								250						50	/					
#8 HLS-B 1000cc c̄ 1 mill. U. Aq. Penicillin																			/			50		
PER SHIFT	450cc Ⓥ								250cc Ⓥ								100 cc Ⓥ							

INTAKE 24 HOUR SUMMARY

OUTPUT IN cc PER HOUR	7	8	9	10	11	12	1	2	3	4	5	6	7	8	9	10	11	12	1	2	3	4	5	6
VOIDED																								
CATHETER	50	30	35	75	35	45	20	35	20	35	17	35	55	38	35	80	40	40	8	40	35	16	45	80
EMESIS																								
OTHER Specific Gravity	1.023																1.023							
PER SHIFT	325cc								315 cc								304 cc							
OUTPUT 24 HOUR SUMMARY	944 cc																							
STOOLS	No								No								No							

ST. JOHN'S MERCY MEDICAL CENTER / ST. LOUIS, MISSOURI

ACUTELY ILL PATIENT RECORD

2

FORM 533

Fig. 18-2 (cont.)

use of silver nitrate has been somewhat restricted on some burn units because of esthetic and economic considerations related to its staining property. Effective means of dealing with the problems of staining have been developed in the past three years, so that it is practical to use silver nitrate and have a stain-free, attractive burn unit.

Substances which are relatively non-porous will take only a surface stain. These stains can be removed by soap and water, household cleansers, or any of the commercial silver nitrate removers, within a few minutes during the daily housekeeping activities. Materials used in this burn unit include a non-porous flooring (Tytron, Monsanto Chemical Co.) and a paint-like substance applied to walls (Liquid Tile, Architectural Finishes, Inc.); each of these non-porous substances is stain resistant, easily cleaned, durable, and attractive.

Linens can be maintained relatively stain-free if they are laundered in a special formula while the silver nitrate stain is still damp. The laundry department at St. John's Mercy Medical Center has developed a formula for stain treatment that costs only about 5¢ per 100 pounds of laundry.

The expense involved in using stain-resistant materials is reasonable in view of the esthetic value of an attractive burn unit.

19 Fluid Balance in the Patient With Digestive Tract Disease

CHARACTER OF GASTROINTESTINAL SECRETIONS

The average daily volume of gastrointestinal secretions is approximately 8,000 ml., as compared to a plasma volume of 3,500 ml. Most of these secretions are reabsorbed in the ileum and proximal colon; only about 150 ml. of relatively electrolyte-free fluid is excreted daily in the feces.

Gastrointestinal secretions consist of saliva, gastric juice, bile, pancreatic juice and intestinal secretions. Their average daily volume and pH are listed in Table 19-1. The electrolyte content of these secretions is presented in Table 19-2.

Table 19-1. Average Daily Volume of Gastrointestinal Secretions and Their Usual pH

Secretion	*Volume (ml.)*	*pH*
Saliva	1,500	6-7
Gastric juice	2,500	1-3
Pancreatic juice	700	8.0-8.3
Bile	500	7.8
Small intestine	3,000	7.8-8.0

Table 19-2. Electrolyte Content of Gastrointestinal Secretions Expressed in Milliequivalents per Liter

Secretion	Na^+	K^+	Cl^-	HCO_3^-
Saliva	9	25.8	10	10-15
Gastric juice (fasting)	60.4	9.2	84	0-14
Pancreatic juice (fistula)	141.1	4.6	76.6	121
Bile (fistula)	148.9	4.98	100.6	40
Small intestine (suction)	111.3	4.6	104.2	31

Weisberg, H.: Water, Electrolytes, and Acid-Base Balance, ed. 2, p. 143. Baltimore, Williams & Wilkins, 1962.

With the exception of saliva, the gastrointestinal secretions are isotonic with the extracellular fluid; in addition, material entering the gastrointestinal tract tends to become isotonic during the course of its absorption. Many liters of extracellular fluid pass into the gastrointestinal tract, and back again, as part of the normal digestive process. This movement of water and electrolytes is sometimes referred to as the "gastrointestinal circulation."

FLUID IMBALANCES ASSOCIATED WITH THE LOSS OF GASTROINTESTINAL FLUIDS

Loss of gastrointestinal fluids is the most common cause of water and electrolyte disturbances. This fact becomes evident when one considers the large volume of fluids in the gastrointestinal tract and the many ways in which they can be lost from the body. Vomiting, gastrointestinal suction, diarrhea, fistulas and drainage tubes are some of the abnormal ways in which these fluids can be lost; fluids trapped in the gastrointestinal tract, as in intestinal obstruction, are physiologically *outside* the body. Any condition that interferes with the absorption of fluids from the gastrointestinal tract can cause serious water and electrolyte disturbances.

Vomiting and Gastric Suction

The absorption of gastric secretions and ingested fluids is hindered by vomiting and gastric suction. To understand the imbalances likely to occur with these conditions, it is helpful to review the normal characteristics of gastric juice, which is the most acid of the gastrointestinal secretions, with a pH of from 1 to 3; occasionally, the pH is higher than 3. The main electrolytes in gastric

Table 19-3. Possible Abnormal Fluid Exchange of Adult in 24-Hour Period

Entrances	*Exits*	*Water (ml.)*	*NaCl (Gm.)*
G.I. Tract	*G.I. Tract*		
Gastric Gavage	Saliva	500- 1,500	2-8
Duodenal Gavage	Vomiting	100- 6,000	0.5-40
Enemas	Suction Drainage, Intubation or Fistula	100- 6,000	0.5-40
	Diarrhea	500-17,000	2-80
	Rectal Mucorrhea ("Pseudodiarrhea")	350- 2,000	1-9
	Primary or Secondary Malabsorption Syndrome	100-14,000	0.5-75

Weisberg, H.: Water, Electrolyte and Acid-Base Balance, ed. 2, p. 140. Baltimore, Williams & Wilkins, 1962.

juice are hydrogen, chloride, potassium and sodium. Imbalances most often associated with the loss of gastric juice include:

Fluid volume deficit
Metabolic alkalosis (base bicarbonate excess)
Potassium deficit
Sodium deficit

FLUID VOLUME DEFICIT When a large volume of water and electrolytes is lost from the body, fluid volume deficit results. Note in Table 19-3 that 100 to 6,000 ml. may be lost in 24 hours from vomiting or suction. Since the gastric secretions are greatly reduced when the stomach is at rest, the patient should receive nothing by mouth during gastric suction or persistent vomiting. If the suction or vomiting is prolonged, and fluid replacement therapy is inadequate, fluid volume deficit will result. Consequently, the nurse should be alert for the following symptoms indicating the presence of fluid volume deficit:

Dry skin and mucous membranes
Longitudinal wrinkling of the tongue
Oliguria
Acute weight loss—in excess of 5%
Body temperature drop
Exhaustion

METABOLIC ALKALOSIS Excessive loss of gastric juice by vomiting or gastric suction causes metabolic alkalosis, because hydrogen and chloride ions are lost from the body. Loss of chloride ions causes a compensatory increase in bicarbonate ions. The base bicarbonate side of the carbonic acid–base bicarbonate ratio is increased and the pH becomes alkaline. The nurse should be alert for symptoms of metabolic alkalosis when the patient has sustained a prolonged loss of gastric juice by vomiting or gastric suction. These symptoms include:

Slow, shallow respiration (compensatory respiratory reaction to retain CO_2 and to correct alkalosis)
Muscle hypertonicity and tetany (due to decreased calcium ionization in alkalosis)
Changes in sensorium
- Personality changes may be the first symptoms to appear
- Previously placid patient may become irritable and uncooperative
- Patient may be disoriented

POTASSIUM DEFICIT Gastric juice is rich in potassium. A prolonged loss of this fluid frequently leads to potassium deficit, particularly if potassium replacement therapy is inadequate. The nurse should be alert for symptoms of potassium deficit. These include:

Muscular weakness
Gaseous intestinal distention
Soft, flabby muscles
Carphologia (aimless plucking at bedclothes)
Paresthesia and flaccid paralysis of extremities

Weak, irregular pulse
Respiratory failure
Heart block and cardiac arrest (as late symptoms)

SODIUM DEFICIT The sodium content of gastric juice is relatively high. The nurse should be aware that gastric suction or prolonged vomiting can lead to sodium deficit, especially if plain water is drunk. Symptoms of sodium deficit include:

Anorexia, apathy, sometimes great apprehension
Abdominal cramps
Hypotension (declines further when sitting or standing)
Syncope with position change
Rapid, thready pulse
Oliguria, low specific gravity of urine
Cold skin, particularly in the extremities
Decreased body temperature, unless infection is present
Hand veins fill slowly
Fingerprinting on sternum

OTHER IMBALANCES Prolonged vomiting or gastric suction can result in magnesium deficit, an imbalance not as common as those listed above. The magnesium concentration in gastric juice is 1.4 mEq./L. In addition, the body conserves magnesium well. However, its continued loss by suction or vomiting, plus its dilution with magnesium-free replacement fluids, can result in symptoms of magnesium deficit. These include:

Hyperirritability
Gross tremors (may occur in any extremity but are most common in the arms)
Confusion and disorientation
Tachycardia
Hypertension
Hallucinations, usually visual (may be auditory)
Carphologia
Abnormal sensitivity to sound (hyperacusis)
Convulsions (usually generalized and not preceded by an aura)

Another imbalance is ketosis of starvation; unless adequate parenteral nutrition is provided for the patient with prolonged vomiting or gastric suction, ketosis of starvation will occur. Due to the absence of carbohydrate, the body must use fat for energy purposes. As a result of increased fat utilization, ketone bodies accumulate in the blood. Because ketones are strong acids, they can convert metabolic alkalosis into metabolic acidosis. The odor of acetone on the breath indicates starvation ketosis; other symptoms of metabolic acidosis include deep, rapid respiration and weakness.

NURSING IMPLICATIONS The nurse should be alert for symptoms of the imbalances described above, report their occurrence to the physician, and in addition, should attempt to minimize the loss of water and electrolytes by vomiting and gastric suction. When the nurse is in charge of patients with vomiting, she should:

1. Discourage oral intake, particularly water, if vomiting is persistent and frequent. Ingested substances stimulate gastric secretions. If the substance is hypotonic, electrolytes will move from the extracellular fluid into the stomach. When the stomach is emptied by vomiting, water and electrolytes from the gastric secretions and extracellular fluid are lost. Obviously, oral intake while vomiting persists promotes water and electrolyte depletion.
2. Report vomiting early so that appropriate treatment can be started before water and electrolyte losses become serious. Medications to relieve nausea may prevent further vomiting. Nutrition by the parenteral route allows the stomach to rest.
3. Administer p.r.n. medications, as prescribed, to relieve nausea.
4. Measure or estimate as accurately as possible the amount of vomitus lost from the body so that lost water and electrolytes can be replaced by parenteral fluids. All fluids lost and gained by the body should be recorded on the intake-output record. (Nursing responsibilities in measuring and recording fluid intake and output are discussed in Chapter 12.)

5. Measure body weight daily to detect significant changes in fluid balance. Daily weights are helpful in detecting fluid volume deficit, particularly if vomitus has not been measured. A patient on a starvation diet should lose about one-half pound a day, whereas a loss in excess of this amount probably implies a fluid volume deficit. A weight gain implies fluid volume excess if the patient is on a starvation diet. (Nursing responsibilities in measuring daily weights are discussed in Chapter 12.)
6. Report substantial improvement in the patient's condition early so that he can be returned to oral intake as soon as tolerated. (Dietary considerations for the patient with vomiting are discussed in Chapter 14.)

Important nursing actions in the care of the patient with gastric suction are as follows:

1. Irrigate the tube with an isotonic electrolyte solution, such as isotonic solution of sodium chloride, or as prescribed by the physician. Lytren can be employed. Plain water is unsuitable as an irrigating solution; because it is hypotonic, water causes gastric secretions to increase in order to render it isotonic. The irrigating water is sucked out along with electrolytes from the gastric secretions and from the extracellular fluid.
2. Record the irrigating solution volume as intake and whatever is recovered as output.
3. Prohibit intake of water or other electrolyte-free solutions, for the same reason as described under 1. Ice chips made from a suitable electrolyte solution, such as isotonic solution of sodium chloride, lactated Ringer's solution, or Lytren, may be administered if prescribed by the physician.
4. Measure and record the amount of fluid lost by suction, as well as all other fluid gains and losses.
5. Measure daily weight variations to help detect early fluid volume deficit or excess.

Diarrhea, Intestinal Suction and Ileostomy

FLUID VOLUME DEFICIT Intestinal hypermotility shortens the opportunity for absorption of intestinal fluids and thus results in increased fluid loss in bowel movements. The hypermotility can be caused by a disease process, such as ulcerative colitis, or by the frequent use of an irritant cathartic. The liquid stools expelled as a result of hypermotility contain water and electrolytes derived from secretions, ingested food and fluids, and extracellular fluid brought into the bowel to render ingested substances isotonic. Note in Table 19-3 that as much as 17,000 ml. can be lost in 24 hours from diarrhea. Obviously, prolonged diarrhea is a serious threat to water and electrolyte balance. The amount of fluid lost in intestinal suction averages around 3,000 ml. daily. Thus, the nurse should be alert for symptoms of fluid volume deficit when the patient has sustained large fluid losses from the intestinal tract. (Symptoms of fluid volume deficit are listed in the discussion of gastric suction and vomiting.)

METABOLIC ACIDOSIS Intestinal juice varies in composition according to the area of the intestine in which it was formed. However, the intestinal secretions are all alkaline, including pancreatic juice and bile, which are mixed with intestinal juices in the intestines. The chief electrolytes in intestinal juice include sodium, potassium, bicarbonate and chloride.

The intestinal secretions are alkaline because of the preponderance of bicarbonate ions. Loss of bicarbonate results in a compensatory increase in chloride ions; the base bicarbonate side of the carbonic acid–base bicarbonate ratio is lightened and the pH is decreased. Symptoms of metabolic acidosis (primary base bicarbonate deficit) include:

Shortness of breath on exertion (mild deficit)
Deep, rapid breathing (moderate or severe deficit)
Weakness and general malaise
Stupor progressing to coma

SODIUM DEFICIT Intestinal secretions have a high concentration of sodium; excessive loss of these secretions results in sodium deficit. (Symptoms of sodium deficit are listed in the discussion of gastric suction and vomiting.)

POTASSIUM DEFICIT Relatively large amounts of potassium are contained in the intestinal fluid; therefore, potassium deficit occurs frequently with diarrhea, prolonged intestinal suction, and recent ileostomy. (Symptoms of potassium deficit are listed in the discussion of gastric suction and vomiting.)

NURSING IMPLICATIONS The nurse should be alert for symptoms of fluid imbalances likely to occur in the presence of diarrhea, ileostomy or intestinal suction.

Important nursing actions in the care of the patient with *diarrhea* include:

1. Discourage oral intake, particularly irritating foods apt to stimulate peristalsis. Less fluid is formed when the intestinal tract is at rest.
2. Report diarrhea early so that appropriate treatment can be started before water and electrolyte losses are severe. Medications to reduce peristalsis may relieve diarrhea. Nutrition by the parenteral route allows the intestinal tract to rest.
3. Administer p.r.n. medications as prescribed to prevent diarrhea.
4. Measure, or estimate as accurately as possible, the amount of liquid feces lost from the body so that lost water and electrolytes can be replaced by parenteral fluids. All fluids lost and gained by the body should be recorded on the intake-output record.
5. Measure body weight daily to detect significant changes in fluid balance. Daily weights are helpful in detecting fluid volume deficit, particularly if the liquid stools have not been measured.
6. Report substantial improvement in the patient's condition early so that he can return to oral intake as soon as tolerated.

(Dietary considerations for the patient with diarrhea are discussed in Chapter 14.)

Important nursing considerations and actions in the care of the patient with recent *ileostomy* include:

1. Measure and record the fluid lost by ileostomy, as well as other fluid losses and gains by the body.
2. Be alert for symptoms of water and electrolyte disturbances in the immediate postoperative period; potassium deficit is the most frequent imbalance. Other imbalances may include sodium deficit and fluid volume deficit. Patients with ileostomies are more likely to develop water and electrolyte disturbances when their stomas first begin to function, as shown by a comparison of the amount of water and electrolytes lost in a 24-hour period in the early postoperative period, with the amounts lost in a similar period after the ileostomy has adapted. Fluid loss from a recent ileostomy may be as high as 4,000 ml. in 24 hours; each liter of the fluid may contain 130 mEq. of sodium and 16 mEq. of potassium. (Potassium loss from a recent ileostomy may range from 4 to 98 mEq. per liter.) An adapted ileostomy usually loses no more than 500 ml. in 24 hours; each liter of fluid may contain 46 mEq. of sodium and 3 mEq. of potassium.

Nursing responsibilities in the care of the patient with *intestinal suction* include:

1. Irrigate the tube with an isotonic or hypotonic electrolyte solution, or as instructed by the physician. Plain water should never be used to irrigate intestinal suction tubes, particularly those located low in the intestines, since plain water is injurious to the mucosa of the ileum. In addition, it promotes increased secretion of intestinal juice and causes electrolytes to be withdrawn from the extracellular fluid in an attempt to render it isotonic. The irrigating solution is sucked out with electrolytes from the intestinal juice and from the extracellular fluid.
2. Record the irrigating solution volume as

intake and whatever is recovered as output.

3. Prohibit the intake of water or other electrolyte-free solutions in liquid or solid form, for the same reason as described in number 1. Ice chips made from a suitable electrolyte solution, such as isotonic solution of sodium chloride or Lytren, may be administered if prescribed by the physician.
4. Measure and record the amount of fluid lost by suction, as well as all fluid gains and losses by the body.

Prolonged Use of Laxatives and Enemas

The prolonged use of laxatives and enemas results in serious water and electrolyte disturbances, particularly potassium deficit. Other possible deficits include sodium deficit and fluid volume deficit.

Cathartics increase the water and electrolyte output through the fecal route, by hastening the excretion of fecal contents and thus reducing the absorption time. Irritant cathartics cause hypermotility of the bowel by irritating the bowel mucosa. Saline cathartics draw water from the extracellular fluid into the bowel. The distended bowel produces mechanical stimulation and the large amount of fluid is propelled out of the bowel. A large fluid volume deficit can result from continued use of saline cathartics, which interfere with electrolyte absorption from the intestines.

Enemas also deplete body water and electrolytes, particularly if plain water is used. Electrolytes from the extracellular fluid enter the bowel to make the water isotonic. Then the water and electrolytes are excreted by propulsive movements initiated by distension of the bowel with water.

The nurse should teach patients to avoid the repeated use of cathartics and enemas; when frequent bowel irrigations are indicated, an isotonic electrolyte solution should be used. (A number of measures to help patients overcome the habitual use of laxatives and enemas are described in Chapter 14.)

Fistulas and Drainage Tubes

Gastrointestinal fluids can also be lost through fistulas, whereby deficits of sodium, potassium, chloride, or bicarbonate may result, depending on the area in which the fistula is located.

An educated guess as to the content of the fluid and imbalances likely to accompany its loss can be made by reviewing the usual electrolyte content of the fluid in the region of the fistula. (See Table 19-3.) For example, fluid from a pancreatic fistula has a high sodium content—as much as 185 mEq./L. Thus, one would expect a sodium deficit to result unless adequate sodium replacement is carried out. Because pancreatic juice is alkaline, one would expect metabolic acidosis to accompany its loss from the body. When in doubt, the physician may choose to test the fluid's pH and electrolyte content.

In addition to pH changes, fistulas can cause a serious contraction of extracellular fluid volume. For example, a duodenal or jejunal fistula may drain 3 to 6 L. daily; a pancreatic fistula may drain 2 L. daily.

If possible, the nurse should attempt to measure the fluid lost by way of a fistula. If not, she should try to estimate the volume as accurately as possible. Statements as to how much of a dressing was saturated, as well as extent of gown and linen saturation, help the physician plan fluid replacement therapy.

A large volume of bile can be lost after cholecystectomy when a T-tube is inserted. The nurse should measure this drainage the same as she does drainage obtained by gastrointestinal suction. The physician has to know the amount lost from the body in order to replace the water and electrolyte losses with parenteral fluids. The nurse should be alert for symptoms of sodium deficit when large volumes of bile are lost, especially if sodium is also being lost by gastric suction. Bile has an alkaline pH, so one would anticipate metabolic acidosis if the bile loss is prolonged.

Trapped Gastrointestinal Fluids

Fluids trapped in an obstructed bowel, or in the peritoneal cavity, are "lost" because they are not available for use by the body. Yet, they cannot be directly measured as one measures fluid losses caused by vomiting or suction. Trapped fluids present a problem in planning fluid replacement therapy. Gastrointestinal conditions associated with fluid accumulation in the body include gastrointestinal obstruction, peritonitis and cirrhosis of the liver.

GASTROINTESTINAL OBSTRUCTION Gastrointestinal obstruction is accompanied by serious imbalances in water and electrolytes, the nature of which depends on the site of the obstruction.

If the *pylorus* is obstructed, gastric contents cannot enter the intestines and are lost by vomiting; the patient may develop metabolic alkalosis. This imbalance occurs because excessive amounts of hydrogen and chloride ions are lost in vomiting.

If the *upper small intestine* is obstructed, the patient will vomit intestinal juices and gastric juice. The loss of acid and alkaline fluids may be approximately equal; this prevents serious disturbances in pH.

If the obstruction is in a *distal segment* of the *small intestine*, the patient may vomit larger quantities of alkaline fluids than of acid fluids. (Recall that secretions below the pylorus are mainly alkaline.) Thus metabolic acidosis can result from a low intestinal obstruction.

If the obstruction is *below the proximal colon*, most of the gastrointestinal fluids will have been absorbed before reaching the point of obstruction. Solid fecal material accumulates until symptoms of discomfort develop. Reverse peristalsis may cause vomiting of a fecal nature (which can be severe) late in bowel obstruction.

Small intestinal obstruction traps gastrointestinal fluids and gas proximal to the obstruction. Large quantities of water and electrolytes continue to be secreted into the bowel lumen, even in the absence of oral intake. Also, the increased pressure within the distended bowel draws fluid from the plasma and the tissues. Decreased selectivity of the intestinal membrane allows plasma proteins to enter both the intestinal lumen and the gut wall. Due to distention, the mucosa of the bowel above the obstruction is greatly stimulated to secrete more fluid. The edematous bowel wall is not able to absorb the large fluid volume; thus, the distention becomes progressively greater. Ten liters or more of fluid can collect in the bowel, resulting in severe extracellular fluid volume deficit. Plasma volume is substantially reduced and hypovolemic shock often ensues. In addition to fluid, the gut is distended by gas, mostly from swallowed air. Stasis of the gut also causes accumulation of gas produced by bacterial action and diffusion from the bloodstream.

Blood loss from a strangulated hernia may be great. The volume of blood sequestered into an infarcted bowel segment may be approximately 10 per cent of the total blood volume for every 24 hours of obstruction. A reduced circulating blood volume causes hypotension, rapid thready pulse and decreased renal blood flow with azotemia and oliguria. Death may result unless the blood volume is restored.

Nursing Implications The nurse should frequently observe the vital signs of patients with gastrointestinal obstruction. A fall in blood pressure with an increased pulse rate indicates further contraction of the plasma volume and oncoming circulatory collapse. Such findings should be quickly reported to the physician. Fluid administration before surgery aims at stabilizing the vital signs sufficiently to withstand the stress of surgery. Balanced electrolyte solutions, plasma and whole blood are frequently used replacement fluids. (Nursing responsibilities in parenteral therapy are described in Chapter 16.) The hourly urinary output should be observed; oliguria or anuria are indications of inadequate fluid replacement. Urinary specific gravity is high when fluid replacement is inadequate. When possible, the urinary output should be at least 50 ml. per hour before surgery.

Recall that the volume of fluid trapped in the intestine can only be estimated. Weight measurements are also valueless in detecting the amount of fluid trapped in the bowel. Careful observation of vital signs, the patient's appearance, urinary volume, and specific gravity are significant.

PERITONITIS Peritonitis involves the loss of extracellular fluid into the peritoneal cavity as an inflammatory exudate, causing fluid volume deficit.

Calcium deficit can also occur in generalized peritonitis and acute pancreatitis, because large amounts of calcium are immobilized in the diseased tissues and exudates, for reasons unclear.

CIRRHOSIS OF THE LIVER WITH ASCITES

Ascites results from a combination of factors: (1) mechanical obstruction to venous outflow from the cirrhotic liver; (2) increased capillary permeability; (3) hypoalbuminemia; (4) hormonal effects. Water and electrolyte disturbances that may occur in cirrhosis of the liver are summarized in Table 19-4.

Symptoms of cirrhosis are variable but may include the following:

weakness and fatigue

anorexia, nausea, vomiting, diarrhea or constipation
(blood from the portal vein backs into the gastrointestinal organs and interferes with their normal activity)

abdominal fullness
(at first due to flatulence, later to ascites)

weight loss
(may be masked by excessive fluid retention)

enlarged liver
(at first the liver may be enlarged with fatty tissue, later it becomes small, hard and nodular)

enlarged spleen
(spleen is engorged with venous blood from the portal system)

low grade fever

jaundice

edema due to hypoalbuminemia

putrid, fecal odor to the breath

hypoglycemia
(glycogen metabolism impaired)

spider angiomata
(dilated superficial vessels resembling small bluish-red spiders may appear in the skin of the face and trunk)

palmar erythema

enlarged male breasts and atrophy of testicles
(caused by the liver's inability to deactivate estrogen)

embarrassed respirations if the amount of ascites is large
(however, if a high ammonia level is present, hyperventilation may occur)

Portal hypertension causes enlarged abdominal veins, esophageal varices and internal hemorrhoids
(these may be sites of profuse hemorrhage)

increased bleeding tendencies, due to vitamin K deficiency and decreased prothrombin formation

deficiency of vitamins A, C and K caused by inadequate formation, utilization and storage by the liver

intensified reaction to certain medications, caused by the liver's inability to detoxify them
(morphine and barbiturates should be avoided in patients with advanced liver disease)

greater susceptibility to infection, secondary to decreased formation of antibodies by the liver

elevated ammonia level at first causes dullness, drowsiness, loss of memory, slow, slurred speech and personality changes—later, these may progress to confusion and disorientation, and finally, to stupor and coma

"hepatic flap" is caused by a high ammonia level—this tremor is characterized by spasmodic flexion and extension at the wrists and fingers, as well as lateral finger twitching
(hepatic flap can be elicited in susceptible patients by elevating the arms, hyperextending the hands, and spreading the fingers)

Patients with ascites are treated with low sodium diets and diuretics; accurate intake-output records and weight charts are helpful to the physician in planning the degree of sodium restriction and the diuretic regimen. Dietary restriction of sodium to less than 200 mg. daily prevents additional fluid retention in most patients. Without the need for frequent paracentesis, protein is conserved and a high caloric, moderately high protein, vitamin supplemented diet may be better utilized. If dietary sodium restriction alone does not suffice, diuretic therapy

Table 19-4. Water and Electrolyte Disturbances in Cirrhosis of the Liver with Ascites

Water and Electrolyte Disturbance	*Cause*
Sodium and water retention	Aldosterone level elevated (recall that aldosterone causes Na retention, which in turn causes water retention) (the liver normally inactivates aldosterone and prevents its excessive buildup in the body; however, the cirrhotic liver does not perform this function well)
Low plasma sodium level (which may occur)	Antidiuretic hormone level elevated (due to failure of the liver to inactivate ADH) (recall that ADH causes the kidneys to retain water) Frequent paracentesis Severe dietary Na restriction (sometimes Na intake is reduced to less than 100 mg. daily to control ascites) Na moves into the cells to replace K loss (K loss is the result of diuresis, malnutrition, or hyperaldosteronism)
Decreased plasma protein level (hypoalbuminemia results in reduced plasma osmotic pull)	Albumin lost in ascites (1 L. of ascites contains as much albumin as 200 ml. of whole blood) (Normally, blood flowing into and out of the liver has the same volume. In cirrhosis, however, the volume of hepatic venous outflow is reduced by one-half. This mechanical blockage leads to the formation of an ultrafiltrate of blood which escapes into the abdominal cavity) Decreased protein synthesis due to liver dysfunction
Generalized edema	Reduced plasma protein level allows fluid to leave the plasma space and enter the tissue space Excessive aldosterone and ADH levels cause fluid retention Portal hypertension causes increased hydrostatic pressure and thus edema of the lower extremities
Potassium deficit (severe potassium deficit is often a late manifestation of liver disease)	Aldosterone level elevated (recall that aldosterone causes K loss) Poor dietary intake due to anorexia and nausea Prolonged use of potassium-losing diuretics
Elevated blood ammonia level (ammonia ties up glutamic acid which is necessary for brain tissue functioning, and it interferes with glucose oxidation, upon which the brain relies for energy)	Failure of the diseased liver to convert ammonia to urea (The kidneys produce ammonia and normally the liver converts it to urea; the urea is subsequently excreted by the kidneys. Failure of the damaged liver to convert ammonia to urea causes the ammonia level to rise.) Occurrence of gastrointestinal hemorrhage causes the intestine to digest blood proteins, in turn causing the ammonia level to rise
Respiratory alkalosis (which may occur if the ammonia level is high)	A high ammonia level acts as a respiratory stimulant and may induce hyperventilation
Magnesium deficit (which occurs in some cases of alcoholic cirrhosis)	Poor dietary intake Alcohol produces Mg diuresis
Calcium deficit may occur	Possibly due to inadequate storage of vitamin D by the diseased lever

may be necessary. It is best not to use thiazide or mercurial diuretics daily because of the danger of potassium deficit. Potassium supplements may be given when hypokalemia is a problem. An aldosterone blocking agent may be used in conjunction with other diuretics when advanced disease causes more resistant fluid retention. (Recall that an aldosterone blocking agent, such as spironolactone (Aldactone), causes sodium excretion and potassium retention.) Eventually, patients with ascites become refractory to diuretics and require paracentesis to relieve symptoms of intra-abdominal pressure and respiratory distress.

As much as 20 L. of ascitic fluid may accumulate in one week; unfortunately, its removal only causes more to form. Paracentesis further depletes the body of protein, sodium and water. The patient should be observed for symptoms of circulatory collapse following the removal of a large volume of fluid by paracentesis, since a rapid shift from the plasma to the ascitic fluid space may follow the procedure; acute sodium depletion may also follow paracentesis. There is reaccumulation of ascitic fluid with flow of water and sodium from the interstitial fluid and secondarily from the plasma into the abdominal cavity, reducing plasma volume and sodium concentration. Water is retained in excess of sodium and further dilutes its concentration in plasma. The nurse should be alert for pallor, weak, rapid pulse and hypotension following the removal of a large amount of fluid by paracentesis. No more than 3 to 5 L. of ascitic fluid should be removed at a time. Albumin is sometimes administered intravenously to correct hypoalbuminemia; however, the quantity that is practical to give is often ineffective in restoring a normal plasma albumin level.

A low plasma sodium level is an indication to restrict the patient's water intake; the amount of water restriction must be prescribed by the physician. Fluids must be evenly spaced over the waking hours to avoid excessive thirst and discomfort. Severe edema may also necessitate fluid restriction.

Bleeding in the gastrointestinal tract increases ammonia formation (caused by digestion of blood proteins) and may precipitate hepatic coma. The nurse should be alert for gastrointestinal bleeding in the stool (melena) and in the vomitus (hematemesis). Sometimes enemas or cathartics are used to rid the intestine of blood and thus decrease ammonia formation. Ammonia formation caused by excessive bacterial growth in the small bowel can be decreased by the administration of bowel sterilizing antibiotics, such as neomycin. Constipation contributes to the accumulation of ammonia and must be prevented. (Ammonium chloride should not be used in diuretic therapy since it elevates blood ammonia level.)

Impending hepatic coma is an indication to temporarily eliminate protein from the diet. A decrease in protein intake results in decreased ammonia formation; as the patient improves, more protein can be added to the diet. Thiazide diuretics may increase ammonia formation and contribute to the development of hepatic coma. (Loss of potassium, caused by diuresis, apparently increases the tendency to ammonium accumulation.)

20 Fluid Balance in the Patient With Urological Disease

INTRODUCTION

The kidneys excrete water, electrolytes, and organic materials and conserve whatever amounts of these substances the body requires. They act both autonomously and in response to blood-borne messengers, such as the mineralocorticoids and antidiuretic hormone. Failure of renal function causes a variety of water and electrolyte disturbances.

ACUTE RENAL FAILURE

Etiology

Acute renal failure implies a pronounced reduction in urine flow, lasting for days or weeks, in a previously healthy person. The condition can be caused by:

Severe and prolonged shock
Severe fluid volume deficit
Hemolytic blood transfusion reaction
(lysis of red blood cells results in renal vasoconstriction and tubular blockage with hemoglobin)
Severe crushing injuries
(severely crushed muscles release large amounts of myoglobin into the blood stream; myoglobin can block the tubules and might also produce vasoconstriction)
Nephrotoxic chemicals
(such as lead, arsenic, and carbon tetrachloride)
Endotoxemia
Renal vascular occlusion

Patients with these conditions should be observed for the possible development of acute renal failure. The nurse should measure the urinary output carefully, as well as all other fluid losses and gains. A reduced urinary output may be due to excessive fluid loss through another route, or to inadequate intake; or, it may be due to acute renal failure. A urinary output under 400 ml. in the adult represents oliguria and should be reported.

Acute renal failure can be divided into two phases—oliguria and diuresis.

Oliguric Phase

PATHOLOGIC PHYSIOLOGY AND SYMPTOMS
The first manifestation of acute renal failure is decreased urinary output, usually appearing within a few hours after the causative event. Anuria is rare; instead, a 24-hour output of about 50 to 150 ml. is the rule for the first few days. After this time, the urine output gradually increases. The oliguric phase may last one day or several weeks; the average duration is 10 to 12 days in severe cases.

The nurse should be alert for symptoms of the major problems of this phase: they include potassium excess, fluid volume excess, metabolic acidosis, and uremia. Other problems include calcium deficit, sodium deficit and anemia. Death is usually due to cardiac arrest caused by potassium excess or pulmonary edema caused by fluid volume excess.

POTASSIUM EXCESS Potassium excess usually occurs in the oliguric phase. Recall that the kidneys normally excrete 80 per cent or more of the potassium lost daily from the body. When the kidneys are not functioning, potassium excretion is greatly reduced. If no protein or potassium is ingested, and if sufficient calories are supplied to prevent endogenous cellular catabolism, it is unlikely that serious potassium excess will develop during the first few weeks of oliguria. However, patients with massive crushing injuries or large quantities of necrotic tissues may have a rising plasma potassium concentration despite no intake of protein and potassium, since catabolized necrotic tissue releases potassium into the extracellular fluid. The presence of acidosis augments the intracellular to extracellular shift of potassium, thereby hastening potassium buildup in the plasma.

Recall that the normal plasma potassium level is 5 mEq./L. When this level is doubled, death may occur, due to cardiac arrest. (Excessive potassium causes weakness and dilatation of heart muscle, and cardiac arrest in diastole.)

The nurse should be alert for the symptoms of potassium excess. They include:

- Anxiety and restlessness
- Muscular weakness progressing to flaccid paralysis (primarily affects limbs and respiratory muscles)
- Respiration decreased as a result of respiratory muscle weakness
- Decreased pulse rate, finally resulting in bradycardia
- Cardiac arrhythmias
- Falling arterial blood pressure
- Cardiac arrest and death

A plasma potassium concentration of 6 mEq./L. is a cause for concern; a concentration of 7 mEq./L. demands immediate treatment. (See discussion of treatment.)

FLUID VOLUME EXCESS Fluid volume excess is a frequent problem during the oliguric phase. Symptoms include elevated venous pressure, distention of the neck veins, edema, puffy eyelids, bounding pulse, and shortness of breath. It is usually due to the excessive administration of fluids, either orally or intravenously. Hypertension, pulmonary edema and congestive heart failure are complications of fluid volume excess. Pulmonary edema is manifested by severe dyspnea, moist rales and frothy sputum.

METABOLIC ACIDOSIS Metabolic acidosis is the result of the retention of acid metabolites normally excreted in the urine; their accumulation in the bloodstream causes the pH to drop. Decreased food intake causes increased utilization of body fats and the accumulation of ketonic acids in the bloodstream. These acids further decrease the pH.

Metabolic acidosis causes a compensatory increase in pulmonary ventilation, which causes the elimination of large amounts of carbon dioxide from the lungs with a resultant decrease in the carbonic acid content of the blood. The pH is partially corrected by this mechanism. Anorexia, weakness, apathy and coma may also be symptoms of metabolic acidosis.

Vomiting commonly occurs with the development of uremia. If vomiting occurs at the time metabolic acidosis is developing, it is possible that the metabolic alkalosis accompanying vomiting may help to counteract acidosis. However, because gastric hypoacidity frequently occurs with uremia, vomiting may not have a significant effect on the pH. Extensive diarrhea contributes to the development of metabolic acidosis.

SODIUM DEFICIT The plasma sodium concentration may be normal or below normal. Contributing to sodium deficit is the administration of excessive amounts of water, which dilutes the plasma sodium. It may also be due to a shift of sodium into the cells, particularly if acidosis is present. Occasionally sodium deficit becomes severe as a result of excessive loss of sodium in vomiting, diarrhea, or as a result of treatment with certain cation exchange resins, such as Carbo-Resin. Symptoms of sodium deficit include:

- Anorexia
- Apathy or apprehension
- Abdominal cramps
- Syncope on changing positions
- Hypotension
- Rapid thready pulse
- Cold skin
- Convulsions (if sodium deficit is due to excessive water intake)

CALCIUM DEFICIT The plasma calcium concentration may be below normal; calcium deficit may be related to the increased concentration of phosphorus in the bloodstream. (Phosphorus is a constituent of one of the retained metabolic acids.) A reciprocal relation exists between calcium and phosphorus so that an increase in one causes a decrease in the other.

Calcium deficit does not usually present symptoms of tetany, probably because the decreased blood pH of metabolic acidosis favors calcium ionization. (Recall that calcium ionization increases in acidosis and decreases in alkalosis.) Chvostek's sign may be positive even though other symptoms of calcium deficit are not present. If metabolic alkalosis develops as a result of treatment with alkaline fluids, calcium deficit becomes manifest with the development of muscle twitching and convulsions.

The major significance of calcium deficit is that it enhances the toxic effects of potassium on the heart. (Recall that calcium and potassium have antagonistic actions on heart muscle.) Sodium deficit also enhances potassium toxicity because sodium is mildly antagonistic to potassium.

ANEMIA Normochromic, normocytic anemia of unknown etiology usually occurs. It is possibly due to increased blood destruction and erythropoeisis. The hematocrit may fall below 20 per cent, and the hemoglobin below 7 Gm. The degree of anemia seems to be related to the level of azotemia.

URINE CHANGES The urine is usually bloody for the first few days, becoming clear about the end of the oliguric phase. If renal failure is due to hemolytic blood transfusion reaction, the urine has a port wine color. A low specific gravity ranging from 1.002 to 1.010 characterizes the oliguric phase. (Oliguria with a low specific gravity differentiates acute renal failure from severe dehydration, which is characterized by a low urinary volume with a high specific gravity.)

UREMIA If therapy fails to relieve oliguria and uremia progresses, nausea, vomiting, diarrhea, abdominal distention and mild ulcerations of the gastrointestinal tract may occur. Cerebroneuromuscular complications may produce irritability, disorientation, stupor, convulsions and coma. The administration of an anticonvulsant, such as diphenylhydantoin (Dilantin), may be necessary to prevent fatal seizures.

Treatment

Because acute renal failure is a self-limiting condition, treatment is aimed at maintaining life long enough for the injured renal tubules to heal and resume function.

FOOD AND FLUID INTAKE

Carbohydrates *At least* 100 Gm. of carbohydrate should be administered daily; this amount decreases endogenous protein catabolism by approximately one-half and also helps prevent ketosis. Such catabolism is harmful, since it releases potassium and nitrogenous products into the extracellular fluid; plasma levels of these substances rise. Administered glucose forms glycogen, essential for restoration of cellular potassium stores.

Oral carbohydrate intake should be encouraged if nausea and vomiting are not present. Sometimes these symptoms can be relieved by dimenhydrinate (Dramamine) or diphenhydramine (Benadryl). (Hard candy supplies carbohydrates.) High carbohydrate, low protein foods are occasionally added to the diet; examples of such foods include rice, sweet or Irish potatoes, cornmeal and toast. High caloric intake decreases endogenous protein catabolism.

Intravenous carbohydrate administration is necessary if oral intake is impossible. A hypertonic carbohydrate solution must be used to supply the necessary amount of carbohydrate and to avoid excessive fluid administration. A 20 per cent glucose solution may be administered by slow drip over the 24-hour period. One liter of 10 per cent glucose in water can be used to supply 100 Gm. of carbohydrate if the patient requires as much as 1,000 ml. of water.

Insulin The addition of insulin to the carbohydrate solution can serve to increase its utilization and promote further removal of potassium from the extracellular fluid. The patient should be observed for signs of hypoglycemia after the administration of a concentrated carbohydrate solution, particularly if insulin has been added to it. The pancreas is stimulated to secrete insulin due to the high carbohydrate intake, and sudden discontinuing of the infusion may result in an excessive supply of insulin; 200 or 300 ml. of a 5 per cent glucose solution may be administered following the concentrated solution to counteract this effect.

An emergency measure for the treatment of potassium excess is the administration of 50 ml. of 50 per cent dextrose with 20 units of regular insulin intravenously every 3 or 4 hours.

Restriction of Potassium and Protein Intake High potassium foods should be excluded from the diet because the nonfunctioning kidneys are unable to excrete potassium. Foods to avoid include meats, legumes, nuts, milk, fresh fruits, fruit juices, tea and coffee.

The diet should be low in protein. Four Gm. of protein furnish 1 Gm. of urea, hence a high protein intake adds to the severity of the uremia. In addition to urea, protein foods provide potassium, sulfates, phosphates and water.

High Fat, High Caloric Diet Fat provides less water of oxidation than carbohydrate or protein; thus it is least likely to cause an excessive fluid volume. Frozen butter balls, ranging in size from 5 to 15 Gm., are frequently administered to achieve a high caloric intake. Some are prepared with powdered sugar to increase palatability and caloric value.

Tube feedings composed of Lipomul, glucose, vitamins and water have been administered to patients with acute renal failure to increase caloric intake. Use of tube feedings can be hazardous, however, when frank uremia is present, because of the possibility of producing gastric bleeding.

The aim of the diet in uremia is to give as many non-protein, non-electrolyte calories as possible.

Restriction of Fluid Intake The amount of fluid administered must be carefully planned to suit the patient's needs, with the body considered as a closed system; excessive fluid intake should be avoided. The physician calculates a fluid dose that will just replace fluid losses from the body; insensible losses are approximately 500 to 600 ml. The rest of the fluid dose matches the urinary output of the previous day and other losses, such as from vomiting or diarrhea. The nurse must keep an accurate account of fluid gains and losses, because an inaccurate record could lead to a fluid overdose and fluid volume excess with its dangerous sequelae. (Nursing considerations in measuring and recording fluid intake and output are discussed in Chapter 12.)

Accurate daily body weight measurements are also necessary for determining the desired fluid dose. (Nursing considerations in obtaining accurate body weight measurements are discussed in Chapter 12.) With decreased food intake, the patient can be expected to lose about one-half pound daily. Failure to lose this amount implies fluid retention; on the other hand, a loss in excess of this amount implies excessive loss of body fluid.

The nurse should check the fluid intake orders carefully and avoid administering an excessive amount. All routes of fluid gain should be considered when recording the daily fluid intake. For example, fluid retained from an enema counts as part of the daily intake.

Alkalinizing Fluids When acidosis is manifested by frank Kussmaul respiration, stupor, or coma, alkalinizing fluids, such as sodium bicarbonate or sodium lactate are administered. Indiscriminately used, these fluids may cause volume excess, congestive heart failure and pulmonary edema.

Mannitol The intravenous administration of 50 to 100 ml. of 25% mannitol is usually advocated early in acute renal failure. Mannitol acts as an osmotic diuretic and increases urinary output. It is thought that an increased urinary flow helps flush out the clogged tubules.

Sodium Administration Sodium deficit is usually treated by limiting the water intake. Occasionally hypertonic solution of sodium chloride is administered to correct a severe sodium deficit produced by excessive vomiting or diarrhea. Hypertonic solution of sodium chloride should be administered with caution because it can easily result in fluid volume excess with congestive heart failure and pulmonary edema.

Calcium Administration Calcium deficit can be treated with calcium gluconate by the oral or intravenous route—orally if nausea and vomiting are absent, intravenously in all other cases. Ten ml. of a 10 per cent calcium gluconate solution is the recommended intravenous dose for an adult. Calcium can cause pronounced improvement in electrocardiograph changes produced by potassium excess, even though the plasma potassium concentration is not changed.

Calcium may be indicated when alkalinizing fluids are given to treat acidosis, since symptoms of calcium deficit may be induced by an increase in blood pH. (Calcium ionization is decreased when alkalinity of the extracellular fluid increases.) Restoration of a normal pH may disclose a calcium deficit that was not evident when the plasma pH was below normal.

Blood Administration Packed red blood cells may be administered if the hematocrit drops below 20 per cent, the hemoglobin drops below 7 Gm., or obvious blood loss occurs.

Pus Drainage and Debridement of Necrotic Tissue If the patient has dirty wounds, undrained pus collections, or necrotic tissue, the plasma potassium concentration rises as a result of catabolism. To prevent severe potassium excess, it is important that necrotic tissue and pus be removed.

Cation Exchange Resins Cation exchange resins may be used to increase potassium excretion from the bowel. The resins may be taken by mouth, if tolerated, or may be instilled as a retention enema. When the resin is administered orally, the solution in which it is suspended should be recorded as part of the daily fluid allowance. While the cation exchange resins are given to remove potassium ions from the intestinal tract, they also remove other cations, such as sodium, calcium and magnesium. It may be necessary to replace these ions if the resins are used for more than a few days. Such patients should have regular electrolyte studies.

Sodium polystrene sulfonate (Kayexalate) is a sodium-potassium exchange resin. During its use, sodium ions are partially released by the resin in the intestine and replaced by potassium ions from the body. Hypokalemia may occur if the effective dose is exceeded; it is necessary, therefore, to determine the plasma potassium level daily. Since sodium is released in the intestine during electrolyte exchange, the resin should be administered with caution to patients with heart or renal failure. (Signs of excessive sodium retention include hypertension and edema.) The average adult oral dose of sodium polystrene sulfonate is 15 Gm., 1 to 4 times daily in a small quantity of water or syrup. Sorbitol, a nonresorptive cathartic, may be given to combat constipation. The resin may also be given as an enema; each adult dose, usually 30 Gm., is administered in 150 to 200 ml. of water. Best results are achieved when the emulsion is warmed to body temperature before use. The enema should be retained for 4 to 10 hours, if possible, and followed by a cleansing enema. The enema vehicle administered with the cation exchange resin should be measured before instillation and after expulsion, with the amount absorbed by the bowel counted as part of the daily fluid allowance.

Cation exchange resins are of most value as a preventive rather than an emergency measure to reduce severe potassium excess.

Diuretic Phase

PATHOLOGIC PHYSIOLOGY AND SYMPTOMS

The diuretic phase begins when the 24-hour urine volume approaches 1 L. a day, usually around the tenth day after onset; in some instances, it may not occur for 14 to 21 days. During this phase, the partially regenerated tubules are unable to concentrate urine, and the glomerular filtrate is excreted virtually unchanged. Thus, the patient's condition does not improve in the first few days of the diuretic phase; indeed, uremia may be more severe during this period than at any other time. Convulsions, stupor, nausea, vomiting, hematemesis, bloody diarrhea, or hemorrhage may occur. The reason for the severity of the uremia lies in the rapid contraction of the total body fluid. For this reason, early and prompt replacement of fluid is needed until the blood urea nitrogen begins to fall. This replacement must be carried out, even though it may cause a persistence of edema and other untoward symptoms. The chief cause of death during the diuretic phase is infection, since the patient has extremely low resistance.

The amount of urinary output depends on the treatment the patient received during the oliguric phase. If fluid overloading was allowed, the urine volume may be more than 5,000 ml. daily. If the patient was well managed, the urine volume is not excessive.

Treatment

Treatment during the diuretic phase depends on the amount of water and electrolytes excreted in the urine. The patient's body weight should be closely observed. If the body weight decreases at a moderate rate, oral fluids are not forced; if, however, it decreases too rapidly, water and electrolytes must be supplied in sufficient amounts to prevent deficits.

Alkalinizing fluids may be administered if acidosis is severe. Since excessive sodium loss may occur during diuresis, the daily plasma sodium level should be observed and replacement carried out if necessary. Potassium replacement may also be required.

If uremia is severe, as indicated by a high plasma potassium level, a high BUN, and pronounced symptoms, dialysis may be indicated.

PERITONEAL DIALYSIS Because of its large surface area, the peritoneum can be used as a dialyzing membrane for the removal of toxic substances, body wastes, water, and electrolytes. Peritoneal dialysis can be used in the treatment of acute renal failure from any cause. While it is only about one-sixth as effective as hemodialysis, it is nevertheless an efficient method for treating renal failure. Its chief advantage is that it can be used in all hospitals, while the artificial kidney is usually available only in large medical centers. Peritoneal dialysis requires only a fraction of the personnel and equipment needed for hemodialysis. Although the physician inserts and removes the peritoneal catheter, the nursing staff is primarily responsible for the care of the patient during the treatment. Peritoneal dialysis can be used in patients with shock when arterial blood flow is insufficient for hemodialysis, and because it is a slower process, biochemical problems do not arise as frequently as in hemodialysis. Nonetheless, careful attention must be given to maintaining fluid and electrolyte requirements, and plasma electrolyte concentrations should be checked at regular intervals. A major disadvantage of peritoneal dialysis is its inefficiency; what can be accomplished with 6 hours of hemodialysis takes 36 to 48 hours with peritoneal dialysis.

It is most often used for supporting patients with acute renal failure, for certain drug ingestions, or during evaluation of patients with chronic renal failure. Indications for dialysis include high plasma levels of potassium and urea, severe metabolic acidosis, pulmonary edema, and deterioration of the patient's general condition.

A solution for peritoneal dialysis must, in most instances, approach the electrolyte composition and tonicity of the plasma so that normal plasma constituents will not be altered. It must be at least slightly hyperosmotic to plasma to prevent its absorption with development of fluid volume excess. Various concentrations of dextrose or sorbitol may be used to render the solution hyperosmotic. Dialysis solutions with 1.5% dextrose are available.* These slightly hyperosmotic solutions are useful in removing abnormal plasma constituents, such as barbiturates, or excessive amounts of normal plasma constituents, such as potassium or calcium. Dialysis solutions are also available with a 7% dextrose concentration.* These more hyperosmotic solutions are useful in removing edema fluid. An intermediate osmotic effect can be achieved with the use of a dialysate containing a 4.25% dextrose concentration. Dialysis solutions are available with and without potassium; potassium is omitted only in cases of hyperkalemia. Solutions containing about 4 mEq. of potassium per liter are used for patients with normal plasma potassium levels. (If the patient has hypokalemia, a solution with a greater than normal potassium concentration may be employed.) Varying concentrations of potassium, depending on the patient's need, may be added to potassium-free solutions. The addition of potassium is particularly important for the

* Inpersol (Abbott Laboratories)
Dianeal (Baxter Laboratories)
Peridial (Cutter Laboratories)

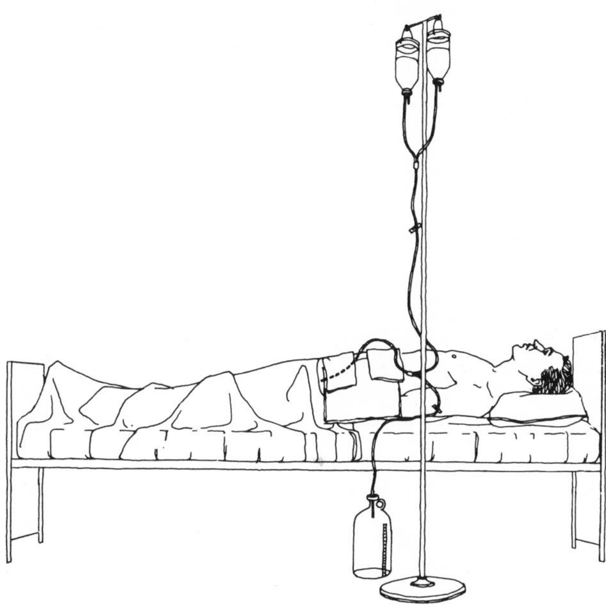

Fig. 20-1. Peritoneal dialysis setup. (Abbott Laboratories: Inpersol. pp. 16-17. North Chicago, Illinois, 1964)

digitalized patient, since the plasma potassium level may fall rapidly during dialysis. (Recall that potassium deficit makes the patient more susceptible to digitalis toxicity.)

It is desirable to warm the dialysis solution to body temperature before administration. The bottles can be warmed by immersion in a warm water bath set at 37°C. (98.6°F.) Rubber bands should be used to hold the wet labels in place; a glass marking pencil can be used to indicate the contents of the bottle. To avoid contamination of the equipment, the outside of the bottles should be dried carefully before use. A warming cabinet is sometimes used to warm the dialysis solution; care should be taken to avoid overheating. Infusion of the dialysate at body temperature is more comfortable for the patient, increases peritoneal clearance, and prevents hypothermia.

Medications should be added before the bottles are hung for infusion. Heparin is added to prevent the formation of fibrin clots (the dose is not sufficient to produce systemic heparinization). Antibiotics may be added to the dialysate if necessary. Extreme care is required to prevent contamination when medications are added; the most frequent serious complication of peritoneal dialysis is peritonitis. Some dialysates are available in single 2 L. bottles; because medications are added to only one container, the opportunity for contamination is reduced. If two separate 1 L. bottles are used, contamination risk can be minimized by adding medications to only one of the bottles. (Solutions from two separate bottles mix quickly in the abdomen.)

Prior to the initiation of peritoneal dialysis, the patient should be given a careful explanation of the treatment; reassurance and support are required throughout the lengthy procedure. The position of choice during peritoneal dialysis is a modified semi-Fowler's. Meperidine (Demerol) may be given one-half hour before the insertion of the catheter to achieve analgesia and sedation.

Before insertion of the peritoneal catheter, the bladder and colon should be emptied to avoid injury. The patient's weight and vital signs should be checked, prior to the procedure, for later reference.

After the abdomen is shaved and prepared, an abdominal paracentesis is performed and a catheter inserted into the peritoneal cavity. Two liters of solution are allowed to enter in about 10 minutes. If the patient complains of discomfort when the fluid is instilled, the flow rate may have to be reduced; the physician should be notified if the pain does not subside. Analgesics may be administered if necessary; lidocaine may be added to the dialysate to alleviate pain. If the pain persists, the physician may need to change the location of the peritoneal catheter. The fluid is left in for 30 to 60 minutes and then drained into a bottle or plastic drainage bag. (Drainage of the fluid from the peritoneal cavity should not take longer than 30 minutes.) To facilitate drainage, it may be necessary to gently massage the abdomen or adjust the patient's position.

The dialysis solution is instilled and drained at regular intervals until the patient shows definite improvement. Peritoneal dialysis is usually performed for 36 to 48 hours in the adult patient.

The nurse should use meticulous technique during peritoneal dialysis to prevent peritonitis. Abdominal dressings should be checked frequently for bleeding or leakage of solution; if present, the physician should be notified. Wet dressings should be changed immediately to minimize the chance of wound contamination. Vital signs should be observed periodically for significant changes. The time each exchange begins and the amount of fluid instilled and removed should be recorded. When the amount of drainage is more than the amount of fluid infused, the patient's cumulative fluid balance is said to be negative. When the amount of drainage is less than the amount of fluid infused, the patient's cumulative fluid balance is said to be positive. The physician should stipulate the limits of positive and negative balance considered desirable for each patient. As a general rule, however, a positive balance exceeding 500 ml. or the negative balance exceeding 1,000 ml. should be reported. The use of hypertonic dialysates, such as those with a 7% dextrose concentration, may cause the amount of drainage to exceed the amount of infused fluid by 500 ml. per exchange. Vital signs should be checked often and the patient observed for signs of shock when hypertonic dialysates are used.

A too vigorous use of dialysis can cause excessive loss or absorption of fluid. Symptoms of fluid volume deficit or excess should be reported. Fluid intake and output from all routes should be measured and recorded. Finally, body weight measurements are invaluable in assessing the patient's state of fluid balance. An in-bed scale is of great value in monitoring weight changes during dialysis. (See the section on weight measurement in Chapter 12.)

CHRONIC RENAL DISEASE

Etiology

Chronic renal disease can result from glomerulonephritis, pyelonephritis, polycystic kidneys, essential hypertension, and urinary obstruction.

PATHOLOGIC PHYSIOLOGY AND SYMPTOMS

Water and Electrolyte Changes Chronic renal failure is characterized by progressive disease with loss of renal tissue. Eventually, renal blood flow and glomerular filtration decrease. The tubules lose their ability to form ammonia and to excrete nonprotein nitrogenous products. One of the earliest regulatory functions of the kidney to fail is the maximal urine concentrating ability. It becomes necessary for the kidneys to excrete a large urinary volume (up to 3000 ml. per day) to rid the body of wastes. Later, the tubules gradually lose their ability to conserve electrolytes as well as water.

Plasma potassium concentrations vary widely in patients with chronic renal failure. Some have normal levels until oliguria and starvation occur. In some cases of chronic nephritis with polyuria, the plasma potassium may be low. Excessive aldosterone production may cause a low plasma potassium level, whereas, excessive dietary protein intake or the administration of stored blood may cause the potassium concentration to rise. High plasma potassium levels do not usually occur until late in chronic renal failure. Metabolic acidosis occurs as a result of the impaired renal excretion of acid metabolites and the inability of the tubules to form ammonia. (Acidosis is often responsible for the patient's early morning nausea.) Although the respiratory mechanism partially corrects the decreased blood pH, it is sometimes necessary to treat the acidosis medically; sodium bicarbonate tablets may be given, in dosages of several grams per day, depending on the severity of the acidosis and on the sodium intake limitations.

Sodium is lost in the urine, but the plasma level usually remains near normal if the patient is not placed on a severely restricted low-sodium diet, or if excessive sodium loss does not occur with vomiting and diarrhea. Some patients retain sodium when it is given in average amounts. Fluid volume excess, hypertension, congestive heart failure and pulmonary edema may result from the excessive administration of salt to such patients. The plasma calcium concentration is decreased, and the phosphorus concentration is increased. Because acidosis is present, tetany is not common. Muscle twitching may occur due to calcium deficit, but convulsions in patients with chronic renal failure are usually of another origin.

Other Changes Anemia occurs in chronic renal failure; its severity is related to the degree of azotemia. Mild anemia does not usually present symptoms. Severe anemia can contribute to the development of congestive heart failure. Anemia also predisposes to acidosis because of the decreased buffer action of the deficient red blood cells.

Mild bleeding, such as bruising or bleeding of gums, may occur early. Severe bleeding into the brain or lungs can develop late. The cause of the bleeding tendency in uremic patients is not known; it is thought to be related to the failure of a platelet factor. Other complications of chronic renal failure include pericarditis, pleurisy, hyperparathyroidism, osteomalacia, osteodystrophy and uremia. Pericarditis and pleurisy are usually late symptoms; they may be associated with myocarditis and pneumonitis. (Hyperparathyroidism is discussed in Chapter 22.)

Demineralization of bone, most often in the hands, may be revealed by x-ray. Chronic negative calcium balance can produce osteodystrophy in the adult; symptoms may include pain and stiffness of the limbs and joints. There is great variability in the extent of osteodystrophy seen among adult patients with chronic renal disease. In childhood, chronic renal insufficiency may cause bone lesions similar to those of vitamin D deficiency rickets.

Uremia is a toxic condition caused by failure of the kidneys to excrete urea, potassium, organic acids and other metabolic waste products. Symptoms of uremia include:

- Chronic fatigue
- Insomnia
- Anorexia
- Intractable nausea and vomiting
- Ammonia odor to breath, unpleasant metallic taste in mouth
- Pruritis (skin is dry and scaly, with excoriations caused by scratching)
- Pale sallow skin (due to urochrome deposition in skin and to anemia)
- Increased bleeding tendency revealed by epistaxis, bleeding gums, easy bruising, petechiae, and conjunctival hemorrhage
- Coarse muscular twitching, first occurring during sleep
- Deep, rapid respirations (a respiratory attempt to compensate for metabolic acidosis)
- Chest discomfort (may be caused by pericarditis or pleurisy)
- Neuropathy (foot drop, impotence, anesthesia, motor weakness and paralysis)
- Hypertensive symptoms such as headache and visual difficulties (visual difficulties due to retinal hemorrhages)
- Uremic frost (urea crystals excreted through sweat glands, heaviest on nose, forehead, and neck)
- Gradual diminution of mental acuity over a period of time, leading to semicoma
- Transient episodes of lucidity or agitated psychotic behavior
- Generalized convulsions

Treatment

FOOD AND FLUIDS Patients with symptoms of chronic renal failure should have their protein intake reduced, a measure which alone may improve symptoms greatly. A caloric intake high enough to prevent endogenous protein catabolism is also indicated. Oral intake may be discouraged by the presence of nausea and vomiting; medication, such as chlorpromazine, may be required. The nurse should seek such an order when necessary to relieve the patient's nausea. Attractive small frequent feedings may encourage eating.

Encouraging activity may also stimulate appetite, provided congestive heart failure requiring bed-rest is not present.

Sodium restriction may be necessary for some patients and harmful to others. Those retaining excessive sodium and water require a low-sodium diet. On the other hand, patients who excrete large quantities of sodium in the urine require a normal diet to prevent sodium deficit. The physician has to determine sodium needs according to test diets and clinical observations, such as excessive weight gain. (Low-sodium diets are described in Chapter 14.) If the plasma potassium level is elevated, foods containing potassium should be eliminated.

Patients with chronic renal failure should be urged to drink from 2,000 to 3,000 ml. of water daily to aid in the elimination of urinary waste products. If the patient is unable to excrete large volumes of water, however, fluid intake should be limited to his needs. In the final stages of chronic renal failure, patients may experience extreme thirst, probably due to cellular dehydration produced by the increased osmotic effect of the high urea level. Such patients may drink themselves into dilutional hyponatremia. Thirst is an unreliable guide to the uremic patient's state of hydration.

DIURETICS Patients with excessive salt and water retention may be helped by diuretics, such as the thiazides or the mercurials. The danger of toxicity from diuretics is reduced by giving them intermittently rather than daily. Patients who require frequent diuretic therapy can be protected from toxicity by alternating drugs every few days.

ALKALINIZING FLUIDS Severe metabolic acidosis may be treated with alkaline fluids such as sodium bicarbonate or sodium lactate, although the danger of giving a sodium salt to a patient with a tendency to sodium retention must be considered. Potassium citrate or potassium bicarbonate can be given to patients who are losing potassium because of excessive production of aldosterone. Daily weight measurements are valuable clues to the body's fluid volume status. Symptoms of increased fluid retention should be reported.

TREATMENT OF CALCIUM DEFICIT When the pH is increased due to the administration of alkalinizing fluids, it may be necessary to administer calcium to prevent tetany. Measures to reduce the high phosphorus level may cause an increased calcium level. Therefore, aluminum hydroxide is sometimes administered to combine with phosphate in the gastrointestinal tract.

BLOOD TRANSFUSIONS Low hematocrit and hemoglobin concentration may necessitate blood transfusion. Symptoms of low hemoglobin include weakness, shortness of breath and anorexia. Blood transfusion may relieve these symptoms if uremia is not present. Stored blood should not be used if potassium excess is a problem. (Recall that stored blood is high in potassium.) Fresh packed red blood cells should be used if fluid volume excess is present.

ANTIBIOTICS Patients with uremia have a low resistance to infection and commonly develop pneumonitis. Urinary tract infections may be the precipitating cause of renal failure. Urinary catheters should not be used unless absolutely necessary because of the danger of infection. Although antibiotics are needed to combat infection, they must be used cautiously in patients with renal failure. It must be remembered that antibiotics which rely upon the kidneys for excretion will be retained. Elevated levels of certain antibiotics may be harmful to the patient; for this reason, it is necessary to decrease the dosage.

DIALYSIS Peritoneal dialysis is generally unsuitable for maintenance of patients with chronic renal failure. Ultimate complications of repeated peritoneal dialysis are infection with subsequent fibrous occlusion of the peritoneal cavity. Patients dislike the repeated insertion of the catheter and the prolonged period of restricted activity. The use of arteriovenous shunts has made long-term hemodialysis available to such patients. Before shunts were available, frequent cannulation of blood vessels rendered them useless and prevented frequent hemodialysis. Although valuable, external A-V shunts are not without problems; they are subject to infections and thrombosis, despite meticulous care. A technique has been described by Brescia et al. for anastomosing the distal radial artery and adjacent vein side-to-side, creating a subcutaneous A-V fistula. This internal shunt has several advantages over external shunts: (1) it allows the patient more freedom; (2) it does not require maintenance care; (3) it decreases the risks of clotting and infection; (4) it is not cosmetically undesirable. A disadvantage to the use of an internal shunt is that two venipunctures with large gauge needles are required with each dialysis treatment. (Hypertrophy of the venous side of the fistula allows access to it by repeated venipunctures.)

NEPHROTIC SYNDROME

Nephrotic syndrome refers to the concurrent occurrence of marked proteinuria, hypoalbuminemia, and generalized edema. Causes of nephrotic syndrome may include inflammatory renal disease (e.g., acute glomerulonephritis), glomerular disease associated with another systemic disease (e.g., secondary syphilis), mechanical disorders (e.g., thrombosis of a renal vein), poisons (e.g., mercury), and miscellaneous causes (e.g., renal transplant). All the causes of nephrotic syndrome involve the glomeruli, and all result in tubular degeneration.

Due to increased glomerular permeability, large amounts of albumin are lost through the kidney, resulting in decreased plasma osmotic pressure. Fluid is lost from the plasma to the interstitial space and also into the potential spaces of the body (such as the abdominal cavity, pleural cavity, and the pericardium). Edema develops first in dependent parts and later becomes generalized. Protein losses in the urine may amount to as much as 30 to 40 Gm. per day; the high protein losses result in malnutrition, and this, in turn, is responsible for muscle wasting. Hyperlipemia (abnormally high blood lipids) is also present; the high concentration of plasma lipids results from failure of the tissues to remove lipoproteins from the plasma, a condition especially apt to occur in nephrotic children.

Sodium retention is also a factor in nephrotic edema; it may be due to decreased glomerular filtration, increased tubular reabsorption, or both. Large quantities of aldosterone may be found in the urine when edema is present.

The administration of intravenous salt-free human albumin temporarily increases the protein osmotic effect of blood and draws the edema fluid into the intravascular space, increasing blood volume and stimulating sodium excretion. Unfortunately, the effects of albumin administration are only transient because the kidneys continue to lose albumin. A high protein diet will be of some benefit.

Sodium restriction helps relieve nephrotic edema, as do mercurial diuretics. ACTH may be used to decrease proteinuria and increase urine output. Although it is thought that ACTH may affect glomerular permeability and inhibit the secretion of ADH, its exact actions in relieving edema are not known.

URETERAL TRANSPLANT INTO THE INTESTINAL TRACT

Electrolyte Imbalances

Ureteral transplants can be made into the sigmoid colon (ureterosigmoidostomy), terminal end of the ileum (ureteroileostomy), or into a segment of the ileum isolated from the intestinal tract (ileal-bladder). Patients with ureteral transplants into the intestinal tract may develop metabolic acidosis and eventually potassium deficit.

Metabolic acidosis occurs when urine is reabsorbed from the intestinal tract. Recall that urine is usually acid (average pH of 6) and has a high chloride content. Absorption of urinary chloride into the bloodstream causes a compensatory decrease in bicarbonate. The decrease in the bicarbonate side of the carbonic acid–base bicarbonate balance causes the blood pH to drop.

Potassium deficit occurs, largely as the result of excessive renal chloride excretion. This can be explained in the following way: urinary chloride is absorbed from the intestine into the bloodstream and must eventually be re-excreted by the kidneys. A cation, such as potassium or sodium, is excreted with chloride. The continued absorption of urinary chloride by the intestine can deplete the body of potassium. Other factors contribute to potassium deficit. Patients with ureteral-intestinal transplants often have diarrhea, a common cause of potassium deficit. Also, it is possible that the dilute (hypotonic) urine stimulates intestinal secretions to achieve isotonicity. (Recall that all substances entering the gastrointestinal tract assume the tonicity of the area of the tract in which they are located, provided they remain there long enough.)

Intestinal secretions are rich in potassium; if the urine is excreted from the intestine before absorption can take place, the potassium of the intestinal secretions is lost with the urine, further depleting the body's potassium stores. In addition to pH decrease, potassium deficit, and perhaps mild sodium deficit, the blood urea nitrogen level is elevated, due to the absorption of urinary urea from the intestine into the bloodstream. The patient with electrolyte disturbances following ureteral transplants may have weakness, intense fatigue, anorexia, nausea and vomiting. When acidosis is severe, hyperpnea is noted.

FACTORS CONTRIBUTING TO THE DEVELOPMENT OF ELECTROLYTE IMBALANCES

Electrolyte disturbances do not occur in all patients with ureteral-intestinal transplants. Persons with normal renal function can withstand the absorption of urine without changes in pH or electrolyte levels. Some degree of renal damage must be present for patients with such implants to develop electrolyte imbalances. Unfortunately, many patients with good kidney function develop renal damage as a result of urinary tract infections caused by intestinal organisms, and *then* begin to develop electrolyte imbalances.

Absorption of urine is increased when the urine remains in the intestine for a prolonged period. Thus, the likelihood of metabolic acidosis is greater in patients with ureteral-sigmoid transplants than in those with implants into the ileum since the sigmoid is larger than the ileum and can accommodate larger volumes of urine before peristalsis is initiated.

Prolonged periods of inactivity, as when the patient is bedfast during an illness, favor unsatisfactory urinary drainage. Stricture of the ileal-bladder stoma can also cause urinary retention. Since exposure of a large area of the intestinal mucosa is associated with a higher urinary absorption than is the exposure of a small area, it may sometimes be better to transplant the ureters into an ileal conduit or onto the abdominal wall.

Treatment

Treatment of the electrolyte disturbances usually consists of the administration of potassium and sodium, as gluconate, lactate, or citrate salts. Patients with ureteral transplants into the intact bowel may require the insertion of a rectal catheter to drain urine when they are confined to bed for a prolonged period. A low acid-ash diet may also be helpful. (See Chapter 14.) The success of treatment is inversely proportional to the degree of renal damage present.

Nursing Implications

To prevent or minimize electrolyte disturbances in patients with ureteral transplants into the intestine, the nurse should:

1. Encourage the patient to drink approximately 3,000 ml. of fluids daily, unless intake is restricted. This amount of fluids ensures frequent emptying of the intestine.
2. Encourage the patient to walk; activity favors emptying of the intestines.
3. Encourage the patient with ureteral transplant into the intact bowel to evacuate every few hours. This practice limits the absorption time of urine.
4. If the patient has an ileal-bladder, see that the ileostomy bag is emptied before it is completely full so that urine drainage will not be hindered or back up into the ureters; the patient should also be instructed on how to dilate his stoma and thus prevent poor urine drainage due to a stricture.
5. Look for and report symptoms of electrolyte disturbances, such as weakness, intestinal distention, soft flabby muscles, deep rapid respiration and disorientation.

21 Fluid Balance in the Patient With Cardiac Disease

ALTERATIONS IN ELECTROLYTE CONCENTRATIONS: EFFECTS ON THE HEART

Electrolytes Affecting the Myocardium

Potassium, calcium, magnesium, and hydrogen ions influence neuromuscular irritability; therefore, deficient or excessive quantities of these ions can alter heart contractions.

POTASSIUM Potassium influences both impulse conduction and muscle contractility; alterations in its concentration may change myocardial irritability and rhythm. The normal plasma potassium concentration is from 4.0 to 5.6 mEq./L.

A deficit of potassium causes increased myocardial irritability; a pronounced deficit may induce cardiac arrest in systole. Adverse effects may appear at a plasma level of 3 mEq./L. Hypokalemia potentiates the action of digitalis and may result in arrhythmias.

Potassium excess, on the other hand, has a depressant action on the heart, causing the heart to become dilated and flaccid and slowing the heart rate. A plasma potassium level of 7 to 9 mEq./L. causes definite slowing of conduction. Elevation of the plasma potassium level to 2 to 3 times normal usually causes death through cardiac arrest during diastole.

CALCIUM The effects of calcium on the heart are almost opposite those of potassium. Thus, calcium deficit depresses the heart in much the same way as does potassium excess. Because the actions of calcium and potassium are antagonistic, the two ions must be present in the proper ratio if normal heart action is to continue. For example, a deficit of calcium renders the myocardium more susceptible to potassium excess. (Conversely, the administration of a calcium solution helps alleviate the cardio-toxic effects of potassium excess.) An excess of calcium causes the heart to go into spastic contraction.

MAGNESIUM A deficit of magnesium may cause ventricular premature beats; ventricular tachycardia may follow. Magnesium excess can cause atrioventricular and intraventricular conduction abnormalities; bradycardia can result when the plasma concentration exceeds the top normal value.

pH Changes

Acid-base disturbances influence cardiac activity. Acidosis causes an increased heart rate because it stimulates the cardio-accelerator center, whereas alkalosis causes a slowed heart rate because it stimulates the vagus nerve. High concentrations of carbon dioxide in the blood can cause cardiac arrhythmias, both auricular and ventricular. If the pH of the extracellular fluid goes down, extracellular potassium goes up; if the pH of extracellular fluid goes up, extracellular potassium goes down. The effects of an excess or a deficit of potassium ions on the myocardium are described above.

ELECTROCARDIOGRAMS

The electrocardiogram (ECG) reflects the sum of all ionic influences on the myocardium. Therefore disturbances in the concentrations of electrolytes alter electrocardiographic tracings (See Table 21-1 and Figures 21-1, 21-2, and 21-3). The ECG renders important diagnostic help in detecting disturbances in electrolyte concentration,

Table 21-1. Effects of Potassium and Calcium Imbalances on the Electrocardiogram

Electrolyte Alteration	*Effect on ECG*
Potassium deficit (Hypokalemia)	Low, rounded, prolonged T waves Prolonged Q-T interval Depression of the S-T segment Negative T waves A-V block Premature contractions Paroxysmal tachycardia Auricular flutter Auricular fibrillation
Potassium excess (Hyperkalemia)	Elevation and peaking of T waves Depression of the S-T segment Widening of the QRS complex Disappearance of P waves Heart block
Calcium deficit (Hypocalcemia)	Prolonged Q-T interval Normal T wave
Calcium excess (Hypercalcemia)	Shortening of the Q-T interval (not diagnostic)

Adapted from Grace, W.: Practical Clinical Management of Electrolyte Disorders, p. 76. New York, Appleton-Century-Crofts, 1960; and Weisberg, H.: Water, Electrolyte and Acid-Base Balance, ed. 2, p. 203. Baltimore, Williams & Wilkins, 1962.

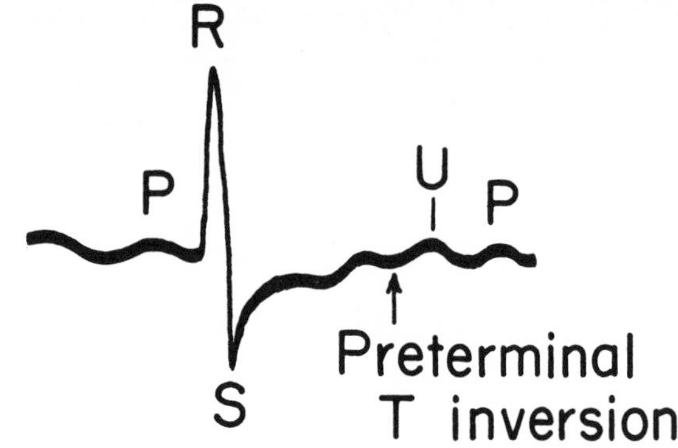

Fig. 21-1. ECG changes produced by hypokalemia. (Sharp, L., and Rabin, B.: *Nursing in the Coronary Care Unit,* Page 93. Philadelphia, J. B. Lippincott Co., 1970)

especially of potassium and calcium. Specific changes in the ECG are often associated with particular electrolyte disturbances, but these changes may also be produced by cardiac disease. Thus, evidence of an electrolyte disturbance on the ECG should be confirmed by plasma electrolyte studies. Changes due to myocardial damage tend to be localized, while changes due to electrolyte disturbances often appear in all leads. Ideally, the ECG should be interpreted by the attending physician because he knows about the patient's clinical condition and history.

Nursing Implications

Frequently, the only information available to the physician interpreting the ECG is that appearing on the requisition filled out by the nurse. The nurse, therefore, should supply as much pertinent information as possible.

Although ECG request forms differ, the typical form has spaces for the following:

Whether the patient is taking digitalis, quinidine, diuretics, or other drugs that influence electrolyte metabolism
The blood pressure reading
Reason for taking the ECG
Clinical diagnosis
Clinical comments

The nurse must understand the reasons behind the questions if she is to fill out the request correctly.

Medications That Can Affect the Electrocardiogram

DIGITALIS To increase the strength of cardiac muscle contractions, digitalis is commonly employed; this results in increased cardiac output. Unless the physician reading the ECG knows that the patient is receiving digitalis, he may make an incorrect interpretation. For example, digitalis affects the Q-T interval, as does myocardial disease. Excessive doses of digitalis cause changes in the T wave. Similar changes are caused by myocardial ischemia, pericarditis, and myocarditis. When digitalis is used in patients with myocardial infarction, it is not always possible to differentiate between the ECG changes caused by the drug and those caused by myocardial damage.

These facts serve to emphasize the point that the physician reading the ECG must know if the

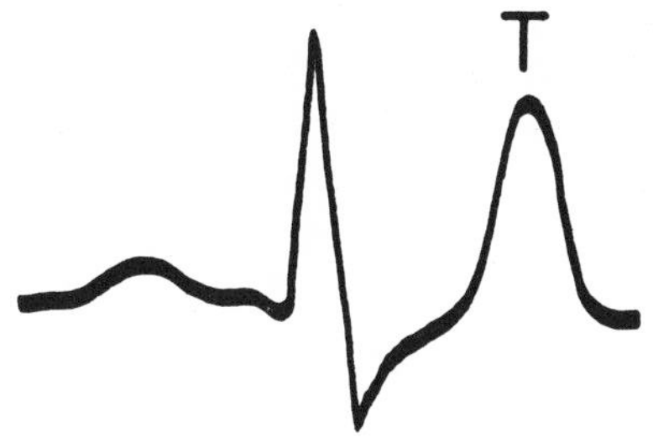

Fig. 21-2. ECG changes produced by hyperkalemia. (Sharp, L., and Rabin, B.: *Nursing in the Coronary Care Unit,* Page 94. Philadelphia, J. B. Lippincott Co., 1970)

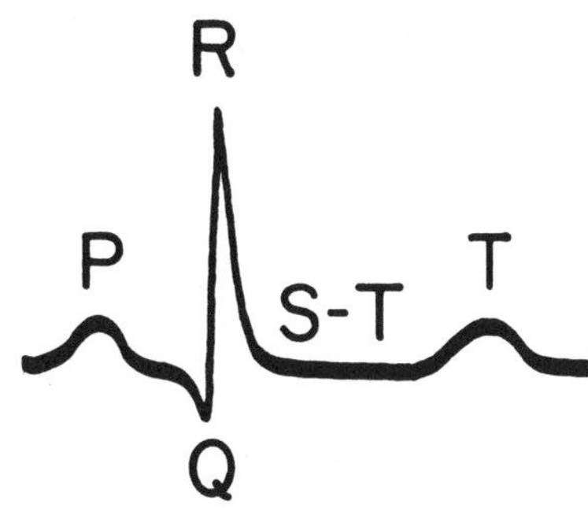

Fig. 21-3. ECG changes produced by hypocalcemia. (Sharp, L., and Rabin, B.: *Nursing in the Coronary Care Unit,* Page 93. Philadelphia, J. B. Lippincott Co., 1970)

patient is taking digitalis. Yet, carelessness in filling out the ECG requisition may result in this essential information being omitted.

QUINIDINE It is important that the use of quinidine be recorded on the requisition. Quinidine produces ECG changes related to the fact that this drug lengthens the repolarization time of cardiac muscle. Recall that quinidine is used to treat cardiac arrhythmias because it depresses the excitability of cardiac muscle and prolongs both the conduction time and the effective refractory period.

Quinidine characteristically increases the Q-T interval, and flattens and broadens the T wave. In high doses, it prolongs the P-R interval and widens the QRS complex.

PROCAINE AMIDE Procaine amide (Pronestyl) has the same antiarrhythmic effect as quinidine. Electrocardiographic signs of cardio-toxicity from overdose of this drug include excessive QRS interval widening and drug-induced arrhythmia.

Clinical Comments and Diagnosis

As emphasized above, the nurse filling out the ECG requisition should state the reason for the ECG and briefly describe the patient's clinical condition. If the patient has experienced chest pain, then the nature of the pain and its location should be briefly described. The presence of dyspnea or symptoms of "indigestion" should also be recorded, as should the presence of electrolyte imbalances or suspected imbalances. Losses of electrolytes from vomiting, diarrhea, gastric suction, etc. should be noted. (Potassium deficit readily results from such body fluid losses.)

If the diagnosis has been established, it should be recorded; frequently, the diagnosis may give hints as to the patient's electrolyte status. For example, acute renal failure or chronic nephritis cause potassium excess. Diabetic acidosis is often associated with potassium deficit. Acute pancreatitis or accidental removal of parathyroid tissue during thyroidectomy can cause calcium deficit.

CONGESTIVE HEART FAILURE

The nurse should have a basic understanding of the pathologic mechanisms involved in congestive heart failure so that she can base nursing care on sound physiologic principles.

Pathologic Mechanisms

It was once thought that the primary disturbance underlying congestive heart failure was the failure of the heart as a pump. Now it is recognized that congestive heart failure stems from many factors, including disturbances involving the following organs:

Heart
Adrenal cortex
Central nervous system
Kidneys
Vascular network
Liver

THE HEART The incomplete emptying of the heart causes an increase of venous blood volume at the expense of arterial blood volume. Decreased arterial volume apparently stimulates increased secretion of aldosterone, which, in turn causes the retention of sodium and water, thus producing an increase in total blood volume. But because of cardiac weakness and the incomplete emptying of the heart, the venous blood volume increases more than the arterial blood volume. The increased hydrostatic pressure produced by excessive venous blood volume causes a transudation of fluid from the capillaries to the tissues, or edema.

THE ADRENAL CORTEX The secretion of aldosterone may increase to two or three times the normal value in patients with congestive heart failure. Because of the hormone's potent sodium-retaining action, much attention has been focused on it as one of the major causes of edema in congestive heart failure. In addition to promoting sodium retention, aldosterone causes excessive potassium excretion.

THE CENTRAL NERVOUS SYSTEM Antidiuretic hormone (ADH) acts on the distal tubules of the kidneys, causing water retention. This secretion by the posterior pituitary gland is increased in most patients with congestive heart failure. Thus, such patients frequently retain water in excess of sodium.

Statland states that the increased ADH secretion stems from stimulation of the pituitary gland by the volume receptors in the left atrium and the great veins, as well as from the decreased cerebral blood flow caused by decreased cardiac output.

THE KIDNEYS Aldosterone acts on the renal tubules to cause increased retention of sodium and water. ADH acts on the distal tubules to cause increased water retention. Decreased cardiac output causes decreased renal blood flow; the kidneys respond by retaining sodium and water. Contributing to the decreased renal blood flow is the vasoconstriction described below.

THE VASCULAR SYSTEM Widespread vascular spasm tends to compensate for the decreased circulating blood volume caused by weak heart action. The vasoconstriction affects both venous and arterial vessels and is probably due to sympathetic stimulation and the release of norepinephrine. The vascular spasms are particularly pronounced in the kidneys and cause a further reduction in renal blood flow.

THE LIVER The increase in the venous blood volume may, in time, cause liver congestion or cirrhosis, with decreased hepatic function. Normally, aldosterone and ADH are inactivated by the liver. It is possible that the liver congestion of congestive heart failure contributes to edema by preventing the inactivation of these hormones.

Summary of Water and Electrolyte Disturbances Accompanying Congestive Heart Failure

A multitude of water and electrolyte disturbances are associated with congestive heart failure. The probable causes of these disturbances and the disturbances themselves are itemized in Table 21-2.

It is important that the nurse be aware of the water and electrolyte disturbances that can occur with congestive heart failure and with therapy. Such understanding is necessary for meaningful nursing observations. Knowledge of which fluid imbalances may occur enables the physician to institute suitable preventive measures.

Symptoms of Congestive Heart Failure

Congestive heart failure can be caused by a variety of conditions, including myocardial in-

Table 21-2. Water and Electrolyte Disturbances in CHF

Cause	*Water and Electrolyte Disturbance*
Excessive aldosterone secretion Decreased renal blood flow secondary to cardiac failure and vasoconstriction	Increased retention of sodium and water by the kidneys resulting in: Increase in total sodium content of body Increase in total extracellular water volume
Excessive secretion of ADH causes increased retention of water	Relatively greater retention of water than sodium May depress serum sodium to abnormally low levels, even though the total body sodium is above normal
Hydrostatic pressure is increased by the excessive venous blood volume	Shift of fluid from the intravascular compartment to the interstitial compartment with edema
Excessive aldosterone secretion promotes potassium excretion Excessive use of diuretics or prolonged loss of potassium by vomiting or diarrhea represent typical causes of potassium deficit	Potassium deficit
Slowing of the circulation interferes with the excretion of metabolic acids and carbon dioxide Increased liberation of lactic acid from anoxic tissues and failure of the body to metabolize it rapidly	Mild metabolic acidosis
Pulmonary congestion interferes with the elimination of carbon dioxide from the lungs	Respiratory acidosis
Mercurial and thiazide diuretics cause a greater excretion of chloride ions than sodium ions; loss of chloride ions causes a compensatory increase in bicarbonate ions, hence alkalosis	Metabolic alkalosis if mercurial or thiazide diuretics are used extensively
Extensive use of potent diuretics plus severely restricted sodium intake Excessive loss of sodium from other routes, such as repeated paracentesis, vomiting, or diarrhea	Sodium deficit

farction, disease of the valves, hypertension, arteriosclerosis and thyrotoxicosis. Although these conditions differ widely, they produce much the same clinical picture. Characteristic symptoms and their probable causes are listed in Table 21-3.

Additional symptoms may be caused by the various water and electrolyte disturbances that may occur with congestive heart failure and its treatment; these disturbances may include sodium deficit, potassium deficit, respiratory acidosis, metabolic alkalosis, metabolic acidosis, and fluid volume excess. (Descriptions of these imbalances are given in Chapters 8, 9 and 10.)

Clearly, congestive heart failure is a complex illness, demanding highly skilled nursing care. Because fluid imbalances represent a major problem in congestive heart failure, the nurse must make meaningful observations relating to these disturbances; such observations are of great help to the physician as he plans therapy. The major areas of concern to the nurse are pointed out in the following section.

Treatment of Congestive Heart Failure: Nursing Implications

When possible, treatment involves elimination of the underlying disease producing the heart failure. For example, surgical correction of a valvular disorder or removal of a calcified pericardium may restore cardiac function to normal and produce a spontaneous diuresis. Unfortunately, most persons with congestive heart failure have irreversible cardiac damage, such as that caused by myocardial infarction. When the primary disease

Table 21-3. Symptoms of CHF and Their Causes

Symptom	*Cause*
Fatigue with little exertion or at rest	Tissue anoxia due to decreased cardiac output
Troublesome cough producing non-characteristic sputum, although it may at times be brownish or blood-tinged	Transudation of serum into the alveoli causes pulmonary congestion
Dyspnea on exertion	Cardiac output is inadequate to provide for the increased oxygen required by exertion
Elevated venous pressure	Increase in total blood volume Accumulation of blood in the venous system results from incomplete emptying of the heart
Decreased urinary output	Decreased cardiac output and renal blood flow Sodium and water retention caused by excess aldosterone secretion Increased water retention caused by excess ADH secretion
Visible distention of peripheral veins, most noticeable on face, neck and hands	Elevated venous pressure
Edema first appears in dependent parts	Hydrostatic pressure is greatest in dependent parts of the body
Edema later becomes generalized	Progressive cardiac failure causes substantial increase in hydrostatic pressure in all parts of the body
Fever	Complications accompanying congestive heart failure, such as bronchopneumonia, thrombophlebitis, or myocardial infarction Fever may be present even in the absence of complications (Steel feels that the cutaneous vasoconstriction occurring with CHF interferes with normal heat loss from the skin)
Tachycardia	Effort to compensate for decreased cardiac output
Engorgement of the liver and other organs	Decreased cardiac output causes damming of venous blood Increase in total blood volume and interstitial fluid volume
Nausea and vomiting	Edema of the liver and intestines Impulses arising from the dilated myocardium in acute CHF Digitalis toxicity
Anorexia	Potassium deficit Digitalis toxicity
Constipation	Poor nourishment and inadequate bulk in diet Lack of activity Depression of motor activity by hypoxia
Increased respiratory difficulty Dyspnea even at rest Orthopnea	Increased tissue hypoxia due to progressive failure of the heart as a pump
Cyanosis, particularly of lips and nail beds	Venous distention Inadequate oxygenation of blood
Pulmonary edema with severe dyspnea, coughing of pink frothy fluid, cyanosis, shock and death	Increased venous pressure may cause serum and blood cells to transude into the alveoli

cannot be eliminated, the only alternative is to make the most efficient use possible of remaining cardiac function.

REST Rest causes a reduction in the tissue's oxygen need and lightens the burden on the circulatory system. It also produces a physiologic diuresis. Sometimes rest alone is sufficient to alleviate the symptoms of congestive heart failure. The amount of rest required varies with the individual and may range from complete bedrest to only slight restriction of activity.

The prescription of physical rest by the physician must be specific enough to have meaning to the patient. Too often, patients are given ambiguous directions to "rest" or to "take it easy." Such vague statements are not only useless; they may actually be harmful, because each person interprets rest differently. The nurse can help by encouraging the patient to ask the physician specific questions regarding the activity permitted.

Another important nursing responsibility consists in observing such responses of the patient to exercise as pulse and respiratory rate changes. Careful reporting of these observations helps the physician determine the desired amount of activity. Because the patient's condition may fluctuate widely from day to day, the nurse must often use her own judgment in controlling his activity. For example, assume that a patient has been allowed up in a chair for 30 minutes in the morning. Even though this period is permitted, the appearance of dyspnea, chest pain, or a substantially increased pulse rate before the 30 minutes are up indicates that the patient should be put back to bed.

Emotional rest is also important in the management of congestive heart failure. Periods of tension are associated with increased sodium and water retention, while periods of emotional relaxation are associated with diuresis. Nursing efforts should, therefore, be directed toward avoiding emotional problems and achieving a relaxing environment. The importance of emotional rest is not as widely recognized as it deserves to be. A major nursing responsibility is emphasizing the importance of emotional rest to the patient's family and to nonprofessional personnel giving direct patient care. At times, judicious use of sedatives may help promote needed rest and relaxation.

LOW-SODIUM DIET Restriction of sodium ions in the diet is a valuable aid in the management of congestive heart failure. In general, the fewer number of sodium ions in the body, the less water is retained.

The degree of sodium restriction necessary to control edema varies with the severity of the heart failure. Many patients can achieve a sufficiently low intake of sodium simply by not adding salt in cooking or at the table and by avoiding high sodium foods, such as salted crackers, bacon, ham, salted nuts, foods with sodium salt preservatives, and so on. As a rule, restriction of the intake of salt to from 2 to 5 Gm. daily instead of the usual 10 Gm. or more in an average diet is sufficient to control edema. But more drastic sodium restriction to less than 1 Gm. a day—even 250 mg. a day or less—may be required for some patients.

The degree of sodium restriction necessary to control edema also varies with other facets of treatment, such as rest and the use of diuretics. For example, an ambulatory patient requires more severe sodium restriction than a patient at bedrest, because rest in itself encourages diuresis. A patient receiving potent diuretics has much less need of severe sodium restriction than a patient not receiving diuretics. Indeed, drastic restriction of sodium intake can be dangerous in the patient receiving a potent diuretic.

Although dietary sodium restriction is simple in theory, it is frequently difficult to achieve. Many patients fail to adhere to low-sodium diets because they mistakenly believe them to be unpalatable; others lack an understanding of the foods allowed and to be avoided. All too often, the only diet instruction given to the patient consists of handing him a copy of his diet on the day of his discharge from the hospital.

The nurse should make every effort to make the diet acceptable to the patient. First of all, she should give him an explanation of why he must be on the diet. Secondly, the dietitian should discuss the diet with the patient and learn what his food preferences are. The possible use of salt substitutes should be discussed with the physician. All of these contain potassium chloride and, thus, should not be used in the presence of oliguria and severe kidney disease. Additional sessions should be held while the patient is in the hospital in order to increase his knowledge and acceptance of the diet. The nurse should support the dietitian's efforts. In instances where a dietitian is not available, the nurse should carry the full responsibiilty of diet instruction; for this reason, she should have a working knowledge of low-sodium diets. (See Chapter 14 for a more thorough discussion of sodium restricted diets.) Literature concerning these diets is available from the American Heart Association at the request of the patient's physician. Excellent books on the preparation of attractive low-sodium diets are available.

Patients on severe sodium restriction should be observed for symptoms of sodium deficit, especially if they are receiving potent diuretics, or if they are losing sodium through such routes as vomiting, diarrhea, excessive perspiration, or repeated paracentesis.

DIGITALIS Cardiac function is frequently improved by the administration of digitalis, which acts by increasing the strength of the heartbeat and the cardiac output. Edema fluid is mobilized by the improved cardiac function, and diuresis results. Usually the physician attempts to give enough digitalis to reduce the resting apical pulse to 60 to 80 beats per minute.

Excessive doses of digitalis result in the following toxic symptoms:

Aversion to food (which usually precedes other symptoms by 1 or 2 days)
Nausea
Excessive salivation
Vomiting
Abdominal pain
Diarrhea
Headache
Confusion (particularly in elderly patients with arteriosclerosis)
Blurred vision
Yellowish-green "halo" vision, or presence of white dots ("frost") on objects
Bradycardia (due to A-V block)
Variety of arrhythmias, including ventricular tachycardia, in which the heart beats rapidly and irregularly

It is important to differentiate between the combined anorexia and nausea of heart failure and that produced by digitalis toxicity. Patients receiving digitalis should have periodic electrocardiograms to detect early the development of digitalis toxicity. Before administering the drug, the nurse should check the apical-radial pulse for a full minute, noting rate, rhythm, volume, and pulse deficit. The drug should be withheld, and the physician notified when:

The apical pulse is below 60
A marked change in regularity occurs
The apical pulse is above 100

An overdose of digitalis may have a depressant action, causing conduction disturbance and excessive slowing of the heart. It may also cause increased myocardial irritability, producing extrasystoles or tachycardias. The nurse should be alert for a coupled pulse beat (bigeminy) in which the regular beat is followed almost immediately by a weak beat and a pause. A bigeminal pulse is a common sign of digitalis toxicity in adults; bigeminal pulse, and other irregularities, should be reported to the physician. The nurse should also report pulse deficit, caused by failure of the extra systoles to produce a pulse at the wrist. If digitalis is not discontinued, the premature beats can take on the rhythm of ventricular tachycardia and progress to ventricular fibrillation.

Calcium ions enhance the action of digitalis; thus, decreasing the plasma calcium concentration is helpful in counteracting the cardio-toxic effects produced by digitalis. The plasma calcium level can be reduced by the intravenous infusion of disodium edetate (Endrate); this drug ties up excess calcium and removes it from the body. (Conversely, calcium should never be administered intravenously to a digitalized patient.)

Symptoms of digitalis toxicity may be induced by potassium deficit, since this deficit sensitizes the heart to digitalis. The patient maintained on digitalis without toxicity can, in the presence of potassium deficit, exhibit arrhythmias typical of digitalis intoxication. An irregular pulse caused by digitalis toxicity can usually be corrected by the administration of a potassium salt, either by mouth or, if necessary, parenterally. Magnesium has also been reported to correct the toxic rhythms produced by digoxin.

Patients prone to develop potassium deficit (such as those receiving mercurial or thiazide diuretics, or those with vomiting, diarrhea, or poor food intake) should be observed with especial care for signs of digitalis toxicity.

DIURETICS A valuable aid in the symptomatic treatment of congestive heart failure, the primary purpose of diuretics is to promote the excretion of sodium and water from the body. In varying degrees, most diuretics tend also to promote the excretion of potassium. Diuretics that are associated with hypokalemia include the thiazides, the mercurials, furosemide (Lasix), ethacrynic acid (Edecrin) and the carbonic anhydrase inhibitors, such as acetazolamide (Diamox). Mercurial diuretics are used less frequently than the other diuretics because many of them require intramuscular administration and they have more side effects, including cramps, diarrhea, skin rashes and local pain at the injection site. (See Chapter 14 for a more thorough discussion of diuretics.)

Excessive loss of potassium ions during diuretic therapy can be either prevented or corrected by the administration of a suitable potassium supplement, such as K-Lyte, Kaon Elixir, Potassium Triplex or K-Lor. The use of diuretics should be decreased when sodium loss is occurring from another route; a low-sodium diet can take the place of diuretic therapy in many persons. It is less expensive, safer, and, in many respects, more pleasant.

An acidifying agent, such as ammonium chloride, is sometimes given to enhance the effect of mercurial diuretics in resistant cases of edema. Acidifying agents enhance mercurial diuretic action because of the following facts: diuretics cause a relatively great loss of chloride ions from the body. This loss of chloride causes a compensatory increase in bicarbonate, hence metabolic alkalosis. Alkalosis decreases the effectiveness of mercurial diuretics; hence, the rationale for acidifying agents. A mild state of acidosis is often induced through the use of these agents in order to promote maximal effectiveness of the mercurial diuretic. Although relatively safe, ammonium chloride may sometimes cause gastrointestinal symptoms.

Ethacrynic acid (Edecrin) and furosemide (Lasix) are potent diuretics that are effective even after their action has produced hypochloremic alkalosis. They are unusually potent and have a rapid onset. Patients receiving these diuretics should be observed closely for signs of too vigorous diuresis, such as lethargy, weakness, dizziness, anorexia, vomiting, leg cramps, mental confusion, and circulatory collapse.

Potassium conserving diuretics are capable of producing diuresis in congestive heart failure. Spironolactone (Aldactone) is an aldosterone antagonist, which acts by blocking the potent sodium retaining effect of aldosterone on the renal tubules. Aldactone should not be given in conjunction with a potassium supplement because of the danger of potassium excess. (Recall that aldosterone causes potassium loss; therefore, its antagonist permits potassium retention.) Triamterene (Dyrenium) also promotes sodium loss and potassium retention although it has a different mode of action. (It interferes with the exchange of sodium ions for potassium and hydrogen ions.) Again, potassium supplements should not be given because hyperkalemia may result; symptoms of hyperkalemia include paresthesia of the extremities, nausea, weakness and intestinal cramping with diarrhea. If hyperkalemia is severe, cardiac arrest can occur. Only patients with adequate renal reserve should receive potassium conserving diuretics.

Primary nursing responsibilities in the care of the patient with congestive heart failure include keeping an accurate account of fluid intake and output and measuring the weight daily. (See the discussion of both of these procedures in Chapter 12.) The data obtained from these measurements are of inestimable use to the physician as he regulates the dose of diuretics and the degree of dietary sodium restriction for each patient.

FLUID ADMINISTRATION

Oral Intake Water intake is usually not restricted in congestive heart failure unless there is a body sodium deficit or dilution of the serum sodium by the excessive retention of water.

Undue loss of sodium may be caused by the excessive use of diuretics, vomiting, diarrhea, severe diaphoresis, or repeated paracentesis. A drastically reduced sodium intake may predispose to sodium depletion, although persons on low sodium intake for prolonged periods usually develop remarkable sodium conservation, something that does not happen in the case of patients on low potassium intake, since there is no true body conservation of potassium. If the water intake of patients in a mild state of sodium depletion is not reduced, the depressed serum sodium level may become further depressed; a frank state of sodium deficit may then develop. Symptoms of this condition include:

Weakness
Abdominal cramps
Anorexia
Nausea
Vomiting
Inexplicable feeling of impending doom
Prostration
Collapse

The operation of abnormal routes of sodium loss should alert the nurse to search for the symptoms tabulated above, especially if the sodium intake is low and diuretics are being given. Although the total sodium content of the body is elevated in congestive heart failure, water retention caused by excessive ADH hormone secretion may dilute the serum sodium concentration to below normal levels. Moreover, part of the sodium in the extracellular fluid moves into the cells to replace the potassium loss which so often occurs with congestive heart failure. There is no characteristic clinical picture accompanying this state. When it is well developed, however, the usual therapeutic measures fail to reduce the edema that accompanies it.

One of the chief features of intractable heart failure is the inability of the kidney to respond to the usual diuretics. In such instances, treatment may consist of the use of acidifying salts, as described earlier, mercurial diuretics, continued sodium restriction, and restriction of water intake to 1,000 ml. per day. The use of more potent diuretics may be necessary; it has been found that patients refractory to other diuretics often respond successfully to ethacrynic acid (Edecrin) and furosemide (Lasix).

Intravenous Fluids The intravenous route for fluid administration may be necessary in critically ill patients with congestive heart failure. Many physicians are hesitant to administer fluids to such patients for fear of causing circulatory overload and pulmonary edema. While there is little doubt that intravenous administration of fluids to a cardiac patient carries some risk of causing circulatory overload, the fear of this complication has been exaggerated to the point that many cardiac patients receive inadequate fluid therapy. The recent increase in the use of venous pressure monitoring devices has done much to alleviate the problem. Frequent checks of venous pressure during fluid administration give early warning of circulatory overload and serve as guides to the safe administration of needed water and electrolytes.

The nurse should pay careful attention to the volume, speed and composition of fluids administered to the patient with congestive heart failure. The response to fluids should be observed frequently and the flow rate adjusted accordingly. (See Chapter 16 for a more detailed discussion of venous pressure monitoring and nursing responsibilities in intravenous fluid administration.)

Pulmonary Edema The symptoms of acute pulmonary edema include:

Restlessness
Severe dyspnea
Gurgling respirations
Cyanosis
Coughing up of frothy fluid

Welt has pointed out possible causes of pulmonary edema other than administering excessive quantities of fluid or too rapid administration of fluid. Inadequate fluid administration can result in peripheral vascular collapse with tissue anoxia; this condition in itself can precipitate an acute attack of pulmonary edema. Some patients develop pulmonary edema during venipuncture, or shortly after fluids have been started before there has been time for expansion of the circulatory volume. Pulmonary edema in these instances can be explained as a reaction to fear related to the venipuncture. The following illustrative case was related by Welt:*

A patient with chronic renal insufficiency and hypertensive and arteriosclerotic heart disease with failure despite complete digitalization was admitted to the hospital. It was decided to improve her severe anemia with blood transfusion. The nature of the procedure was not explained to her, she had not been sedated, there was a little difficulty with the venipuncture, and when the needle was successfully introduced into the vein she developed severe acute pulmonary edema. The procedure was discontinued and she recovered from this episode in a few hours. Later that day the nature of and indications for the transfusion were explained to her, she was sedated, and tolerated the administration of 1,000 ml. of whole blood with no untoward reaction whatsoever.

In addition to fear of venipuncture, the patient may interpret the need for intravenous fluids as a grave prognostic sign. This is but another reason to take time to explain to the patient what the intravenous administration consists of and why it is being used.

Occasionally, hypertonic solution of sodium chloride is administered to the cardiac patient to correct a sodium deficit. Great care should be taken to infuse the solution slowly in accordance with the order of the physician. A too rapid administration of hypertonic saline results in a dangerous overloading of the circulatory system.

Acute pulmonary edema constitutes a medical emergency that requires quick, intelligent action by the nurse and the physician. The patient should be quickly placed in a high Fowler's position, and oxygen should be started while the physician is being summoned. Best results are achieved when oxygen is given under positive pressure, since this helps prevent further escape of fluid into the lungs. Preparation should be made for intravenous administration of morphine sulfate. Usually one-sixth to one-half grain is ordered in order to relieve the apprehension so characteristic of pulmonary edema. It has also been suggested that morphine may help to reverse pulmonary edema by interrupting reflex arcs set up by the increased venous pressure. Alternating tourniquets may be used to obstruct venous return to the heart; they can remove up to 700 ml. of blood from the circulating volume. The removal of 200 to 500 ml. of blood by phlebotomy may be tried in order to relieve the work load on the heart and to reduce venous pressure. Rapid digitalization improves cardiac function and thus helps relieve pulmonary edema. Either sodium ethacrynate (Sodium Edecrin) or furosemide (Lasix) may be used to treat acute pulmonary edema; they are rapidly effective when given intravenously and produce an intense diuresis.

* Welt, L.: Clinical Disorders of Hydration and Acid-Base Equilibrium, ed. 2, p. 131. Boston, Little Brown, 1959.

ELECTROLYTES IN CARDIAC RESUSCITATION

SODIUM BICARBONATE Metabolic acidosis occurs in cardiac arrest; it is related to the accumulation of lactic acid and other products of anoxic metabolism. Sodium bicarbonate, an alkali, is often used to correct metabolic acidosis; 50 ml. of a 7.5% solution (containing 3.75 Gm.) may be administered by direct venous injection. This amount can be repeated in 5 minutes, if necessary, to restore cardiac activity.

CALCIUM CHLORIDE Calcium chloride may be given intravenously or intracardially to strengthen the cardiac contraction; the dose is usually 10 ml. of a 10% solution. Calcium is especially helpful in treating patients with potassium excess. Recall that calcium and potassium have antagonistic effects; thus, raising the plasma calcium level decreases the cardio-toxic effects of hyperkalemia. (Calcium should *not* be administered intravenously to the digitalized patient because calcium ions enhance the cardio-toxic action of digitalis.)

POTASSIUM CHLORIDE Potassium chloride may be given intravenously to correct arrhythmias caused by digitalis; 40 mEq. of KCl in 500 ml. of 5% D/W may be given over a 2- to 3-hour period.

If the serum potassium level is above 2.5, no more than 10 mEq. per hour or 200 mEq. per day should be given. If the serum potassium level is less than 2.0 and electrolyte changes are evident in the ECG, 40 mEq. may be given per hour with no greater concentration than 60 mEq. per liter of I.V., up to 400 mEq. per day.*

NURSING OBSERVATIONS RELATED TO FLUID BALANCE FOLLOWING OPEN HEART SURGERY

This section was prepared by Catherine A. Smith, R.N., Clinical Specialist in Cardiovascular Nursing, St. Louis, Mo.

One of the most challenging areas of nursing today is the care of the patient undergoing open heart surgery. Due to the magnitude and the severity of the surgical procedure and the emotional trauma endured by both patient and family, a highly skilled nurse is required to adequately meet the demands and requirements that arise.

It is not within the scope of this section to discuss all phases of nursing care of the patient undergoing open heart surgery. Rather, it shall be confined to the nursing responsibilities in relation to disturbances of fluid balance during the postoperative period.

The process of open heart surgery inflicts a tremendous insult upon the body. Extracorporeal circulation is not as effective as normal circulation. The process of hypothermia, together with extracorporeal circulation, affects every organ in the body, producing biochemical changes. Many of these physiological disturbances have not yet been adequately investigated. Those which are known should be familiar to the nurse caring for the patient following open heart surgery.

A good observer is needed at the bedside of these patients, as with any acutely ill patient. There are many symptoms of water and electrolyte disturbances that are apparent to a thoughtful observer. Of all the persons involved in patient care, the nurse is the person in most constant attendance. This places her in the position most favorable to noting beginning changes in body physiology. She has a responsibility to be alert and highly skilled in the observations she makes. It is not her function to diagnose, but rather to be sensitive to meaningful changes and to relate these to the physician.

ACIDOSIS AND THE NEED FOR OXYGEN

Studies have shown that metabolic acidosis frequently occurs following cardiopulmonary bypass and profound hypothermia; this has generally been attributed to hypoxia. This state is manifested by a decrease in blood pH and bicarbonate levels. Therefore, these patients are ideally assessed during the first few postoperative hours with blood pH and bicarbonate studies. The frequency of these determinations is dependent upon the clinical course of the patient.

The nurse, being the person in most constant attendance during the early postoperative period, must be alert for signs of metabolic acidosis. Hyperpnea is a dependable physical sign; it is the increase in the depth of respiration that makes hyperpnea so easy to recognize—there is a tendency to be concerned only about the rate of respiration and to neglect to take note of the depth of respiration. An increase in depth of respiration should be promptly reported to the physician.

The nurse must realize that one of the most common complications following heart surgery with cardiopulmonary bypass is respiratory insufficiency; if untreated, it can proceed to respiratory acidosis. These patients are extremely sensitive to oxygen lack; by the time a patient with previously good color exhibits cyanosis, hypoxia may be at a dangerous level. Therefore, the nurse must be familiar with the signs of respiratory distress and respiratory acidosis so that she can promptly communicate this information to the physician and prompt therapy can be initiated. Signs of respiratory distress may include:

Disturbed facial expression and general behavior of distress

* Sharp, L., and Rabin, B.: Nursing in the Coronary Care Unit, p. 185. Philadelphia, J. B. Lippincott Co., 1970.

Shallow, labored, rapid respiration
Feeble coughing
Restlessness
Tachycardia
Cyanosis

To further faciiltate care of the patient following open heart surgery, the nurse's knowledge should include an understanding of the possible causes of respiratory insufficiency and acidosis, which can occur either when the functional capacity of the lungs is reduced significantly or when the patient is unable to perform sufficient respiratory work to provide adequate ventilation. Some of the causes of decreased functional capacity of the lungs include:

Atelectasis
Hemothorax
Bronchospasm
Pulmonary edema
Pulmonary infections

Some of the causes of the patient's inability to perform adequate respiratory work are:

Shallow breathing due to incisional pain
Respiratory depressant drugs
Inability of the heart to deliver sufficient amounts of blood to the lungs to permit adequate gaseous exchange

Any of these causes can result in lowered arterial oxygen tension and increased carbon dioxide. Frequent blood studies for pO_2 and pCO_2 are desirable in order to detect early changes and to estimate the progression of recovery processes. (See Chapter 12 for a discussion of blood gas studies.)

Considering these causes and ever mindful of the preventive aspect of nursing care, it becomes evident that following open heart surgery the patient must be conscientiously engaged in a systemic regimen of turning, coughing and deep breathing. Coughing can do no harm—it should be begun immediately postoperatively while the patient is still somewhat insensitive to pain due to the residue of anesthetic. Because coughing is an uncomfortable experience for the patient, the nurse should help the patient perform these exercises in such a manner that they are most tolerable and comfortable for him. Kindness, sympathy and an unhurried manner are important. A pillow held firmly over the site of the incision is reassuring and comforting to the patient.

The state of acidosis, whether respiratory or metabolic, has adverse effects upon the myocardium and affects cardiac rate and rhythm, changes in which should be immediately reported to the physician. Following open heart surgery, arrhythmias are not unusual, but they are less frequent when myocardial oxygenation is adequate. Dammann has stated that above-normal levels of arterial oxygen tension in the early postoperative period are helpful in the prevention of harmful arrhythmias. Such levels can be achieved by intermittent positive pressure or hyperbaric therapy.

For this reason, oxygen is customarily given by nasal tube or tent for the first 12 hours postoperatively. After this period, nasal oxygen is discontinued if the patient's condition is satisfactory. If an oxygen tent is used, it is continued until the second or third postoperative day. Oxygen consumption studies are frequently performed at the bedside to evaluate further the patient's oxygen requirements.

In relation to oxygen requirement, the nurse should realize that metabolic demands for oxygen are increased by certain physiologic states. Such conditions as undue restlessness, shivering and pyrexia can substantially increase the need for oxygen and the requirement on cardiac output. Appropriate nursing measures should be taken to avoid or counteract these conditions.

DAILY WEIGHT MEASUREMENT The pattern of daily weights provides an accurate account of fluid loss or retention by the body. The physician relies heavily upon weight changes to prescribe therapy. Candidates for heart surgery are placed on daily weights from their date of admission to the hospital. Daily weights are resumed approximately the second or third day following surgery, after the chest tube has been removed and the movement of the patient to the bed scale is facilitated. (Nursing responsibilities in obtaining daily weight measurements are discussed in Chapter 12.)

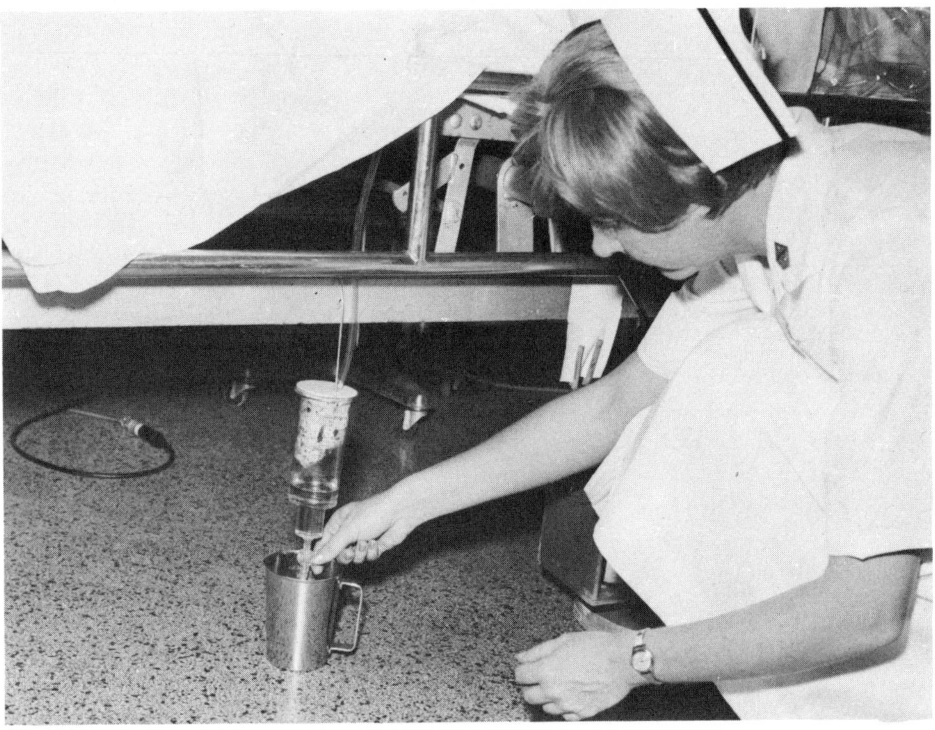

Fig. 21-4. Measuring urine output with Davol Uri-meter.

INTRAVENOUS THERAPY Following open heart surgery, great care and accuracy are required in the management of intravenous fluids. An excessive circulating blood volume can be extremely hazardous; the recently wounded and recuperating heart may be unable to cope with this additional load and pulmonary edema can result. Therefore it becomes evident that intravenous fluid orders must be very clear and specific both to amount and time of infusion. Communication and understanding between physician and nurse cannot be too detailed in this area. Often, however, the physician will order intravenous fluids for a 12- or 24-hour interval. Then it becomes a nursing responsibility to determine the rate at which these fluids should run in order to provide an even distribution over the specified time interval. (See the section dealing with the calculation of flow rate in Chapter 16.)

Each bottle of fluid should be clearly labeled with the time it was begun, the time it is to be completed, and the desired infusion rate. This rate should be checked at frequent intervals—i.e., every 15 to 30 minutes. The importance of the nurse's responsibility in the administration of fluids and the conscientiousness required of her cannot be overstressed.

URINE OUTPUT Since almost every organ system can be affected by the combination of open heart surgery and total body perfusion, deviations from normal urine formation might be anticipated. There is no single factor that will lead invariably to renal complications. Rather, many factors have been noted which singly or in combination predispose the kidneys to serious damage. Among these factors are:

Extracorporeal perfusion rate
Length of the perfusion
Postoperative acidosis

Yeh stated that renal ischemia and nephrotoxins, or their combination, are the most consistent causes of renal failure. He also pointed out that while vasopressor drugs are capable of increasing blood pressure in shock, at the same

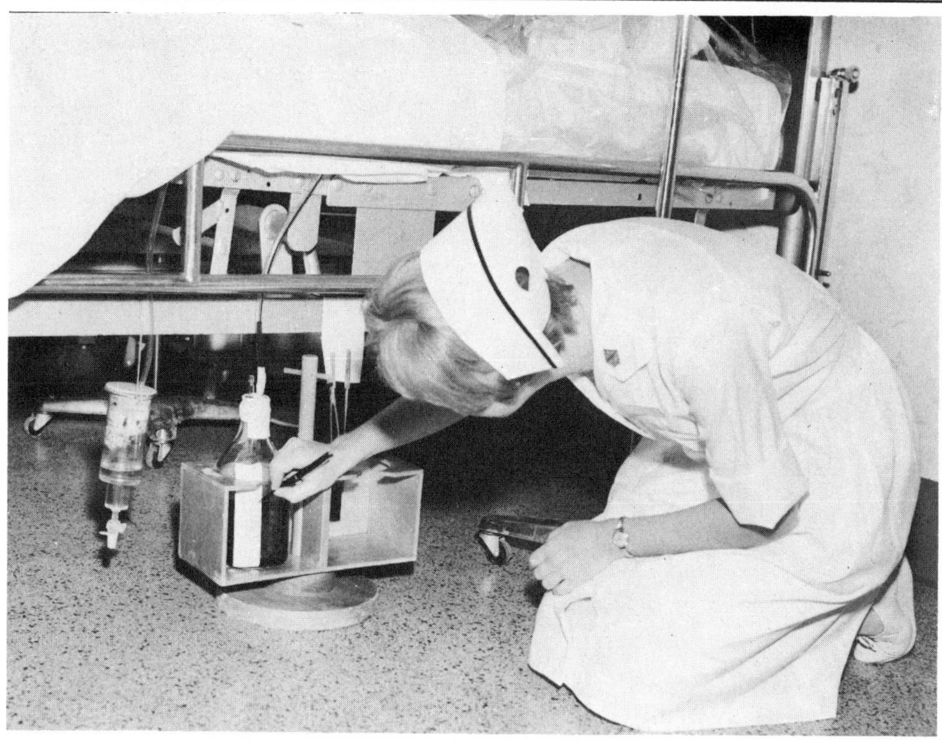

Fig. 21-5. Marking chest tube drainage.

time renal blood flow, renal plasma flow and urine flow can be severely depressed. To aid in the evaluation of kidney function, the BUN is determined daily.

The rationale and details of accurate urine observations should be basic knowledge to the nurse caring for the patient following open heart surgery. In some cases, a Foley catheter will be in place; frequent measurements of urine volume, usually hourly, are of utmost importance. Urine volume should be measured accurately, to the milliliter. (See Figure 21-4.) A vessel with small calibrations should be used. (See discussion of urinary output measurement in Chapter 12.) A urinary output of less than 15 ml. per hour is indicative of inadequate renal function; when the output falls below this figure, the physician should be immediately notified.

Each time the urinary output is measured, a urinary specific gravity test should be performed. (The procedure for determining the specific gravity of urine is described in Chapter 12.) This information will help to determine the state of hydration, as well as the status of kidney function. The average range of urine specific gravity is 1.010 to 1.030.

CHEST DRAINAGE In caring for the patient following heart surgery, the nurse must have an understanding of the principles of water-seal chest drainage. If she possesses a clear understanding of the mechanics of respiration, she can feel perfectly at ease with the water-seal drainage system. The purpose of the system is to drain excess fluid from the operative area and to reestablish normal intrapleural pressure.

The chest tube must be kept patent by regular milking; this should be done every hour, more frequently if necessary. Milking should begin near the patient's chest and continue down the tubing to the bottle, clearing the tubing of any clots. The tubing should be kept free of any kinks, and care should be taken to prevent looping of excess tubing on the floor. (See Figure 21-5.)

The nurse must make certain that the bottle *always* rests below the lowest level of the pa-

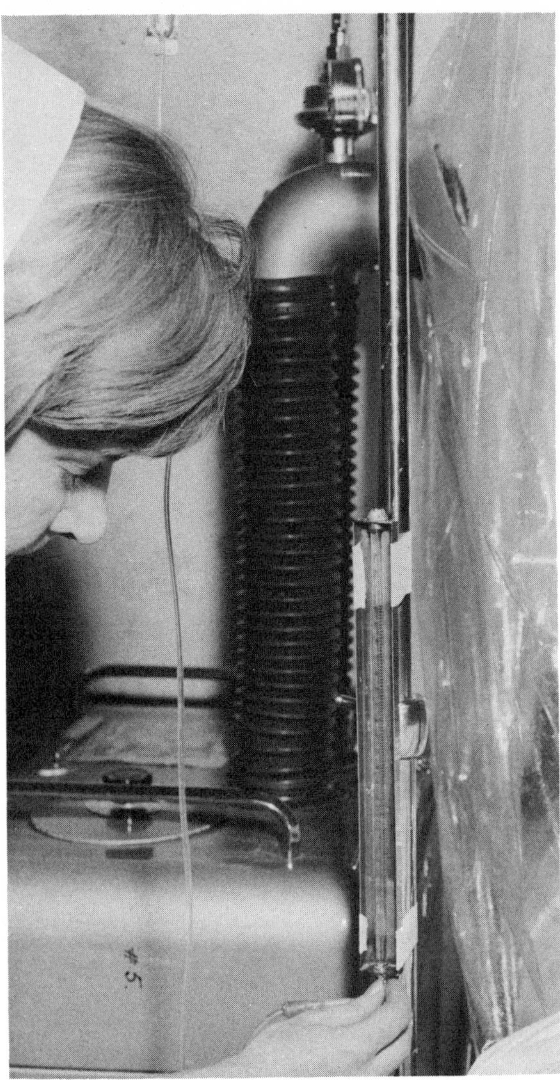

Fig. 21-6. Measuring venous pressure on a spinal manometer.

tient's chest. If the bottle is raised to chest level, negative pressure may suck water into the intrathoracic space. The chest bottle should either be kept in a holder or taped securely to the floor; this will prevent accidentally knocking the bottle over and breaking the water-seal system.

All connections must be secure and well taped. If the drainage bottle should be broken or if the water-seal fails for any reason, the tube should be clamped immediately, near the chest. Two clamps should be kept at the bedside for each chest tube at all times.

The water-seal setup should be observed for the amount and character of drainage. Bright red drainage is expected immediately postoperatively, gradually becoming darker, then more serosanguineous. Any sudden change should be reported immediately. To record the amount of drainage, a piece of adhesive tape should be vertically applied to the bottle so that hourly marks can be made, thus giving an accurate account of fluid loss. For children, the bottle can be placed on a small scale to better indicate small increments of drainage.

The nurse should keep in mind the importance of determining how much the patient has lost in an hour-by-hour pattern. For instance, consider these contrasting records:

300 ml.	First hour	400 ml.
50 ml.	Second hour	50 ml.
50 ml.	Third hour	50 ml.
25 ml.	Fourth hour	25 ml.
50 ml.	Fifth hour	25 ml.
100 ml.	Sixth hour	0 ml.
100 ml.	Seventh hour	10 ml.
150 ml.	Eighth hour	5 ml.
Cause for Concern		No Cause for Concern

Oscillation of the fluid in the tubing should also be noted. When this ceases, it may indicate that the lung has re-expanded or that a clot obstructs the tubing. The tubing should be checked for patency at this time.

There should be adequate tubing to allow the patient to turn freely in bed; he should be turned every 1 to 2 hours. Turning to the affected side will facilitate drainage. Care must be taken that the patient does not occlude the chest tube.

VENOUS PRESSURE All the blood in the body returns to the right atrium of the heart. For this reason, the pressure within the right atrium is known as the central venous pressure. The pressure within the systemic veins depends heavily upon the central venous pressure. If the pressure within the right atrium rises, the pressure within the systemic veins will also rise; thus,

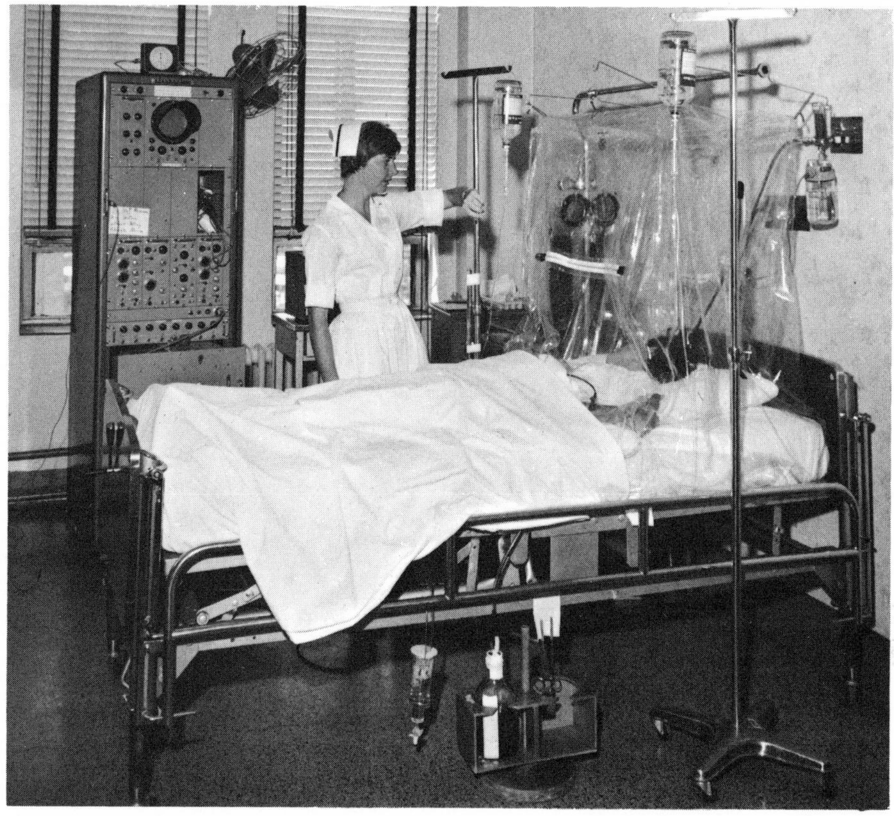

Fig. 21-7. Fluid gains and losses following open heart surgery.

a direct method of measuring peripheral venous pressure gives a reflection of the central venous pressure.

The nurse should realize that venous pressure can be a useful guide in assessing the circulatory status following severe trauma and major surgery. Venous pressure can be affected by several complications.

Hypervolemia The circulatory system is overloaded and the venous pressure tends to be elevated. The work load of the heart is increased. This may lead to peripheral and pulmonary edema and failure of the myocardium.

Hypovolemia The circulating blood volume is inadequate and venous pressure is decreased. This may be due to vasodilation from rewarming of the body after the period of hypothermia used during the surgical procedure. Hypovolemia more commonly results from postoperative bleeding or shifts in fluid volume between the various compartments.

Cardiac Tamponade There is an accumulation of fluid in the pericardial sac that causes compression of the heart and an increased venous pressure.

Congestive Heart Failure The venous pressure will increase.

Venous pressure can be measured by a direct venipuncture and recorded in centimeters of water on a spinal manometer. (See Figure 21-6.) Following open heart surgery, the femoral vein is frequently used to obtain these readings. By means of a three-way stopcock, the venous pressure manometer can remain attached to the intravenous fluids that the patient is receiving continuously. Accurate venous pressure readings are dependent upon a good base line. To obtain this base line, the patient must be in a supine position. One must realize that venous pressure is expressed in relation to the level of the tricuspid valve; therefore, the zero point on the manometer must be on an equal level with the tricuspid valve. This is essentially a midline structure, midway between the anterior and posterior of the body. Initially, this base line will be determined by the physician and the manometer secured at the proper level. The nurse, however, will be responsible for obtaining subsequent venous pressure readings—as frequently as every one-half hour during the immediate postoperative period. For this reason, she should have a thorough understanding of the principles involved in obtaining accurate venous pressure readings. She must realize that any deviation in position of the patient will affect the venous pressure reading. For example, if the patient is turned on his side or the head of the bed is elevated, the venous pressure reading will vary. When using this method, care should be taken not to change the level of a high-low bed once the manometer is in place. Every effort should be made to position the patient so as to obtain an accurate reading. (Venous pressure measurement is discussed in more detail in Chapter 16.)

22 Fluid Balance in the Patient With Endocrine Disease

ROLE OF ENDOCRINE GLANDS IN FLUID BALANCE HOMEOSTASIS

The endocrine homeostatic controls include the adrenals, the parathyroids, and the anterior and posterior pituitary glands.

ADRENAL GLANDS The adrenal mechanism is very closely associated with retention and excretion of sodium, potassium and water; these effects are exerted through the action of the adrenocortical hormones on the renal tubules.

The primary adrenal cortex secretions are mineralocorticoids and glucocorticoids. Aldosterone is the most important mineralocorticoid; cortisol is the most important glucocorticoid.

The chief function of aldosterone is the control of sodium concentration in the body. Its effect on potassium and sodium is 50 times stronger than cortisol's effect on these electrolytes.

The chief action of cortisol is to promote gluconeogenesis and to deposit glycogen in the liver. It also influences protein catabolism. Other effects of the glucocorticoids include control of inflammation, maintenance of gastric acidity, and a mild mineralocorticoid influence on sodium and potassium concentrations.

Androgenic adrenocorticoids (17-ketosteroids) are also produced by the adrenal cortex. These hormones favor a positive nitrogen balance and they oppose the catabolic effects of the glucocorticoids. Sexual effects of these hormones include promotion of hair growth in the pubic and axillary areas.

PARATHYROID GLANDS Parathyroid hormone (parathormone) causes an increase in the plasma calcium concentration, primarily by increasing the rate of bone resorption. Any *decrease* in the plasma calcium concentration causes stimulation of the parathyroid glands; conversely, any *increase* in the plasma calcium level causes parathyroid activity to decrease.

Another function of parathormone is to increase the renal excretion of phosphate ions and thus to lower the plasma phosphate concentration. The plasma phosphate concentration indirectly influences parathyroid activity, since a reciprocal relationship exists between calcium and phosphate ions—a rise in the concentration of one causing a decrease in the other. Thus, when an increase in phosphate concentration causes a reciprocal decrease in the calcium concentration, the decreased calcium concentration causes parathyroid stimulation.

Evidence exists that the parathyroids produce a second hormone, calcitonin, which has an effect opposite that of parathormone; instead of elevating low levels of serum calcium, calcitonin serves to decrease high calcium levels.

PITUITARY GLANDS The anterior pituitary gland secretes several hormones. Some of these, such as the growth hormones, exert a direct effect on the metabolism of water and electrolytes. Others exert an indirect effect by stimulating other endocrine glands whose hormones directly influence metabolism; these include thyroid-stimulating hormone (TSH), adrenocortical stimulating hormone (ACTH), and the gonadotrophic hormones.

The posterior pituitary gland releases a water conserving hormone referred to as the antidiuretic hormone, or ADH. As the name implies, it inhibits diuresis. (It seems more direct to think of it as conserving water.) The release of ADH is influenced by the "osmostat," an auxiliary control located in the plexus of the internal carotid artery. The osmostat is sensitive to changes in osmolarity (electrolyte concentration) of the extracellular fluid.

ENDOCRINE DISORDERS CAUSING FLUID BALANCE DISTURBANCES

It is not within the scope of this chapter to discuss all of the endocrine disturbances causing fluid balance disturbances. A brief discussion of adrenocortical insufficiency and parathyroid disorders is presented. (Diabetes insipidus is discussed in Chapter 23.) Much emphasis is placed on diabetic acidosis because this condition is commonly encountered by the nurse.

Adrenocortical Insufficiency

Adrenocortical insufficiency may be caused by destruction or suppression of the adrenals, or it may be secondary to hypofunction of the pituitary gland. The disease can be either acute or chronic; symptoms are primarily due to decreased aldosterone and cortisol secretion.

WATER AND ELECTROLYTE CHANGES Water and electrolyte disturbances occurring with adrenocortical insufficiency include:

- Sodium deficit
- Potassium excess
- Extracellular fluid volume deficit
- Mild metabolic acidosis
- Hypercalcemia

Decreased aldosterone secretion is largely responsible for the increased urinary excretion of sodium and retention of potassium, although decreased cortisol secretion undoubtedly contributes to these changes as well. Water loss accompanies the increased urinary excretion of sodium and results in extracellular fluid volume deficit. Sodium is lost in addition to water. Hypercalcemia may also occur with adrenocortical insufficiency.

Decreased cortisol secretion causes a delay in water excretion; decreased glomerular filtration rate contributes to this effect. A loss of bicarbonate ions accompanies the sodium loss and a mild metabolic acidosis may result.

OTHER METABOLIC CHANGES Carbohydrate, protein and fat metabolism are impaired by adrenocortical insufficiency. Lack of cortisol causes decreased glyconeogenesis and depletion of the liver glycogen; thus, hypoglycemia can occur. Negative nitrogen balance results from the decreased secretion of 17-ketosteroids. Fat metabolism is slowed due to the reduced secretion of cortisol and corticosterone.

Other abnormalities include a reduced cellular response to injury, leukopenia and a decreased number of neutrophils.

CHRONIC ADRENAL INSUFFICIENCY Symptoms of chronic adrenal insufficiency may include:

- Fatigue out of proportion to activity
- Emotional depression and irritability
- Weight loss (due to fluid volume deficit and negative caloric balance)
- Hypotension (particularly pronounced when patient changes from a supine position to an upright position)
- Chronic gastrointestinal complaints of a vague nature
- Alternating diarrhea and constipation
- Hypoglycemia, noticed several hours after meals (symptoms include hunger, nervousness, sweating, headache, and confusion)
- Poor resistance to infection
- Muscle wasting and weakness
- Pigmentation of skin and mucous membranes common in adults
- Dental caries
- Craving for salt
- Poor reaction to stress (mild adrenal insufficiency may become severe under stress and can lead to vascular collapse)

Treatment consists of daily hormonal replacement therapy. Cortisone is given daily in a dose usually varying between 12.5 and 37.5 mg. This amount must be greatly increased when infection, trauma, diarrhea, inability to eat or other complications occur. Patients should be advised to consult their physician *immediately* when such conditions occur.

A mineralocorticoid is given in addition to cortisone to control sodium and potassium concentrations in the body. Although cortisone causes sodium retention, its effect is too weak to prevent sodium loss during periods of stress. Desoxycorticosterone is available in a long-acting form, Percorten pivalate, that may be given intramuscularly every 4 weeks.

Dietary sodium chloride intake should be consistent with the patient's taste and usually differs little from the average salt content of a normal diet. Salt tablets should be carried to repair sodium loss due to unusual circumstances, such as excessive heat exposure and sweating. Frequent carbohydrate feedings may prevent symptoms of hypoglycemia.

Overtreatment with cortisone may produce unfavorable symptoms such as acne, moon facies, diabetes mellitus, peptic ulcer, bleeding tendencies and hypertension. Overtreatment with mineralocorticoids may cause excessive fluid retention with weight gain and hypertension. The nurse should be alert for these symptoms. Careful recording of fluid intake and output and daily weight measurement are necessary to detect early fluid retention.

The patient should be made aware of the need for systematic medical follow-up in the control of his disease. He should be taught to avoid excessive physical and emotional stress and infections. In addition he should be aware of the symptoms accompanying under- and overtreatment of adrenocortical insufficiency.

Acute Adrenocortical Insufficiency

The nurse should be alert for acute adrenocortical insufficiency, sometimes termed "adrenal crisis," when patients with decreased adrenal function are exposed to stress, such as surgery, trauma, emotional upset or prolonged medical illness. Such a crisis may occur when a patient with chronic adrenocortical insufficiency fails to take his prescribed hormones. (Adrenal crisis as a result of surgery in patients on prolonged adrenocortical hormone therapy is discussed in Chapter 17.)

Symptoms of acute adrenocortical insufficiency include hypotension, thready pulse, nausea, vomiting, confusion and circulatory collapse. The body temperature may rise as high as 105° F.

Treatment consists of the intravenous administration of hydrocortisone as soon as possible. The blood volume should be expanded by the administration of isotonic solution of sodium chloride and glucose, dextran or blood. Vasopressor drugs may be necessary to raise the blood pressure. Sodium deficit should be corrected over a period of several days with hypertonic saline infusions. Glucose should be administered to prevent or correct symptoms of hypoglycemia. Intravenous hydrocortisone replacement therapy is continued until the patient is improved sufficiently to take cortisol intramuscularly, or cortisone when oral intake is tolerated.

The nurse should keep a close watch for changes in the vital signs. A fall in blood pressure and a rapid, thready pulse may indicate inadequate hydrocortisone and fluid replacement therapy. She should also protect the patient from physical and emotional stress, when possible.

Hypoparathyroidism

Underproduction of parathyroid hormone occurs in primary hypoparathyroidism and in the accidental removal of parathyroid tissue during thyroidectomy. Renal tubular damage can interfere with the action of parathyroid hormone and produce symptoms of hypoparathyroidism (pseudohypoparathyroidism). Decreased parathyroid activity results in:

1. Decreased plasma calcium concentration
2. Increased plasma phosphate concentration

Symptoms of hypoparathyroidism are primarily those of neuromuscular irritability produced by a decrease in the serum concentration of ionized calcium. They include:

Numbness of extremities
Tingling of hands, feet, and circumoral region
Mood changes
Voice changes caused by spasms of vocal cords
Muscular spasm, induced by compressing blood supply to area

Abdominal cramps
Diarrhea
Carpopedal attitude of hands
Facial spasm, induced by tapping over nerve course in front of the ear (Chvostek's sign)
Laryngeal spasms
Convulsions

Other symptoms of hypoparathyroidism are influenced by the duration of the parathyroid hormone deficiency and the age at which it developed. For example, cataracts or calcification of various body parts such as the basal ganglia of the brain may occur when hypoparathyroidism has long been present. Formation of new teeth is restricted when hypoparathyroidism occurs in a child, although the degree of hypoplasia depends upon the age at which hypoparathyroidism began.

The danger of the accidental removal of parathyroid tissue during thyroidectomy is always present because the parathyroids are small and resemble fatty tissue. Removal of half of the parathyroid glands usually doesn't present symptoms. (Most persons have four parathyroid glands; some have less and some have as many as seven.) However, removal of three out of four causes symptoms of hypoparathyroidism, until the fourth gland is able to hypertrophy sufficiently to fulfill the function of all of the glands. Tetany may be produced by temporary interference with the parathyroid blood supply following thyroidectomy.

The nurse should be alert for symptoms of deficit of ionized calcium during the postoperative care of patients who have undergone thyroidectomy. Such symptoms usually appear a few days after the operation. Early complaints are of numbness and tingling in the hands and feet. Compression of circulation to the hand while checking the blood pressure may cause spasm of the forearm muscles and palmar flexion of the hand. Other symptoms of deficit, such as general irritability or "jumpiness," may also be noted. It is crucial to detect calcium deficit early so that appropriate hormonal therapy or calcium replacement or both can be started before the onset of laryngeal spasms and convulsions.

Hypocalcemia due to hypoparathyroidism may be treated by the administration of calcium salts. Calcium gluconate given intravenously may control tetany; calcium gluconate or lactate may be administered orally for the same purpose. An increased dietary intake of high calcium foods will also be beneficial.

Dihydrotachysterol is a substance having an action similar to that of parathyroid hormone (parathormone). It increases calcium absorption from the bone and thus causes an increased plasma calcium concentration. It is given daily until symptoms subside, then weekly until symptoms disappear. The patient may then be maintained on vitamin D.

Hyperparathyroidism

Overproduction of parathyroid hormone occurs in primary hyperparathyroidism and in tumors of the parathyroid gland. Increased parathyroid activity results in:

1. Increased plasma calcium concentration
2. Decreased plasma phosphate concentration

Secondary hyperparathyroidism may be found in patients with renal disease, which interferes with excretion of phosphate ions and causes the plasma phosphate concentration to rise. Due to the reciprocal action of phosphate and calcium, the plasma calcium concentration drops. The low plasma calcium level causes stimulation of the parathyroids and eventually produces parathyroid hyperplasia, which causes progressive decalcification of the skeleton, sometimes referred to as "renal rickets."

Symptoms of hyperparathyroidism produced by the diminished neuromuscular irritability stemming from calcium excess include:

Mental confusion
Loss of memory or mental acuity
Lethargy
Weak, sluggish muscles
Constipation
Vomiting
Anorexia
Abdominal pain (may be the most striking symptom)
Prolonged cardiac systole

Other symptoms of hyperparathyroidism are produced by the excess filtration of calcium through the glomeruli. Calcium sediment deposits in the kidneys and produces tubular damage. Polyuria occurs, due to the increased renal solute load and to the damaged renal tubules. Polydipsia (excessive thirstiness) follows excessive water loss through the kidneys. Uremia and hypertension may eventually follow the renal damage imposed by calcium excess.

An early finding in many patients with hyperparathyroidism is x-ray evidence of subperiosteal resorption of the cortex, most clearly seen in the phalanges. Severe hyperparathyroidism causes excessive bone absorption and eventually produces extensive skeletal decalcification. Decalcified bones are easily broken; on x-ray they show "punched out" areas. The bone disorder produced by hyperparathyroidism is sometimes called von Recklinghausen's disease. There is an increased incidence of pancreatitis and gastric ulcers in patients with hyperparathyroidism.

The treatment of hyperparathyroidism consists of surgical removal of the over-active parathyroid tissue. More than one parathyroid tumor may be present and require the excision of several parathyroid glands. Following surgery, hypoparathyroidism may be present until the remaining parathyroid tissue hypertrophies.

Bone recalcification is rapid following removal of parathyroid tumors; symptoms of calcium excess recede. However, irreversible renal damage and skeletal deformities may have developed.

SEVERE DIABETIC ACIDOSIS

Diabetic acidosis occurs when an insulin lack prevents normal glucose metabolism, and body energy needs are met with the catabolism of fats and proteins. Events often associated with the onset of diabetic acidosis include:

- Failure to increase insulin dosage during times of increased need (infections, thyrotoxicosis, trauma, surgery, pregnancy, and periods of undue stress, including emotional stress)
- Omission, or inadequate dosage, of insulin
- Overeating
- Lack of carbohydrate, causing increased utilization of body fats and proteins (may be caused by strenuous exercise or prolonged vomiting)

Diabetic acidosis is a serious condition presenting several water and electrolyte disturbances. The nurse must be aware of the causes and manifestations of these imbalances so that she can detect their early occurrence and cooperate intelligently in their treatment.

Water and Electrolyte Disturbances Prior to Treatment

Insulin must be present for glucose to pass through the cell to participate in cellular metabolism. When insulin secretion is decreased, glucose cannot be utilized; its concentration in the blood stream rises (hyperglycemia). With glucose unavailable, the body must utilize fats and proteins; as the result of catabolism of fats, ketone bodies accumulate. This leads to ketosis (metabolic acidosis).

CELLULAR AND EXTRACELLULAR FLUID VOLUME DEFICIT Hyperosmolarity of the extracellular fluid is produced by the high glucose concentration. Water is drawn from the cells to maintain osmotic equilibrium. When the glucose concentration in the blood exceeds 180 mg. per 100 ml., glucose is excreted in the urine (glycosuria); because 10 to 20 ml. of water are required to excrete each gram of glucose, water loss through the kidneys is increased. Since sodium and chloride reabsorption are hindered by the osmotic diuresis, excessive amounts of these ions are excreted in the urine. The metabolic end-products of protein and fat increase the renal solute load, thus increasing the water loss. (Recall that materials must be in solution before the kidneys can excrete them.)

Insensible water loss by way of the lungs may be doubled due to the deep, rapid respiration accompanying acidosis. Although both water and electrolyte loss are increased in diabetic acidosis, water loss predominates. In severe diabetic acidosis there is a deficit of approximately 100 ml. of water per kg. of body weight. For example, a patient weighing 154 lbs. may have a water deficit of 7 L.; water is lost both from cells and from extracellular fluid.

KETOSIS (KETO-ACIDOSIS) The increased utilization of fat for energy needs causes accumulation of the ketone bodies aceto-acetic acid, beta-hydroxybutyric acid, and acetone. The usual keto-acid plasma level is 1 mEq./L.; it may reach as high as 20 mEq./L. in diabetic acidosis. Due to the increased keto-acid concentration in the blood stream, ketones are excreted by the kidneys (ketonuria). The accumulation of an excessive number of H^+. stemming from the keto-acids causes the blood pH to drop, sometimes to as low as 6.9 or even 6.8. The increase in the number of ketonic anions (negatively charged ions) causes a compensatory decrease in the number of bicarbonate anions (also negatively charged), representing the body's attempt to maintain electrical equilibrium. The bicarbonate level may drop as low as 5 mEq./L.

COMPENSATORY RESPIRATORY ALKALOSIS A fall in blood pH from the normal to not lower than 7.0 causes stimulation of the respiratory center and hyperventilation, which, in turn, causes an increase in blood pH. If the blood pH drops below 7.0, the respiratory center is depressed rather than stimulated. The acidosis is made more severe, due to retention of carbon dioxide by the lungs and the resultant increase in the carbonic acid content of the extracellular fluid. Severe fluid volume deficit can reduce the plasma volume sufficiently to induce circulatory shock. The resultant decreased blood flow to the respiratory center can also produce respiratory depression, even though the blood pH is above 7.0.

EFFECT OF FLUID VOLUME DEFICIT ON RENAL FUNCTION Plasma volume is decreased due to excessive fluid loss from the intravascular compartment. Decrease in the renal blood flow interferes with glomerular filtration. Organic acids, sulfates, phosphates, potassium, magnesium and nonprotein nitrogen waste products are retained by the kidneys, intensifying the metabolic acidosis. The increased retention of potassium, plus its liberation from the cells (due to fluid volume deficit and starvation), elevates the plasma potassium level. Oliguria eventually results when the plasma volume is decreased sufficiently to produce circulatory shock; it is associated with increased blood levels of potassium, urea, uric acid, creatinine, ketones and nonprotein nitrogen products.

CHANGES IN ELECTROLYTE CONCENTRATIONS Destruction of cells releases protein, glycogen, water and potassium; large quantities of potassium pass from the cells to the extracellular fluid. A cellular potassium deficit exists even though the potassium level of the extracellular fluid may be normal or even elevated. In severe diabetic acidosis, a 154 lb. man may develop a total potassium deficit of approximately 500 mEq.

Deficits of sodium and chloride may develop even though hemoconcentration is present; in addition to their loss with glucose diuresis, these electrolytes may be lost because of vomiting, gastric dilatation and paralytic ileus. Because sodium combines with ketonic anions, its excretion is increased. In severe diabetic acidosis, a 154 lb. man may develop a total sodium deficit of approximately 500 mEq., and a total chloride deficit of approximately 440 mEq.

Magnesium and phosphorus are chiefly cellular electrolytes, having actions related to potassium. Cellular deficits of these electrolytes probably develop in the same way as does cellular potassium deficit. A 154 lb. patient with severe diabetic acidosis may develop a total magnesium deficit of approximately 56 mEq., and a total phosphorus deficit of approximately 260 mEq.

Recognition of Diabetic Acidosis

The nurse should be thoroughly familiar with the symptoms of diabetic acidosis. She should be alert for their occurrence in any diabetic patient, but particularly in those with poor diet habits who are careless in their administration of insulin and those with infections or other illness. One of the nurse's greatest responsibilities to the diabetic patient and his family is to teach them the early recognition of diabetic acidosis.

Diabetic acidosis is characterized by a number of readily recognizable signs and symptoms. These with their probable causes are listed in Table 22-1.

Treatment of Diabetic Acidosis

INITIAL EVALUATION A patient with symptoms of diabetic acidosis should be admitted to the hospital for immediate evaluation and treatment. Often the emergency room nurse spends a brief time with the patient before the physician arrives. She should utilize this time to the fullest advantage to expedite diagnosis and treatment.

While obtaining a voided urine specimen for sugar and acetone tests, the nurse should try to get an account of the events leading to the development of symptoms. If the patient is confused and non-responsive, the information may often be obtained from an accompanying family member. The nurse should also ask if any treatment for acidosis was given prior to hospital admission. (Sometimes the physician may instruct the family by phone to give a fast-acting insulin if symptoms of acidosis are present.) The patient should be kept warm with blankets. (If a voided urine specimen cannot be obtained, the physician may later request a catheterized specimen.) The patient may have a dilated atonic urinary bladder; failure to void should not be attributed to renal failure until the bladder is catheterized to check for this disorder. The nurse should use meticulous technique while performing this procedure; infections are particularly dangerous in the diabetic patient.

The nurse should check and record the vital signs at frequent intervals. A low blood pressure and a rapid thready pulse may indicate severe fluid volume deficit with circulatory failure. A change from deep, rapid respiration to rapid, shallow gasping respiration may indicate a severe drop in blood pH (below 7.0) or impaired blood flow to the respiratory center due to fluid volume deficit and circulatory collapse. A temperature elevation probably indicates the presence of an acute infection; the temperature is usually subnormal in the patient with diabetic acidosis. The patient's level of consciousness should be evaluated at frequent intervals; progressive loss of consciousness indicates increasing severity of acidosis. Other symptoms of acidosis should be searched for and noted. (See Table 22-1.)

The nurse should notify the laboratory to draw blood; the physician usually requests tests for blood sugar, bicarbonate or blood pH, acetone and blood urea nitrogen. Intravenous water and electrolytes such as hypotonic saline or a balanced hypotonic electrolyte solution (Butler type) may be ordered. Initial fluids are given to improve the blood volume and blood pressure. Insulin is not usually administered until the blood sugar and urine test results are available. When acetone is found in the urine, or when other pronounced signs of acidosis are present, a dose of quick-acting insulin may be given before the blood sugar test result is obtained. It is imperative that the presence of hypoglycemia be ruled out before insulin is given. Hypoglycemia is characterized by anxiety, sweating, hunger, headache, dizziness, double vision, twitching, convulsions, nausea, pale wet skin, dilated pupils, normal breathing, and normal blood pressure.

INSULIN ADMINISTRATION Since the lack of insulin initiates diabetic acidosis, insulin administration is required to correct it; however, there is some disagreement as to how much, when and how it should be given.

Some physicians prefer to give adults approximately 100 units of regular or crystalline insulin intravenously the first hour, and then 100 units intramuscularly every hour for the next 3 or 4 hours. (Factors influencing the insulin dose include the patient's blood sugar, weight and the duration of his diabetes.) Other physicians prefer to give multiple doses of regular or crystalline insulin, such as 50 units every hour, until acetonuria diminishes. There are valid arguments for both methods.

Insulin can be given intravenously, intramuscularly, or subcutaneously. For maximal rapidity of action, regular or crystalline insulin is

Table 22-1. Signs and Symptoms of Diabetic Acidosis and Their Probable Cause

Sign or Symptom	*Probable Cause*
Polyuria	Osmotic diuretic effect of hyperglycemia (Renal solute load greatly increased due to presence of high glucose concentration and to the increased concentration of metabolic end-products of fat and protein)
Polydipsia	Cellular dehydration causes thirst (Water loss causes hyperosmolarity of the extracellular fluid; water is drawn from the cells)
Glycosuria	Blood glucose level exceeds renal threshold (usually 180 mg./100 ml.)
Acetonuria	Excessive accumulation of ketones in the blood causes increased excretion of ketones in the urine (acetone is a ketone body)
High specific gravity of urine	High renal solute load
Tiredness, muscular weakness	Lack of carbohydrate, potassium deficit; loss of protein from muscles
Face appears drawn and flushed	Fluid volume deficit (sharpening of facial features) Acidosis (flushed color)
Dry tongue and mucous membranes, cracked lips	Fluid volume deficit
Deep, rapid respiration (Kussmaul)	Compensatory mechanism to increase extracellular fluid pH by the elimination of large amounts of CO_2 from the lungs with the resultant decreased carbonic acid content in blood
Nausea and vomiting (Vomitus may be dark brown, due to blood)	Atony of the stomach Bleeding from stretched gastric mucosa
Brownish particles on teeth, lips and gums	Deposited there when vomitus is expelled
Weight loss	Fluid volume deficit, inability to metabolize glucose
Acetone breath odor (odor similar to that of over-ripe apples)	Acetone content of body increases; acetone is volatile and is vaporized in the expired air
Gastric dilatation and paralytic ileus	Neuropathy Water and electrolyte loss
Abdominal pain, rigid abdomen (can simulate appendicitis, pancreatitis, or other acute abdominal problem)	Apparently related to fluid volume deficit (condition improves when deficit is repaired)
Chest pain (may simulate pain of pleurisy)	Apparently related to fluid deficit (condition improves when fluid deficit is repaired); may be due to overactive respiration caused by acidosis
Moaning	Usually associated with abdominal or chest pain
Soft eyeballs, wrinkled cornea	Fluid volume deficit
Low blood pressure	Fluid volume deficit severe enough to decrease plasma volume significantly
Cold extremities, may have purplish appearance	Decreased peripheral blood flow secondary to fluid volume deficit
Body temperature below normal or normal (If fever is present it is almost always associated with the precipitating factor of the diabetic acidosis, such as an infection)	Fluid volume deficit
Oliguria	Fluid volume deficit causes decreased renal blood flow with decreased glomerular filtration rate Atonic urinary bladder may become greatly distended with urine

Table 22-1. Signs and Symptoms of Diabetic Acidosis and Their Probable Cause *(Continued)*

Sign or Symptom	*Probable Cause*
Rapid, shallow, gasping respiration replacing Kussmaul breathing	Drop in blood pH below 7.0 or significantly decreased blood flow to the respiratory center
Laboratory Findings	
Blood sugar:	
(Normal is 80-120 mg./100 ml.)	
Elevated above normal, usually 400-600 mg./100 ml.; may be as high as 2,000 mg./100 ml.	Faulty glucose metabolism causes glucose to accumulate in the blood
Bicarbonate:	
(Normal plasma bicarbonate level is: 25-29 mEq./L. for adults; 20-25 mEq./L. for children)	
Decreased below normal; may be as low as 5 mEq./L.	Ketonic anions cause a decrease in the bicarbonate level
Others:	
NPN elevated	Impaired metabolism and glomerular function
White count elevated, but differential normal	

best, since only they can be given intravenously. Although intramuscular injections are absorbed more quickly than subcutaneous injections, the intravenous route gives the quickest results of all, and is most dependable when there is some question of absorption from intramuscular or subcutaneous injections because of the presence of shock.

The nurse should observe the patient for signs of hypoglycemia, which might occur with the large doses of insulin required to correct acidosis. Other nursing reponsibilities include performing urine sugar and acetone tests accurately, checking insulin orders with great care, and measuring the insulin dosage carefully. The orders for insulin are based on the blood sugar and acetone levels and on the quantities of sugar and acetone in the urine. Orders for insulin may be confusing in the early treatment of acidosis; the nurse should take sufficient time to be certain she carries them out accurately.

In a sense, urine values for glucose and acetone tell the attendant less about the patient's current status than about past events. With aggressive treatment one can produce hypoglycemia in the presence of glycosuria and ketonuria.

The large doses of insulin sometimes needed to correct acidosis may be frightening to the nurse if she is unaware that in ketoacidosis an abnormal serum globulin is present which antagonizes the action of insulin.

FLUID REPLACEMENT THERAPY

1. Early Phase (First 4 Hours). After the initial insulin dose has been given, emphasis is placed on re-establishing the blood volume and repairing extracellular and cellular fluid volume deficits. Repair of the deficient blood volume causes improved renal function and allows the excretion of excess organic acid wastes and metabolic end-products. This may be accomplished by the administration of 2 to 3 L. of isotonic solution of sodium chloride or hypotonic electrolyte solutions during the first 2 to 6 hours.

Isotonic solution of sodium chloride (0.9%) is readily available and is commonly used in the treatment of diabetic acidosis. It expands the extracellular fluid volume and helps replace losses of sodium and chloride. The first 2 L. can be given in 2 to 4 hours if the patient has satisfactory cardiac and renal status. It does not, however, provide free water for cellular hydration and the establishment of urine flow. Moreover, its chloride content exceeds that normally found in plasma; therefore, if used extensively, it can worsen acidosis by imposing a chloride excess. (An excessive number of chloride ions causes a compensatory decrease in the number of bicarbonate ions.) Usually no more than 3 L. of isotonic saline are given in the first 6 to 12 hours, to avoid making the acidosis more severe.

Since the patient with acidosis loses relatively more water than electrolytes, there is much to be said for the administration of hypotonic solutions; a hypotonic solution of sodium chloride with or without added sodium lactate or bicarbonate can be employed.

Another solution sometimes used in the early treatment of acidosis is a mixture of 750 ml. of lactated Ringer's and 250 ml. of distilled water. The use of sixth molar sodium lactate or 1.5 per cent sodium bicarbonate is recommended by some to increase the bicarbonate content of the blood. Unless these solutions are administered cautiously, they may produce alkalosis.

Authorities disagree as to the desirability of using glucose solutions in the early treatment of diabetic acidosis. Some physicians use them from the onset of treatment; others wait at least 4 hours before infusing glucose solutions. Those against the early use of glucose feel that it does nothing more than to add to hyperglycemia and thus increases osmotic diuresis with the resultant water and electrolyte loss from the body. After the first 4 to 6 hours of treatment, danger of hypoglycemia exists, perhaps because the available glucose has been metabolized and there is no glycogen available. Thus glucose may be needed. (One liter of 5 per cent glucose in water is usually covered with 25 units of regular insulin.)

Fructose has been used in the early treatment of diabetic acidosis because it does not require insulin to be metabolized, thus sparing body fat and decreasing ketogenesis. It does not, however, increase glucose utilization.

Potassium administration is contraindicated in the early phase of treatment, since the plasma potassium level is usually elevated due to the liberation of cellular potassium into the extracellular fluid and to poor renal excretion of potassium caused by decreased urinary output. Potassium excess may cause cardiac arrhythmias; if elevated to two or three times the normal level, cardiac arrest may occur. Potassium solutions are best withheld until the plasma potassium level is normal or below normal. The ECG is used frequently throughout therapy to detect changes in potassium concentration. Signs of potassium excess may appear during this phase, or the ECG may remain normal. Only very rarely does a patient show potassium deficit at this time; if so, it is almost always associated with a severe loss of potassium prior to the onset of diabetic acidosis.

2. Second Phase (4-8 Hours). Approximately 4 to 8 hours after the onset of therapy the patient is usually much improved and the need for parenteral fluids is decreased. Usually oral fluids may be tolerated by this time. The rate of intravenous infusion can be considerably slowed. If the blood sugar has fallen substantially, glucose may be given orally to combat hypoglycemia; intravenous glucose in water may also be required.

Although potassium deficit rarely occurs this early, the plasma potassium level has usually dropped sufficiently to allow potassium to be given, by mouth or intravenously, to ameliorate the developing cellular deficit. Oral administration is preferable. Fluids of high potassium content include orange juice, grape juice, milk and real meat broth. (Contrary to common belief, consommé cubes are not rich in potassium.) Intravenous replacement of potassium can be accomplished by use of a Butler-type solution, or it may be added to a suitable fluid in the form of KCl. (Nursing responsibilities in the administration of potassium solutions are discussed in Chapter 16.)

3. Phase of Potassium Deficit (8-24 Hours). Recall that in the early phase of diabetic acidosis the plasma potassium level is normal or elevated, due to the liberation of potassium from the cells during the breakdown of glycogen and protein, and to decreased renal function with excessive retention of potassium. After administration of potassium-free fluids early in therapy, the plasma potassium decreases for the following reasons:

A. The administered fluids dilute the plasma.
B. Re-establishment of the plasma volume improves renal function and increases potassium excretion.
C. Part of the extracellular potassium enters the cells as they take up glucose under

the influence of administered insulin.

D. Formation of glycogen within the cells—involving utilization of potassium, glucose, and water—causes further withdrawal of potassium from the extracellular fluid.
E. Potassium re-enters the cells to help repair the cellular potassium deficit.

Because of the great need for potassium during the later stages of treatment, potassium should be added to parenteral infusions during this period.

Potassium deficit becomes obvious after 8 to 24 hours of treatment, most often between the 10th and 24th hours. The plasma potassium level may fall as low as 2 mEq./L. (recall that the normal plasma K^+ level is 5 mEq./L.). The nurse should be alert for the symptoms of potassium deficit during these hours, including:

Weakness
Flaccid paralysis of skeletal muscles
Paralysis of respiratory muscles, resulting in shallow, gasping respiration and cyanosis
Abdominal distention
ECG changes
Cardiac failure with ashen color
Sudden death (most common 8 to 20 hours after therapy is started)

Potassium should be given as soon as renal function improves and the plasma potassium concentration falls to normal. The cellular potassium deficit takes over a week to replace; yet, even small amounts of potassium taken regularly help ward off a severe deficit. Fluids mentioned above should be encouraged. Oral replacement of potassium is safer than intravenous replacement; if the patient tolerates oral fluids better, they can be enriched with potassium additives. (K-Lyte, an effervescent potassium preparation, is palatable and well tolerated.)

Summary of Fluid Therapy Aims In the first 24 hours of treatment of diabetic acidosis, the aim is to replace 80 per cent of the total water, sodium and chloride loss. Cellular electrolytes are not assimilated as rapidly as extracellular ones; therefore, only 50 per cent of the potassium and magnesium deficit, and 25 per cent of the phosphate deficit, are replaced on the first day. In addition to replacing past and concurrent losses, daily maintenance needs must be met.

GASTRIC LAVAGE Some physicians routinely perform a gastric lavage on all patients with diabetic acidosis. Others do so only when the patient has demonstrable signs of gastric dilatation, such as nausea, vomiting and epigastric distress.

Removal of gastric contents makes the patient more comfortable; it relieves abdominal distention, vomiting and nausea. Oral intake is made possible earlier. The danger of aspirating gastric contents is less when the distended viscus is emptied, but the hazard of inducing alkalosis should not be disregarded.

CLEANSING ENEMA A cleansing enema may be ordered to relieve abdominal distention caused by intestinal atony.

OTHER THERAPY The patient should be restored to his usual diet as quickly as it is tolerated. After recovery from diabetic acidosis, long-acting insulin can be resumed, with supplemental doses of fast-acting insulin as indicated by urine test results. An excellent opportunity exists for teaching the patient while he is still in the hospital how to prevent future bouts of acidosis.

Nurse's Role in Preventing Diabetic Acidosis

Because the nurse is actively involved in teaching diabetic patients, she is in a splendid position to help prevent diabetic acidosis. She should keep the basic learning principles in mind when teaching self-care to diabetics. The rate of learning of the individual must be considered; so must the knowledge he already possesses concerning the disease. Physicians sometimes present explanations far beyond the patient's comprehension. Rather than risk the embarrassment of asking for a more simplified explanation, the patient may pretend to understand—this can lead to serious difficulties.

It is important for the patient to gain a clear understanding of his condition and of his responsibilities to himself. Time and effort devoted to effective teaching of the diabetic patient pays off handsomely when it helps prevent diabetic acidosis.

Failure to teach the diabetic the importance of (1) taking the prescribed amount of insulin daily, (2) reporting conditions that may alter the need for insulin, (3) adhering to the prescribed diet, (4) performing urine sugar and acetone tests accurately, and (5) seeking medical follow-up as indicated, predisposes to diabetic acidosis.

INSULIN ADMINISTRATION The omission of insulin injections or inadequate insulin doses are common causes of diabetic acidosis. It is not unusual to admit a patient in diabetic acidosis who comments, "I've been vomiting and unable to eat for the past few days and didn't need my insulin." He has assumed that when he does not eat he should omit insulin injections. This common assumption is not true. The body needs insulin, although in modified doses and perhaps a different type, even when the patient is not eating. The nurse should make it clear that insulin should never be omitted without specific direction from the physician. When unable to eat, the patient should contact his physician for instructions. The once-daily injection of long-acting insulin may be temporarily reduced or discontinued, until the patient is able to eat again. Instead, frequent doses of quick acting insulin may be given as indicated by findings of urine sugar and acetone tests. If food intake is decreased for a prolonged period, the patient should be admitted to the hospital for parenteral fluid therapy and observation. It must be remembered that the nausea and vomiting experienced by the patient may be signs of developing diabetic acidosis. If so, failure to take insulin accelerates the development of acidosis.

A number of factors can result in the administration of too little insulin. An inadequate insulin dose may be due to failure to properly mix protamine zinc, NPH, or Lente insulin vials prior to drawing up the insulin. Insulin that is too old or has been spoiled by freezing or overheating is ineffective. Continued injection at the same site may produce inflammation, hypertrophy, or atrophy of the local tissue. Further insulin injected into these areas is not well absorbed and results in an inadequate insulin dosage. The diabetic with poor vision may draw up an inadequate amount of insulin because of difficulty in reading the insulin scale. (Sometimes such a patient may draw up, undetected, a large air bubble which decreases the amount of insulin contained in the syringe.) Drawing up insulin on the wrong scale also causes an inaccurate dosage; for example, drawing up U-40 insulin on a U-80 scale results in half the desired dose. (Of course, poor vision and faulty technique can also cause insulin overdosage.) The diabetic who is poorly controlled at home should be observed for faulty technique in drawing up and administering his insulin.

DIABETIC DIET Eating more than permitted by the prescribed diet is a frequent cause of diabetic acidosis. While this may be due to poor emotional acceptance of the disease, it may also be due to lack of adequate understanding of the diet.

When possible, the diabetic patient should receive his diet instructions during frequent sessions with a dietitian. The nurse should have sufficient understanding of the diet to supplement the dietitian's instructions. Sometimes, in the absence of a dietitian, the nurse must carry the entire responsibility of diet instruction. Few nurses are so well acquainted with diabetic diets that they will not profit from a review prior to teaching the patient.

Urine Testing

Physicians rely heavily on urine sugar and acetone tests to serve as guides in prescribing insulin. The time and frequency of urine tests, as well as the method to be used, should be indicated on the order sheet. Some physicians order "spot checks" (tests of individual urine specimens) at regular intervals. These are usually done on arising, before lunch, before the evening meal, and at bedtime; sometimes they are done two hours after meals. Other times the physician may prefer fractional, or group, urine testing. Fractional urines are usually collected in four parts according to the time of day: before breakfast to just before lunch; before lunch to just before the evening meal; before the evening meal to bedtime; from bedtime until the next morning. Testing of fractional urines helps the physician find the time of day glucose excretion is highest. This information is helpful in prescribing the appropriate type and amount of insulin.

If the tests are performed improperly, or reported incorrectly, the physician will receive false information and the insulin dose is likely to be incorrect.

GENERAL CONSIDERATIONS

1. It is best to use the second of double-voided specimens, particularly when the patient has severe diabetes. After the first specimen is obtained, the patient is encouraged to drink a glass of water; after 30 to 45 minutes, a second specimen is collected. The second specimen is desirable for urinary sugar testing, because it reflects the glucose spill-over into the urine at that time (while the first specimen reflects an indefinite accumulation).
2. Directions given by the manufacturers of the various tests should be followed closely. Although this sounds simple, recent studies have shown that hospital personnel commonly perform urine tests inaccurately. This is a matter of concern for two reasons: (a) control of the hospitalized diabetic is difficult to achieve without the aid of accurate urine testing; (b) personnel performing urine tests inaccurately are hardly in a position to teach patients to perform these same tests.
3. The record used for charting urine test results should indicate the test method used. Unless instructions are clear, various nurses on the unit may use the method they like best; the use of different testing methods for the same patient leads to much confusion. Some nurses use plus marks interchangeably between tests—this, of course, is not accurate. For example: a two-plus on Tes-Tape indicates a sugar concentration of 1/4%, while a two-plus on Clinitest indicates a sugar concentration of three times this amount (3/4%). (See Table 22-2 for a comparison of results in some of the more commonly used tests for urinary sugar content.) When regular insulin is ordered on a sliding scale, based on urinary sugar content, the physician should indicate the specific test he wants used. For example, a typical order might read:

   Give 5 units of regular insulin if Clinitest is one-plus
   Give 10 units of regular insulin if Clinitest is two-plus
   Give 15 units of regular insulin if Clinitest is three-plus
   Give 20 units of regular insulin if Clinitest is four-plus
4. Clean receptacles should be used to collect the specimen; failure to thoroughly rinse out the urinal or bedpan between voidings can cause inaccurate results.
5. It is wise to check the material in the test apparatus for changes from its normal appearance. For example, Clinitest tablets that are disintegrating and have changed to a dark color are not suitable for use and should be discarded. When in doubt, materials can be tested for effectiveness with a nondietetic cola beverage; ordinary table sugar will not produce a positive reaction.
6. Good lighting is necessary for reading test results; this is particularly important when eyesight is impaired. Diabetics with extremely poor vision should have someone else read the test results for them. The color comparison chart should be in good condition—faded charts can lead to inaccurate readings.
7. The test results should be compared with the appropriate color comparison chart. Patients switched to a different form of testing may be unaware that each test method has its own chart; unless instructed otherwise they may continue to use the old chart with the new test.
8. The nurse should be aware that the amount of sugar spilled into the urine depends on the blood sugar level and the renal threshold. Most individuals spill

Table 22-2. Comparison of Degrees of Sugar Content Indicated by Various Urine Tests

Tes-Tape	*Diastix*	*Clinitest (5-drop method)*
0% Negative	0% Negative	0% Negative
	1/10% Trace	1/4% Trace
1/10% (+)	1/4% (+)	1/2% (+)
1/4% (++)	1/2% (++)	3/4% (++)
1/2% (+++)	1% (+++)	1% (+++)
2% (++++)	2% (++++)	2% (++++)

Clinitest (2-drop method)	*Clinistix*
0% Negative	"Light" generally indicates 1/4% or less
Trace	"Medium" generally indicates 1/4 to 1/2%
1/2%	"Dark" generally indicates 1/2% or more
1%	
2%	
3%	
5%	

sugar into the urine when the blood sugar content exceeds 180 mg. per 100 ml. of blood. However, some persons have an elevated renal threshold; that is, the blood sugar may be above normal while the patient continues to have negative tests for sugar in the urine. On the other hand, some have a low renal threshold and spill sugar into the urine while the blood sugar level is near normal or is within the normal range. A urine-glucose value is significant only when the patient's renal threshold for glucose is known. It is helpful to check an occasional blood sugar at the same time as a urine sugar.

TESTS FOR URINARY SUGAR Various tests are available to detect and measure urinary sugar content; among these are Clinitest, Tes-Tape, Clinistix and Diastix.

Clinitest Clinitest* reagent tablets utilize the copper-reducing reaction to measure the amount of sugar in the urine. The method for testing with Clinitest tablets is as follows:

(1) Place 5 drops of urine and 10 drops of water in a clean test tube
(2) Drop in one Clinitest tablet
(3) Observe the reaction carefully for the rapid pass-through phenomenon (if the solution passes through orange to some shade of brown, it indicates that more than a 2% sugar concentration is present, and this should be recorded without reference to the color chart)
(4) Wait 15 seconds after the boiling stops; shake the tube gently and compare the solution with the color chart provided with test (Clinitest's color reaction ranges from blue, no sugar, through shades of green and brown to orange, 2% sugar)

Because the pass-through phenomenon is not well understood, it is a common source of error. To help decrease the frequency of this error, a variation of the Clinitest method has been devised. Two drops of urine, instead of five, are mixed with 10 drops of water; the resulting solution is less concentrated and the urinary sugar content must exceed 5% before the pass-through phenomenon can occur. (Although it is possible to observe the pass-through reaction using the two-drop method, it isn't very likely.) Even though the two-drop method is superior to the five-drop method for patients who commonly run high urine sugars, it may present some problems. A special color chart must be obtained from the manufacturer because the results are different from those of the five-drop method. The two charts appear similar and may be easily confused unless one is aware of their differences. Because the two-drop chart is used infrequently, it must be specially requested.

Clinitest tablets are extremely hygroscopic and thus should not be exposed to moisture; tablets wrapped in foil should be used immediately upon opening. Glass bottles containing Clinitest tablets should be kept tightly closed; after opening, tablets in glass bottles should be used on a regular basis and not stored for an extended period of time. Tablets with a dark blue color should be discarded.

Clinitest registers a color change in response

* Ames Company, Division of Miles Laboratories, Inc., Elkhart, Indiana.

to other reducing agents besides glucose when they are present in concentrations of 1/4% or more. However, such substances are generally not present in sufficient quantities to cause false positives or elevated readings. A partial list of medications that may produce false positive results with Clinitest include:

ascorbic acid (in large doses)
probenecid (Benemid®)
penicillin
isoniazid
sodium cephalothin (Keflin®)
cephalexin monohydrate (Keflex®)
nalidixic acid (NegGram®)
para-aminosalicylic acid

Clinitest is not the method of choice for urine testing in patients with tuberculosis because the antituberculosis drugs are reducing agents.

Clinitest detects not just glucose, but all sugars in the urine (lactose, galactose, fructose, maltose, and pentose). Therefore, it should not be used for urine testing in the last trimester of pregnancy when lactosuria may be present. (Lactose has no effect on Diastix, Clinistix, or Tes-Tape.)

Tes-Tape Tes-Tape* is a roll of yellow test paper impregnated with a dye and an enzyme, glucose oxidase. In the presence of sugar, this enzyme reacts and releases the dye. Tes-Tape is considered specific for glucose determination. The method used for testing with Tes-Tape is as follows:

(1) Collect the urine specimen in a clean container
(2) Tear off about 1½ inches of the test paper and moisten it uniformly with urine (the tape held between the fingers should be kept dry because the hands may carry traces of sugar)
(3) Remove the test strip from the urine and wait one minute; the tape should be held during this period (laying the tape down could result in its contamination if the surface contains traces of sugar)
(4) Compare the darkest area on the test strip with the color chart on the Tes-Tape dispenser (if the tape indicates 1/2% or higher, wait an additional minute and make a final comparison)

The tape remains yellow if the test is negative; intermediate amounts of sugar produce various shades of green, and a concentration of 2% causes the tape to turn blue. Note that this color reaction is very different from that of Clinitest. Tes-Tape is more convenient than Clinitest, but Clinitest is probably more accurate in showing the precise amount of sugar present in the urine. The expiration date on the Tes-Tape package should be checked. Once opened, Tes-Tape cannot be made air-tight and should be kept in a dry place.

Diastix Diastix** reagent strips are used for the semiquantitative determination of glucose in urine. The method for testing with Diastix is as follows:

(1) Urine specimen should be freshly voided and well mixed—the container should be absolutely clean and free from cleansers and disinfectants (refrigerated urine specimens should be allowed to reach room temperature before testing)
(2) Dip the reagent end of the strip in the urine specimen for two seconds, or pass it through the urine stream
(3) Tap the edge of the strip against the side of the urine container or sink to remove excess urine
(4) Exactly 30 seconds after removing the strip from the urine, compare the reagent side of the strip to the closest matching color block (disregard color changes that occur after 30 seconds)

This test may detect minute quantities of glucose in the urine (as low as 1/100% to 1/10%). It, then, may show a trace of sugar when the Clinitest is negative. (Recall that Clinitest shows trace at 1/4%.)

Diastix is designed primarily for use at home

* Eli Lilly and Company, Indianapolis, Indiana.

** Ames Company, Division of Miles Laboratories, Inc., Elkhart, Indiana.

by late-onset diabetic patients who are unlikely to encounter ketonuria. This test is not recommended when there is a likelihood of ketonuria because moderate to large amounts of acetoacetic acid may depress the color response. (Patients treated with a biguanide type of oral hypoglycemic agent may show ketonuria in the absence of marked glycosuria.)

Diastix reagent strips should be kept in a cool, dry place, but not in the refrigerator; the bottle should be kept tightly closed. Prior to use, the test area on the strip should match the negative color block on the color chart; if it doesn't, the strip should be discarded.

Clinistix Clinistix* reagent strips undergo a color change when moistened with urine containing glucose. The method for urine testing with Clinistix is as follows:

(1) Moisten the red end of the Clinistix by passing it once through the urine stream or by dipping it in a fresh urine specimen collected in a clean container
(2) Remove immediately from the urine (prolonged immersion may cause leaching of the reagents)
(3) Exactly 10 seconds after wetting, compare the test area with the color block on the Clinistix bottle label

Clinistix is a specific for glucose. "Light" generally indicates 1/4% glucose concentration or less. (The minimal concentration of glucose detectable by Clinistix ranges from as little as 1/100% to 1/10%.) "Medium" generally indicates glucose in amounts of 1/4% to 1/2%. "Dark" generally indicates 1/2% glucose concentration or more. Large amounts of ascorbic acid or acetoacetic acid have definite inhibitory effects on the color development.

Clinistix should be stored in a cool, dry place, and protected from exposure to direct light, excessive heat or humidity. Discolored strips should not be used. The test end of the strip should not be handled, nor should it be laid on the work surface with the reagent area downward.

TESTS FOR KETONURIA All diabetics should be taught how to test for ketonuria. It is a good practice to test for ketones periodically regardless of the urinary glucose concentration. Of course, the consistent presence of large amounts of sugar in the urine is an indication to test for ketones regularly. Ketonuria tests should especially be performed in diabetic children, difficult to control adult diabetics, the pregnant diabetic, and in the conversion from insulin to oral hypoglycemic agents.

The ketones present in the urine of the uncontrolled diabetic include acetoacetic acid, acetone, and beta hydroxy-butyric acid. Ketonuria may provide the clue to the early diagnosis of diabetic acidosis. Two common tests used to detect ketonuria include Acetest and Ketostix.

Acetest Acetest* detects both acetone and acetoacetic acid in the urine. The colorimetric chart provided with this test has three colors ranging from lavender to deep purple, representing small, moderate, or large amounts of ketones. If the test is negative, the tablet remains buff colored. The method for testing is as follows:

(1) Place an Acetest tablet on a clean surface, preferably a piece of clean white paper
(2) Put one drop of urine on the tablet
(3) Read the reaction at 30 seconds against the color chart (failure of the drop of urine to completely absorb within this period indicates that the tablet has been exposed to moisture and may give a faulty reading)

Ketostix Ketostix* reagent strips are also used to test for acetoacetic acid and acetone in urine. The method for testing is as follows:

(1) Dip the test area of the strip in fresh urine or pass it briefly through the urine stream and remove it immediately
(2) Tap the edge of the strip against the container to remove excess urine
(3) Fifteen seconds after wetting, compare the color of the test area with the color chart (the shade of lavender or purple developed at 15 seconds indicates the

---

* Ames Company, Division of Miles Laboratories, Inc., Elkhart, Indiana.

concentration of ketones in the urine). Ignore color developing on the test area after 15 seconds

Ketostix strips should be protected from moisture, direct sunlight, and heat. Discoloration of the test area of the strip is an indication to discard it.

Recognition of Diabetic Acidosis

Failure of the patient to recognize the early symptoms of uncontrolled diabetes and early diabetic acidosis leads to delay in instituting treatment. The longer the patient goes without treatment, the less are his chances for recovery.

The nurse should stress the importance of being alert for symptoms of acidosis, particularly when an infection, disease, or emotional upset is present. She should also point out that when such symptoms occur, the attending physician should be notified immediately. Manufacturers of insulin preparations provide excellent literature for diabetics; many useful facts are contained in these booklets. For example, symptoms of acidosis and hypoglycemia are described in a clear and simple fashion. The patient should be given copies of such literature for use during teaching sessions and for reference at home. A member of the patient's family should also be taught to recognize symptoms of acidosis.

23 Fluid Balance in the Patient With Neurologic Disease

REGULATION OF FLUID BALANCE BY THE CENTRAL NERVOUS SYSTEM

Respiratory Center and pH Regulation

The amount of carbon dioxide given off by the lungs is controlled by the respiratory center in the medulla. Recall that carbon dioxide is crucial in the carbonic acid–base bicarbonate buffer system. Alkalinity and pH of the extracellular fluid increase when an excessive amount of carbon dioxide is exhaled. On the other hand, the acidity of the extracellular fluid increases and the pH decreases when too much carbon dioxide is retained.

Chemoreceptors found in the aortic arch and in the carotid sinus send stimuli to the respiratory center. Chemical stimuli that increase respiration include:

Increased CO_2 content of blood (up to an arterial concentration of 9%)
Decreased plasma pH
Hypoxia

The inhalation of carbon dioxide in a concentration of less than 9 per cent stimulates the respiratory center and increases respiration by increasing the concentration of carbonic acid and decreasing the pH of the plasma. If the concentration of carbon dioxide in the inspired air is greater than 9 per cent, however, the nervous receptors are unable to respond. Instead of increased respiration, there is decreased respiration and carbon dioxide narcosis. Clinically, this is of crucial import.

A fall in plasma pH causes an increase in rate and depth of respiration, which blows off excess carbon dioxide; however, if the plasma pH falls below 7.0, pulmonary ventilation is depressed, and the acidosis becomes more severe. A reduction in the available oxygen causes hypoxia and increased respiration. Pathologic conditions can cause depression or stimulation of the medullary respiratory neurons and can thus alter plasma pH. (See the section dealing with changes in pulmonary ventilation.)

Influence of Central Nervous System on Osmotic Balance

The central nervous system influences water loss from the kidneys, the skin, and the lungs. It controls the desire to drink, as well as the motor ability to do so. Emotions influence water balance by affecting the drinking pattern; for example, neuroses sometimes cause compulsive water drinking.

Hyperosmolarity stimulates the hypothalamus to release ADH, the secretion of which is also influenced by volume receptors in the left atrium and pulmonary veins.

CLINICAL CONDITIONS

Brain infections, tumors, or trauma can cause a diversity of fluid balance problems, depending on the area of the brain involved. Injury to the hypothalamus and the brain stem presents the most problems, because many metabolic functions are controlled in these areas. Many brain injuries interfere with the patient's ability to recognize thirst, as well as his ability to drink. The desire to eat and the ability to do so may also be affected. Recall that inadequate intake of food and fluids is responsible for a number of fluid imbalances.

Often, water and electrolyte balance is the most critical factor in determining the survival of the neurologic patient. For this reason, the nurse should become acutely aware of common problems so that she can aid in their early detection and correction.

HYPERTHERMIA The heat control center is located in the hypothalamus. Direct injury to this area, or pressure exerted by edema or masses in other areas of the brain, can cause a body temperature elevation. The extent of the elevation provides an important clue to the seriousness of the brain injury. For example, a slight concussion may result in a temperature of 101° F. or less. A more severe head injury may quickly be followed by a high temperature. Cerebral vascular accidents cause temperature elevations that are roughly proportional to the severity of the accident; a rise in temperature in a neurologic patient is an ominous sign. Of course, fever may be due to other causes, such as pneumonia, urinary tract infection, or dehydration (sodium excess).

Patients who have recovered from encephalitis, or those with cerebral damage from birth injuries, may have faulty temperature regulation. Multiple sclerosis is sometimes associated with low, irregular fever. In addition, an injury to the upper cervical spinal cord often results in high, irregular fever. Finally, surgical operations in the area of the third ventricle sometimes cause pronounced hyperthermia.

Fever should be reduced by pharmacologic or physical means. An automatically regulated hypothermic blanket can be most helpful in reducing temperature; sponging with ice water or alcohol is less effective. Fever speeds up body metabolism. (See the discussion of fever in Chapter 14.) Because of the increased energy expenditure, the patient needs more calories and water. Yet, as mentioned above, a neurologic patient is often unable to recognize thirst and hunger. Moreover, impaired motor function may interfere with the mechanics of drinking and eating. Thus, at a time when the need for food and fluids is great, the patient may be unable to respond with increased intake. Because fever resulting from brain lesions may continue for weeks or even months, careful attention must be paid to meeting the patient's need for food and fluids.

Nursing Implications Too often, the nurse falsely assumes that all patients experience normal thirst and appetite and are capable of reacting to their needs for fluids and food. She should remember that confused or unconscious patients do not have this capacity. Thus, she must help assess and meet their nutritional needs.

If the patient is unable to take oral fluids, other routes of intake are available. For example, a patient with difficulty in swallowing may not be able to drink sufficient fluids, yet his fluid requirement can easily be met with tube feedings. A patient with nausea and vomiting can neither take fluids orally nor by gastric tube, but he can be provided with parenteral fluids. Keen observations by the nurse help the physician determine which replacement route is best and thus minimize the duration of the period of inadequate intake.

All confused or unconscious patients should be placed on careful intake-output measurements. Fluid loss by all routes, such as sweating, vomiting, or diarrhea, should be carefully recorded. Body temperature checks should be made every 4 hours—oftener if indicated—to detect elevations. Evaluation of fluids lost from the body serves as a basis for fluid replacement; inadequate fluid replacement eventually results in fluid volume deficit.

It is often difficult to determine the urinary output of neurologic patients, since many of them are incontinent. Because of time-consuming bed changes, the nursing staff is often misled into thinking that incontinent patients have large urinary outputs. Failure to assess the urinary output accurately may lead to inadequate fluid replacement. To avoid guesswork, seriously ill patients should have indwelling urinary catheters. The insensible water loss caused by fever can be assessed by accurate daily weight measurements, which also give an indication of total fluid balance status. (See Chapter 12 for further discussion of nursing responsibilities in fluid intake-output records and body weight measurements.)

Fever often occurs in a patient with cerebral edema, presenting the physician with a difficult problem: the patient needs fluid replacement, yet the danger of increasing cerebral edema may contraindicate such therapy.

Pathologic Conditions Affecting the Respiratory Center

Pathologic conditions of the central nervous system can cause stimulation or depression of the respiratory neurons, thus altering plasma pH.

HYPERVENTILATION Neurologic conditions associated with overstimulation of the respiratory center include:

Meningitis
Encephalitis
Brain tumor
Fever

Hyperventilation results from the overstimulation of respiratory neurons. Increased pulmonary ventilation causes excessive elimination of CO_2, resulting in respiratory alkalosis. A mixture of 5 per cent CO_2 and 95 per cent O_2, breathed for a short period by the patient with cerebral damage, helps relieve the symptoms of respiratory alkalosis.

HYPOVENTILATION Neurologic conditions associated with depression of the respiratory center include:

Direct trauma to the respiratory neurons in the medulla
Pressure on the respiratory neurons secondary to tumor, hemorrhage, or brain abscess
Bulbar poliomyelitis

Hypoventilation results from the depression of respiratory neurons. Retention of excessive amounts of CO_2 causes respiratory acidosis. Hypoventilation, which is far more dangerous than hyperventilation, presents these hazards:

Hypoxia
Respiratory acidosis
Increased CO_2 retention with dilation of the cerebral blood vessels and a rise in intracranial pressure

Hypoventilation due to medullary depression may necessitate the use of a mechanical respirator. Treatment should also be aimed at eliminating the cause of respiratory center depression.

Nursing Implications The nurse should be alert for changes in respiration. She should check the respiratory rate, depth, and rhythm and should watch for symptoms of respiratory acidosis when breathing is suppressed. These include:

Disorientation
Weakness
Coma, if acidosis is severe

The nurse should also watch for symptoms of respiratory alkalosis when the rate and the depth of respiration are increased. These symptoms include:

Light-headedness
Numbness, tingling of fingers and toes
Circumoral paresthesia
Tinnitis
Blurring of vision
Convulsions
Unconsciousness

Some of the symptoms, such as disorientation, weakness, convulsions, coma and blurred vision, may be caused by other conditions, such as brain tumors or cerebral vascular accidents. Such symptoms should be evaluated in the light of the patient's history and neurologic status.

The physician usually orders frequent pH and bicarbonate tests to help evaluate the patient's electrolyte status. These tests help distinguish between symptoms of electrolyte disturbance and those of neurologic origin.

SODIUM EXCESS AFTER BRAIN INJURY Sodium excess is the most frequent electrolyte disturbance following brain injury. It is usually caused by inadequate water intake. Recall that thirst and the motor activities necessary to respond to it are often affected by neurologic trauma.

High protein tube feedings (which are average in sodium content) are contraindicated during the first week after brain trauma. Because of the stress response that follows trauma, the patient is unable to anabolize protein normally. The renal solute load is increased, resulting in excessive water loss, which eventually produces sodium excess. Fever and hyperventilation cause additional water loss and further contributes to sodium excess.

The neurologic patient with respiratory depression may require prolonged mechanical ventilation. Even with humidification, there may be a tendency for the ventilator to remove water and produce hypernatremia. If this occurs, the increased water loss must be replaced; the actual amount required is determined by the clinical condition, urine volume, urine specific gravity, and accurate body weight measurement. Sometimes the converse will occur; the common use of nebulizers with respirators has increased the hazard of water retention. A recent study showed that approximately 20% of the patients treated with prolonged mechanical ventilation developed water retention, hyponatremia, and pulmonary edema. (See Chapter 24.) The nurse should keep accurate intake-output records (including the water contribution from nebulizers). Accurate daily weight measurements should also be made to help detect water deficit or water overloading.

Nursing Implications The nurse should be alert for symptoms of sodium excess when the water intake is deficient or when excessive water loss occurs. Symptoms of sodium excess (water deficit) include:

Dry, sticky mucous membranes
Flushed skin
Oliguria
Urine specific gravity above 1.030
Fever
Plasma sodium above 147 mEq./L.

Fever after neurologic trauma calls for a check of the serum sodium level.

Efforts should be made to supply adequate water, by mouth if possible. If tube feedings are necessary, the nurse should carefully record the amount of water given, plus the total volume of the tube feeding mixture. Few tube feeding mixtures supply adequate water; additional amounts should be given between feedings. The nurse should consult with the physician to determine the desired total intake and to learn of necessary restrictions. The physician may order a specific volume for the 24-hour period in order to prevent or minimize cerebral edema and elevation of the intracranial pressure. If a specific fluid intake is not established, the nurse should give fluids in amounts sufficient to keep the tongue moist and the skin turgor normal.

It may be necessary to use the intravenous route to supply water if the patient is vomiting or has diarrhea. Recall that in Chapter 16, 5 per cent dextrose in water was described as an excellent solution for meeting water needs in most situations. However, any condition likely to be associated with cerebral edema and increased intracranial pressure contraindicates use of this solution. The infusion of an isotonic solution of dextrose raises intracranial pressure, partly because dextrose passes into the cerebrospinal fluid and increases its osmotic pressure. An apparently acceptable solution for supplying water to the brain injured patient is 2½% dextrose in 0.45% saline. Electrolytes, even in small quantities, interfere with the elevating effect of dextrose on cerebrospinal fluid pressure.

SODIUM DEFICIT FOLLOWING BRAIN INJURY

Brain injury may be followed by sodium deficit if excessive water has been given, especially when the patient is perspiring heavily or vomiting. In addition, sodium deficit may occur because of cerebral salt-wasting. Water overdose can be corrected by withholding water until the excess water is excreted; cerebral salt-wasting, however, represents a more difficult problem.

Cerebral Salt-Wasting Involving the urinary excretion of large amounts of sodium, despite an existing sodium deficit, the mechanism of cerebral salt-wasting is not known; the salt-wasting may be caused by inappropriate production of ADH, which causes renal retention of water without concurrent retention of sodium and results in sodium deficit through dilution. It is observed most often in patients with cerebral vascular accidents, although it has been seen in patients with encephalitis, brain tumor, head injury and bulbar polio. The frequency with which cerebral salt-wasting occurs is not known. The possibility of its presence should always be considered.

Sodium replacement is required in patients with cerebral salt-wasting; the amount of sodium needed to overcome symptoms of sodium deficit varies with the individual. The salt-wasting may be temporary, since it sometimes disappears when the neurologic condition is relieved.

Nursing Implications The nurse should be alert for symptoms of sodium deficit when the patient is losing large amounts of sodium and drinking large quantities of sodium-free fluids. Any patient with a cerebral vascular accident, brain tumor, head injury, encephalitis, or bulbar polio may develop cerebral salt-wasting, with the following symptoms of sodium deficit:

Listlessness
Absence of thirst
Loss of appetite
Nausea and vomiting
Headache
Giddiness
Unless corrected, circulatory collapse with increased pulse rate, decreased blood pressure, pale skin, shock, and death

An important nursing responsibility in caring for patients with salt-wasting is the recording of all routes and types of fluid intake and output.

DIABETES INSIPIDUS Diabetes insipidus results from interruption of the hypothalamohypophyseal tract by a variety of lesions, so that the posterior pituitary gland no longer secretes ADH adequately. Causes include brain tumors, head injuries, encephalitis and vascular disease. Sometimes the disease is of an idiopathic origin (no demonstrable etiology).

Symptoms of diabetes insipidus include polyuria and polydipsia; polyuria is caused by the decreased secretion of ADH. (Recall that antidiuretic hormone causes the body to conserve water; a deficiency of this hormone results in an abnormally high water loss into the urine.) Urinary output is usually 4 to 6 L. per day, although it may be as great as 12 to 15 L. The large urinary loss of water causes the body fluid osmolarity to rise and produces thirst; as a result, a large volume of water is consumed. Urinary specific gravity is low, remaining between 1.002 and 1.006. There is a tendency to "wash out" an excess of electrolytes; to offset this, the patient has an increased desire for salt in the diet.

The polyuria of diabetes insipidus must be differentiated from that caused by chronic renal disease, diabetes mellitus, and compulsive water drinking. Chronic renal disease is characterized by a low urinary specific gravity, in addition to other urine abnormalities. The urine of the patient with diabetes insipidus is normal except for the large volume and low specific gravity. In diabetes mellitus, the urine volume is large but has a high specific gravity (due to the presence of sugar). The differential diagnosis presenting the most trouble is between diabetes insipidus and compulsive water drinking.

Compulsive water drinking is usually caused by a neurosis. It is most frequent in women from 40 to 60 years of age, while diabetes insipidus is more common in younger men. The primary disturbance in compulsive water drinking is excessive water intake; polyuria occurs secondarily. Recall that polyuria occurs first in diabetes insipidus; excessive water drinking follows to prevent dehydration. In compulsive water drinking, intake depends largely upon the emotional state of the individual, and therefore, fluctuates greatly from day to day. Water intake in diabetes insipidus remains rather constant from day to day.

Several tests have been devised to help diagnose diabetes insipidus. For example, if water can be withheld long enough to cause concentration of the urine to a specific gravity of 1.010, the patient probably doesn't have diabetes insipidus. However, it is difficult to withhold fluids from the patient with diabetes insipidus, even temporarily, without causing a water deficit or even peripheral vascular collapse. Another test consists of the administration of hypertonic solution of sodium chloride. In the normal individual, this procedure stimulates ADH secretion and thus decreases urinary volume. The individual with diabetes insipidus is unaffected by extracellular osmolar changes; the only mechanism capable of decreasing urinary volume in such patients is the administration of pitressin (vasopressin). The administration of pitressin produces a more concentrated urine in the patient with diabetes insipidus than can be achieved with water restriction.

Posterior pituitary extracts or vasopressin are

used to conserve about 90% of the water which would otherwise be lost by way of the kidneys of the diabetes insipidus patient. A small amount of powdered posterior pituitary gland or synthetic vasopressin may be insufflated into the nose several times daily, or pitressin tannate in oil (0.2 to 0.4 ml.) may be injected every two to three days. A potential complication of the parenteral administration of pitressin, either diagnostically or therapeutically, is water intoxication (excessive retention of water with subsequent sodium dilution). Although the patient with diabetes insipidus usually decreases his water intake when the polyuria is controlled, the compulsive water drinker may not. The patient who has received an overdose might be unable to rid his body of water that he had drunk, resulting in water overload. Urinary volume and fluid intake should be measured and compared to detect excessive water retention. Early symptoms of water intoxication include listlessness, drowsiness and headache; later, convulsions and coma may develop.

Nursing Implications The nurse should be alert for polyuria and polydipsia in patients with brain tumor, head injury, vascular disease, or cerebral infection. An accurate intake-output record is helpful in detecting these symptoms—it also reveals the drinking pattern. (Recall that the drinking pattern helps differentiate between diabetes insipidus and compulsive water drinking.)

If diabetes insipidus is present, provision should be made for an easily accessible water supply. In addition, the patient should be as close to the bathroom as possible. Fluid balance is remarkably well maintained in the patient with diabetes insipidus, as long as he has access to as much water as he wants.

ELEVATED INTRACRANIAL PRESSURE

Causes Elevated intracranial pressure occurs when the rate of cerebrospinal fluid formation is increased or when the rate of absorption of cerebrospinal fluid is decreased. Brain tumors may produce either or both of these effects. Any irritation to the meninges, such as an infection or tumor, causes large quantities of fluid and protein to pass into the cerebrospinal fluid system; the added volume causes a rise in intracranial pressure. A large hemorrhage can directly increase intracranial pressure by compressing the brain. The formation of arachnoidal granulation, caused by hemorrhage or infection, can interfere seriously with cerebrospinal fluid absorption and thereby increase intracranial pressure. An excessive fluid intake can precipitate cerebral edema and increased intracranial pressure in some patients with cerebral disease or injury. Water, ingested orally or as a 5 per cent dextrose in water solution intravenously, may raise intracranial pressure. Carbon dioxide causes dilation of the cerebral vessels, and the increased blood flow resulting from the dilation may produce an abrupt elevation of intracranial pressure; indeed, it may cause papilledema.

Symptoms The nurse should be alert for the symptoms of elevated intracranial pressure in all patients with cerebral abnormalities. Symptoms of elevated intracranial pressure include:

- Changes in level of consciousness
- Progressive rise in blood pressure (usually there is a greater rise in the systolic blood pressure than in the diastolic pressure, resulting in an increased pulse pressure)
- Slowed bounding pulse
- Slowed respiratory rate
- Persistent dull headache, most severe in morning
- Projectile vomiting (may or may not be preceded by nausea)
- Dimming of vision, due to papilledema (edema of the retina surrounding the region of exit of the optic nerve)

Treatment

Hypertonic Glucose. Once commonly used to reduce intracranial pressure, hypertonic glucose solutions are now used sparingly in most hospitals. Infusion of hypertonic glucose increases the intravascular osmotic pressure, withdrawing water from the edematous brain and from the cerebrospinal fluid space. Although the intracranial pressure is reduced, the reduction is not sustained and the pressure rises again. The reason for this lies in the fact that hypertonic glucose increases the osmotic pressure of the cerebrospinal fluid, causing it to attract water by osmosis.

Some authorities feel that hypertonic glucose does more harm than good.

*Hypertonic Urea.** The intravenous administration of a hypertonic solution of urea produces a significant and well sustained decrease in intracranial pressure in patients with cerebral injury or space-occupying lesions. Not metabolized, urea is rapidly excreted by the kidneys, carrying with it large quantities of water and sodium. It can be prepared in concentrations of 4 or 30 per cent. The 30 per cent solution is usually employed for the reduction of intracranial pressure.

The usual dose ranges from 1 to 1.5 Gm./kg. body weight. After the solution has been prepared it should either be used immediately or stored in the refrigerator for no longer than 48 hours. Intravenous urea should be administered slowly; the rate should not exceed 3 to 4 ml. per minute. The effect becomes maximal in 30 to 90 minutes and disappears in about 6 hours. Because urea has a pronounced diuretic effect, an indwelling urinary catheter should be used in comatose patients to assure bladder emptying; the catheter also facilitates accurate measurement of urinary output. Headache, nausea and vomiting, syncope, and disorientation have been reported after intravenous administration of urea.

Since urea in a 30 per cent concentration is an irritating hypertonic solution, it may cause phlebitis and pain. Extravasation of the solution causes sloughing of the surrounding tissues. Because venous thrombosis may occur, the infusion should be started in a large vein, with the needle carefully anchored. Because of the danger of thrombosis, veins in the lower extremities of the aged should not be used.

Contraindications to the use of urea include severe renal or hepatic damage, pronounced extracellular fluid volume deficit or active intracranial bleeding. If the solution is given to patients with kidney disease, the BUN should be checked frequently to determine if renal function is adequate to eliminate the infused urea as well as that produced endogenously. Urea should be administered with great caution to patients with liver impairment since there may be a significant rise in the blood ammonia level. Intracranial bleeding may be reactivated when cerebral edema is reduced by the use of urea.

Adrenal Corticoids. Adrenal corticosteroids may be used to reduce cerebral edema. At first they may be given intravenously in large amounts and then either by mouth or intramuscularly. The effect is less rapid than that achieved with urea, but is more prolonged.

Mannitol. Mannitol is an osmotic diuretic capable of relieving elevated intracranial pressure when given intravenously as a 20 per cent solution. The relatively high total dose is 1.5 to 2 Gm./kg. of body weight. This amount may be given over a period of 30 to 60 minutes, provided the patient has normal cardiac and renal function. Sometimes mannitol is given less rapidly—500 ml. of 20 per cent mannitol over a 90-minute period, for example. Because of the diuretic effect of mannitol, a catheter should be inserted into the bladder before the mannitol is administered. Although 20 per cent mannitol is chemically stable, it may crystallize when cooled excessively. If this occurs, the bottle should be warmed to 50° C. in a water bath, then cooled to body temperature before being administered.

The nurse should obtain a specific order concerning the rate of administration of the solution. If a large amount of mannitol is given rapidly, the patient may complain of headache, a sensation of chest constriction and chills. The increased intravascular fluid volume, caused by the drawing of water into the bloodstream, may cause pulmonary edema or symptoms of water excess (sodium deficit). (Symptoms of pulmonary edema are described in Chapter 21; those of water excess are described in Chapter 17.) The nurse should make every effort to observe the patient closely during the administration of mannitol, especially when it is given at a rapid rate. The site of injection should be observed frequently, since extravasation of mannitol can cause swelling and thrombophlebitis.

* Ureaphil (Abbott Laboratories, North Chicago, Illinois).

24 Fluid Balance in the Patient With Respiratory Disease

The primary function of the lungs is to provide the body tissues with proper amounts of O_2 and to excrete correct quantities of CO_2. Another critical role is that of H^+ control (acid-base balance) and water balance. Alveolar ventilation is responsible for the daily elimination of about 13,000 mEq. of H^+, as opposed to the 40 to 80 mEq. excreted daily by the kidneys. It is obvious that pulmonary dysfunction will produce a rapid change in the plasma H^+ concentration. In contrast, the H^+ excess of renal failure may not be evident until several days after onset.

The lungs can be regarded as organs of body homeostasis, since they regulate the carbonic acid level of the extracellular fluid through exhalation or retention of carbon dioxide.

Under the control of the medulla, the lungs act promptly to correct systemic hydrogen ion changes, which are synonymous with acid-base disturbances. Thus, when the ketosis of starvation produces metabolic acidosis, the medulla signals the lungs to exhale carbon dioxide by means of deep, rapid respiration. When loss of hydrochloric acid through prolonged vomiting produces metabolic alkalosis, the medulla orders the lungs to retain carbon dioxide by means of slow, shallow respiration.

The disruption of normal pulmonary function can produce water and electrolyte imbalances. For example, blockage of the bronchi and of the alveolar-capillary membrane in bronchiectasis results in the inadequate elimination of carbon dioxide from the lungs, with increased carbonic acid concentration in the extracellular fluid and respiratory acidosis. High fever, with its associated hyperventilation, causes an excessive elimination of carbon dioxide from the lungs, and a decreased carbonic acid concentration in the extracellular fluid resulting in respiratory alkalosis.

The lungs remove large quantities of water from the body as water vapor. (Recall that the daily insensible water loss from the lungs is about 300 ml., varying with the environmental humidity and the depth and the rate of respiration.) Abnormal conditions, such as sustained hyperpnea, excessive formation of mucus or of purulent secretions, or continued coughing greatly increase the water loss.

HYPOVENTILATION

Hypoventilation results in carbon dioxide retention and inadequate oxygenation.

Hypercarbia

Hypercarbia (increased CO_2 concentration in arterial blood) signals the medulla to increase respirations. (Another term for hypercarbia is hypercapnia.) Symptoms that may occur with the sudden development of hypercarbia include: increased pulse and respiratory rate, increased blood pressure, dyspnea, dizziness, sweating, feeling of fullness in the head, palpitation, mental clouding, muscle twitching, convulsions, and unconsciousness. However, patients with chronic pulmonary disease who gradually accumulate CO_2 over a prolonged period (days to months) may not develop these symptoms because compensatory changes have time to occur. Comroe* cites an example of an emphysematous patient, kept alive with oxygen therapy for more than a year, who was mentally alert even when his arterial pCO_2 was 140 mm. of Hg (recall that the

* Comroe, J.: Physiology of Respiration, Chicago, Year Book Medical Publishers, Inc., 1965.

normal arterial pCO_2 is 35 to 38 mm. Hg). Yet a rapid rise of arterial pCO_2 to 140 mm. Hg would surely produce unconsciousness.

An elevated pCO_2 increases cardiac rate and force of contraction, whereas sudden reduction of pCO_2 from very high levels may lead to ventricular fibrillation. Carbon dioxide excess produces cerebral vasodilation and increased cerebral blood flow. The increased blood volume in the rigid cranium may produce increased cerebrospinal fluid pressure and papilledema. Extremely high pCO_2 levels result in total anesthesia and death.

Excessive CO_2 retention, of course, produces respiratory acidosis. The plasma pH drops below normal because the increase in CO_2 causes the carbonic acid content of the blood to increase. (See the discussion of respiratory acidosis in the next section of this chapter.)

Hypoxemia

Acute hypoxemia (reduced oxygen content in the arterial blood) causes an increase in pulse rate as the heart attempts to compensate for inadequate tissue oxygenation by supplying more blood. An O_2 test may be helpful in assessing the patient's oxygen need; that is, pulse rate usually decreases by 10 or more beats per minute within the first few minutes after O_2 administration if the patient was indeed hypoxic. Other signs of hypoxemia include confusion, agitation, and an anxious facial expression.

Some observers regard cyanosis as the most characteristic clinical sign of hypoxemia. The term "cyanosis" means blueness of the skin; it is caused by an excessive amount of deoxygenated hemoglobin in the skin blood vessels. Deoxygenated Hb. has a strong blue color that is readily visible when present in a large concentration. Cyanosis only becomes discernible when the arterial oxygen saturation drops below 80%. (Normal arterial oxygen saturation is 95%.) A number of factors influence the degree of cyanosis: one such factor is the thickness of the skin; for example, cyanosis is readily observable in newborn babies because they have thin skin. Cyanosis is often noted first in the lips and fingernails where the capillaries are numerous and the tissues over them are thin and transparent. Another factor influencing the ability to observe cyanosis is the rate of blood flow through the skin. In shock, cyanosis may not be noted because the surface vessels are constricted and contain little blood. It is difficult to detect cyanosis in patients with severe anemia because there is sufficient oxygen available to saturate the small amount of Hb. present. Patients with severe anemia and shock may suffer fatal tissue anoxia without the warning of cyanosis; such patients may display only skin pallor. Recognition of cyanosis also involves a subjective component of color perception. There is apt to be inconsistency among observers describing the same patient, or even in a single individual watching the same patient over a period of hours.

OXYGEN ADMINISTRATION Even though O_2 is required to correct hypoxemia, only as much as is needed should be given. The inordinate elevation of arterial pO_2 can produce pulmonary edema (due to damage of the linings of the bronchi and alveoli). Exposure to 100% O_2 at normal atmospheric pressure for a day or so can produce substernal distress that is aggravated by deep breathing and a decrease in vital capacity. These symptoms disappear when air is breathed for a few hours. (Animals exposed continuously to 80–100% O_2 die of pulmonary edema.) Breathing 50% O_2 for long periods does not seem to cause pulmonary damage.

Frequent measurement of arterial blood gases is necessary to ensure that only enough O_2 is administered to maintain a satisfactory pO_2. It is generally considered safe to give as much O_2 as is necessary to keep arterial pO_2 at 80 mm. Hg.

Various methods are available for O_2 administration. The nasal cannula supplies an O_2 concentration of 25–35% at a flow rate of 8 liters per minute. The nasal catheter supplies a higher concentration, between 30 and 50%, at a flow rate of 8 L. per minute. A tightly fitting oxygen mask supplies an O_2 concentration of up to 90–95% at 8 L. per minute. The Venti-Mask is a specially constructed device that delivers a low concentration of O_2 (either 24 or 28%) and is used for administering O_2 to emphysema patients.

The danger of administering a high O_2 concentration to a patient with an elevated pCO_2 is discussed later in the chapter under CO_2 narcosis.

Dyspnea

Dyspnea refers to difficult breathing. Patients with pulmonary disease often complain of "shortness of breath" or of being "unable to get their breath." It is a subjective symptom that cannot be measured objectively. Several factors enter into the development of dyspnea: one such factor is an abnormality of the respiratory gases in the body fluids, particularly hypercarbia, and to a lesser extent, hypoxemia; other factors include the patient's state of mind and the degree to which the respiratory muscles must work to achieve adequate ventilation. When one consciously controls breathing rate and depth, the sensation of dyspnea is apt to occur.

Nursing Implications

In summary, hypoventilation results in a decreased pO_2, an elevated pCO_2, and a decreased plasma pH (respiratory acidosis). These blood gas changes are indications for the nurse to try to improve pulmonary ventilation. Depending on the circumstance, such actions may include:

Turning the patient from side to side at frequent intervals to allow for gravitational drainage of mucus from the various lung segments

Placing the patient in Fowler's or Semi-Fowler's position to allow for greater chest expansion

Suctioning the patient as necessary to rid the respiratory tract of excessive secretions

Increasing activity, as outlined by the physician, to promote ventilatory and circulatory improvement

Performing other functions as prescribed by the physician, such as postural drainage, chest tapping, and intermittent positive pressure breathing treatments

Table 24-1. Conditions apt to be Associated With Respiratory Acidosis

1. Emphysema
2. Pneumonia
3. Asthma
4. Cardiac failure with pulmonary edema
5. Partial airway obstruction
6. Partial respiratory paralysis
7. Opiates or sedatives in excessive doses
8. Tight abdominal binders or dressings
9. Abdominal distention from ascites and bowel obstruction
10. Pain in the chest or upper abdomen, resulting in splinting of the diaphragm
11. Semicomatose states, as in cerebrovascular accidents
12. Improperly regulated respirator, causing too shallow or too slow breathing
13. Pneumothorax
14. Prolonged open-chest and open-heart operations

RESPIRATORY ACIDOSIS

Pathologic Mechanism and Symptoms

Respiratory acidosis is caused by any clinical situation that interferes with pulmonary gas exchange, thus producing primary retention of carbon dioxide with a resultant increase in carbonic acid concentration of the extracellular fluid. (See Table 24-1.)

Respiratory acidosis may be associated with no obvious clinical signs except dyspnea out of proportion to effort. (Hyperpnea at rest may be another sign.) Other indications of inadequate pulmonary ventilation include cyanosis and tachycardia, although respiratory acidosis can occur without cyanosis. The hydrogen excess of acidosis leads to loss of cellular potassium. The serum potassium level increases; conduction blocks and ventricular fibrillation may follow.

The symptoms of respiratory acidosis may be difficult to detect; the nurse should be alert for their occurrence when the patient has a condition prone to be associated with respiratory acidosis.

Chronic Pulmonary Diseases Associated With Respiratory Acidosis

Chronic pulmonary diseases, such as bronchiectasis, asthma, pulmonary fibrosis, or emphysema may cause respiratory acidosis. A factor common to all these conditions is chronic interference with gas exchange, resulting in primary retention of carbon dioxide with an increase of carbonic acid in the extracellular fluid. Because emphysema is by far the most common cause of respiratory acidosis, it will be discussed as a separate entity.

EMPHYSEMA

Pathologic Mechanism and Symptoms Emphysema involves chronic obstruction to the flow of air into and—even more important—out of the lungs. The chronic airway obstruction causes overdistention of the lungs with air. As a result, the alveoli become enlarged and eventually rupture and coalesce.

Conditions that may contribute to airway obstruction include respiratory infections, smoking, and breathing polluted air. Nevertheless, the precise etiology of emphysema and the exact site of the obstruction are not known. The disease is most common in older persons, particularly males who have done manual labor. Poor ventilation and interference with gaseous exchange at the alveolar level produce hypoxia and hypercarbia.

Retention of carbon dioxide causes a weighting of the carbonic acid side of the carbonic acid–base bicarbonate balance. As a result, this ratio becomes more than 1 to 20, and the balance is tipped in favor of acidosis. The pH of the blood is more acid than normal; the bicarbonate level is increased since the body retains bicarbonate ions to balance the excessive quantity of carbonic acid. Thus, both the carbonic acid content and the bicarbonate content of the blood increase. If the ratio of carbonic acid to base bicarbonate becomes stabilized at 1 to 20, the pH of the extracellular fluid will be normal. For example, if the carbonic acid concentration is 1.60 mEq./L. instead of the normal 1.35 mEq./L., and if the base bicarbonate is 32 mEq./L. instead of the normal 27 mEq./L., the pH will still be 7.4—that is, normal—because the 1 to 20 ratio prevails. This condition is sometimes referred to as "compensated respiratory acidosis." However, if the body compensatory mechanisms fail and the 1 to 20 ratio is upset, the extracellular fluid pH will drop below normal. The condition is then referred to as "uncompensated respiratory acidosis." In compensated respiratory acidosis, the plasma pH will be normal. In uncompensated respiratory acidosis, the plasma pH will drop below normal.

The emphysematous patient may fluctuate between compensated and uncompensated acidosis. For example, a respiratory infection may tip his delicate state of balance and precipitate uncompensated respiratory acidosis.

The symptoms of emphysema with respiratory acidosis may include:

- Chronic fatigue
- Dyspnea, first noted on exertion
- Moderate cyanosis, early
- Respiration with a prolonged expiratory phase accompanied by wheezing or a blowing sound
- Large barrel-shaped chest
- A chest that appears to be held in permanent inspiration, so that the shoulders appear elevated and the neck shortened
- Use of accessory respiratory muscles in breathing
- Chronic productive cough
- Dull headache
- Severe cyanosis in the terminal stages
- Coma, if acidosis is severe

Treatment Ideally, the treatment of respiratory acidosis should consist of eliminating the underlying pulmonary disease. Unfortunately, this is not possible in emphysema. For this reason, treatment is directed toward maximal relief of pulmonary obstruction and the improvement of pulmonary ventilation.

Bronchodilators, such as isoproterenol (Isuprel), help to reduce bronchial spasms and thus improve pulmonary ventilation. Best results are obtained when the patient first exhales completely and then inhales the medication directly into the respiratory tract. Bronchodilators may be administered by means of a positive pressure device, such as the Bennett or Bird respirator, or by means of a hand nebulizer; the nurse should learn how to use this equipment. She should teach the patient how to continue his treatments after he is discharged from the hospital.

Sputum may be thick in the emphysematous

patient and difficult to expectorate. For this reason, an expectorant may be given to liquefy the sputum and make it easier to cough up. Acetylcysteine (Mucomyst) is a safe and effective mucolytic agent that liquefies both purulent and nonpurulent secretions. It is particularly useful in any sort of pulmonary disease in which viscid or inspissated mucous secretions are present. It may be administered by nebulization, by intratracheal instillation, or by direct application. Quibron is a bronchodilator-expectorant combining the effectiveness of theophylline plus the expectorant action of glyceryl guaiacolate. Given by mouth, it is useful for the symptomatic treatment of bronchospastic conditions, including pulmonary emphysema.

An absolute increase in the number of circulating red blood cells occurs in emphysematous patients as a result of hypoxia. Total blood volume also increases. For this reason, phlebotomy may be useful as a therapeutic measure.

Patients with excessive respiratory secretions may be helped by postural drainage, which brings secretions up high enough so that they can be eliminated by coughing. Breathing exercises which utilize the abdominal muscles help the lungs empty and aid in the elimination of carbon dioxide. The nurse should supplement the educational efforts of the physical therapist and the physician, and encourage the patient to practice these exercises.

Antibiotics may be necessary when a respiratory infection occurs. Unfortunately, the patient with emphysema is highly susceptible to such infections, particularly during the winter. Although ideally the patient should move to a mild climate during the fall and winter seasons, this is rarely possible. Hence, the patient should be taught to avoid exposure to respiratory infections, sudden chilling, and unnecessary exposure in damp or cold weather. If, in spite of these precautions, he develops a respiratory infection, he should immediately report that fact to his physician. The secretions of respiratory infections cause further obstruction to pulmonary ventilation in the emphysematous patient. Respiratory acidosis can occur readily, and the patient may become seriously ill in a short time.

ACUTE RESPIRATORY ACIDOSIS The development of acute respiratory acidosis demands special measures. Bronchial aspiration may be necessary to rid the respiratory tract of mucus and purulent secretions. A mechanical respirator, used cautiously, may improve pulmonary ventilation. Overzealous use of a mechanical respirator may cause such rapid excretion of carbon dioxide that the kidneys will be unable to eliminate the excess bicarbonate ions with sufficient rapidity to prevent alkalosis and convulsions. For this reason, the elevated carbon dioxide concentration should be decreased slowly.

Fluid volume deficit accompanying respiratory acidosis may be treated by the intravenous administration of a Butler-type solution containing balanced quantities of extracellular and cellular electrolytes, plus carbohydrate, or with sixth molar lactate. Oxygen can be administered to relieve severe hypoxia; it should be administered with caution to the patient with respiratory acidosis.

PREVENTION OF CARBON DIOXIDE NARCOSIS DURING OXYGEN THERAPY

Carbon Dioxide Narcosis *Carbon dioxide narcosis may be produced by excessive oxygen administration to a patient with chronic respiratory acidosis.* Chronic elevation of the carbon dioxide content of the extracellular fluid causes the respiratory center to become insensitive to carbon dioxide. (Recall that while the respiratory center is normally extremely sensitive to changes in carbon dioxide concentration and that a slight elevation causes respiratory stimulation, arterial carbon dioxide concentration of over 9 per cent causes respiratory depression.) Hypoxia becomes the main stimulus to respiration when the carbon dioxide mechanism is not functioning. A reduction in arterial oxygenation stimulates respiration, and an elevation of arterial oxygenation removes the stimulus. Thus, if oxygen is administered in sufficient quantities to raise arterial oxygenation, respiration will decrease. Decreased respiration favors carbon dioxide retention. Eventually, carbon dioxide narcosis will result unless the situation is reversed.

The nurse should be alert for the occurrence of carbon dioxide narcosis when oxygen is administered to a patient with respiratory acidosis. Symptoms may include:

Drowsiness
Irritability, depression, or euphoria
Warm, flushed skin
Respiratory depression
Tachycardia (arrhythmias may develop)
Hallucinations
Muscular tremors of face or extremities
Blood pressure, normal or elevated
Convulsions
Paralysis of extremities
Deep coma

Safe Oxygen Administration Oxygen therapy should be used cautiously in patients with chronic respiratory acidosis. It is important to give no more than a 30 or 40 per cent concentration of oxygen in air; a higher concentration may produce serious respiratory depression.

Continuous oxygen therapy is dangerous and should be avoided; oxygen is best given intermittently to patients with chronic respiratory acidosis. Best results are obtained when oxygen is administered with an intermittent positive pressure device, which both furnishes oxygen and—more importantly—increases carbon dioxide elimination. To avoid impending carbon dioxide narcosis, the physician may order frequent checks of the carbon dioxide content of the plasma. If this rises excessively, oxygen should be discontinued.

Acute Pulmonary Conditions Associated With Respiratory Acidosis

MECHANICAL OBSTRUCTION WITH A FOREIGN OBJECT Mechanical obstruction of the respiratory tract with a foreign object prevents air flow into the lungs and results in severe anoxia. In addition, air flow from the lungs is interrupted. The sudden retention of carbon dioxide causes acute respiratory acidosis; it can also cause a mild rise in blood pressure.

Ventricular fibrillation and potassium excess are common causes of death in patients with acute respiratory acidosis. Treatment consists of the intravenous administration of a sixth molar sodium lactate solution.

Sudden relief of the obstruction, such as may be produced by tracheotomy, causes hyperventilation and may result in alkalosis and tetany, as carbon dioxide is rapidly eliminated from the lungs. The bicarbonate level remains temporarily high. (Recall that the kidneys cannot excrete bicarbonate ions as rapidly as the lungs excrete carbon dioxide.) Rapid correction of acidosis may cause ventricular fibrillation, probably due to potassium excess.

Apnea may also follow the sudden release of a respiratory obstruction through tracheotomy, possibly because of hypotension and decreased blood flow to the respiratory center. The blood pressure should be checked immediately before and also after tracheotomy to detect hypotension. If hypotension occurs, the physician may request that a vasopressor be given.

Other acute pulmonary conditions that may be associated with respiratory acidosis include pulmonary edema, atelectasis, open chest wounds, and severe pulmonary infections.

OTHER CONDITIONS ASSOCIATED WITH RESPIRATORY ACIDOSIS

Overdoses of Drugs Overdoses of morphine, meperidine or a barbiturate result in depression of respiration and increased retention of carbon dioxide. Before administering a drug of this class, the nurse should carefully check the dose, as well as the time when the drug was last given. In addition, the rate and depth of respiration should be observed before and after administration of the drug.

Pain Severe pain, particularly in the abdomen or thorax, results in splinting of the chest and shallow respiration. Carbon dioxide is retained and respiratory acidosis may develop. Judicious use of analgesics is indicated to relieve pain and to allow the patient to breathe more efficiently.

Weak Respiratory Muscles Weakening of the respiratory muscles may be caused by such conditions as poliomyelitis or spinal cord injuries. Adequate pulmonary ventilation is not possible; an excessive amount of carbon dioxide is retained by the lungs, and respiratory acidosis may develop.

Inaccurate Regulation of Mechanical Respirators Inaccurate regulation of a mechanical respirator may result in excessively shallow and slow respiration. Excessive carbon dioxide is retained by the lungs, causing respiratory acidosis.

Inhalation Anesthesia The use of inhalation anesthetics, such as cyclopropane or ether, may be associated with hypoventilation and carbon dioxide retention. Mild carbon dioxide retention may be well tolerated for a while, particularly if hypoxia is not present. However, respiratory acidosis may develop as soon as 15 minutes after the start of inhalation anesthesia; it is most likely to occur in patients with chronic pulmonary disease, such as emphysema.

A patient may have normal color and still develop respiratory acidosis, particularly during an operation when the anesthetized patient is given oxygen. While the use of oxygen therapy to produce tissue oxygenation is good, if measures are not taken to increase the exhalation of carbon dioxide (such as with a positive pressure breathing device), an excessive amount of carbonic acid may form in the extracellular fluid and cause respiratory acidosis. The first indication of acidosis may be the development of ventricular fibrillation, probably due to potassium excess. Carbon dioxide retention potentiates vagus nerve activity so that minor stimuli, such as tracheal suction, may cause cardiac arrhythmias. Positioning the patient on the operating table in such a way that normal respiratory excursions are prevented contributes to the development of respiratory acidosis.

Excessive Carbon Dioxide Inhalation Inhalation of carbon dioxide in concentrations exceeding 9 per cent depresses the medullary respiratory center and produces an increased alveolar carbon dioxide content. This, in turn, causes an increased plasma carbonic acid level and acidosis. For example, a patient in an oxygen tent from which carbon dioxide is poorly absorbed may breathe excessive quantities of carbon dioxide.

Orthopedic Deformities Restriction of respiratory excursions by spinal deformities may result in carbon dioxide retention and acidosis, even though the lungs are normal.

HYPERVENTILATION

Hyperventilation causes an excessive loss of CO_2 and thus a decrease in the carbonic acid content of the blood. Unless the kidneys can eliminate bicarbonate (HCO_3) sufficiently to maintain a normal carbonic acid–base bicarbonate ratio, respiratory alkalosis will result. (See the discussion of respiratory alkalosis in the next section.) In addition to an excessive loss of CO_2, hyperventilation causes an increased insensible water loss, a fact that must be considered in supplying an adequate fluid replacement.

RESPIRATORY ALKALOSIS

Pathologic Mechanism and Symptoms

Respiratory alkalosis may be caused by any condition that causes an increased excretion of carbon dioxide through the lungs, with a resultant decrease in the carbon dioxide concentration of the extracellular fluid. Hence, a decrease in the carbonic acid side of the carbonic acid–base bicarbonate ratio occurs.

Symptoms vary in respiratory alkalosis. They may be only those of the underlying disease process, or they may be absent. Sometimes, the patient may appear to be short of breath. He may use his upper chest muscles and accessory respiratory muscles during respiration; he may complain of pain and tenderness of the left side of his chest. Alkalosis may cause increased neuromuscular excitability because of the decreased ionization of calcium. (Recall that calcium ionization is decreased in alkalosis.) Anoxia may occur because alkalosis inhibits the release of oxygen from oxyhemoglobin. The most characteristic clinical picture of respiratory alkalosis is represented by the hyperventilation syndrome:

- Dizziness or light-headedness
- Inability to concentrate
- Numbness and tingling of hands, feet, mouth, and tongue
- Tinnitus
- Blurred vision
- Palpitation of the heart
- Sweating
- Dry mouth
- Stiffness, aches, and cramps of muscles

Positive Chvostek's sign
(tapping the facial nerve in front of the ear causes the facial muscles about the mouth to contract)
Positive Trousseau's sign
(compression of the brachial artery for 1-5 minutes causes the muscles of the hand and wrist to go into spasm)
Twitching and convulsions
Loss of consciousness
(fainting may occur without symptoms of tetany)

Hyperventilation causes decreased cerebral blood flow; light-headedness, convulsions, and unconsciousness may be partly due to cerebral ischemia. Symptoms of alkalotic tetany are more likely to occur if the respiratory alkalosis developed rapidly. The nurse should be alert for these symptoms in any patient having a condition likely to be associated with respiratory alkalosis.

Conditions Associated With Respiratory Alkalosis

The most common cause of respiratory alkalosis is the hyperventilation that accompanies emotional upsets. Treatment consists of making the patient aware of his abnormal breathing practices. He should be made to realize that this breathing pattern causes his symptoms; he can be shown how to relieve his symptoms by holding his breath or breathing into a large paper bag. Such measures cause an accumulation of carbon dioxide in the lungs and relieve the alkalosis. A sedative may be required to relieve hyperventilation in very anxious patients; if alkalosis is severe enough to cause fainting, the increased ventilation will cease and respirations will revert to normal.

Hyperventilation can result from hypersensitivity of the respiratory center, such as occurs with meningitis and encephalitis. Respiratory alkalosis develops because excessive amounts of carbon dioxide are blown off by the lungs. The inaccurate regulation of a mechanical respirator, causing too deep and too rapid respiration, results in excessive carbon dioxide elimination—hence, respiratory alkalosis.

Overdoses of salicylates cause excessive stimulation of the respiratory center and hyperventilation. Alkalosis may occur early in salicylate intoxication; later, by the time the patient arrives at the hospital, metabolic acidosis may predominate. Other causes of hyperventilation include high fever, exposure to high environmental temperatures, and oxygen lack. If the hyperventilation is prolonged, respiratory alkalosis may supervene.

STUDY OF BLOOD GAS CONCENTRATIONS

Clinically, blood gas quantities may be roughly assessed by observing various signs in the patient. For example, insufficient oxygenation of blood results in cyanosis. A decrease in the pulse rate and respiratory rate after a few minutes of oxygen administration demonstrates that hypoxemia was present. Elevation of the arterial blood CO_2 concentration causes increased respirations, as does an increased hydrogen ion concentration. However, despite the help obtained from these observations, it is frequently necessary to do blood gas analyses in seriously ill patients.

Blood gas analysis includes measurement of hydrogen, oxygen tension and carbon dioxide tension in arterial and venous blood. These measurements are expressed as pH, pO_2, and pCO_2 respectively. (See Table 24-2.)

Unclotted blood is used to measure blood gases. Most blood gas analyzers require 2½ ml. of blood—some require only ½ ml. or less. Arterial samples are more revealing than venous samples. Arterial blood samples are usually obtained from an indwelling catheter in the brachial, radial, femoral or temporal artery. If a catheter is not in place, a femoral punch may be performed to obtain an arterial blood sample. In some hospitals the nurse is not permitted to draw blood samples, particularly when an arterial punch is required. She may often obtain samples from indwelling catheters, however. When venous samples are used, it is best to obtain the blood from a central vein; blood from peripheral veins should not be used for blood gas studies because they do not indicate true values of pH, pO_2, and pCO_2. The changing blood gas values must be

Table 24-2. Blood Gas Values

Blood Specimen	*pH*	*pCO_2*	*pO_2*	*O_2 Saturation*
arterial	(7.38-7.42) 7.41 average	35-38 mm. Hg	95-100 mm. Hg	90-95%
venous	(7.35-7.45) 7.36 average	40-41 mm. Hg	35-40 mm. Hg	60-85%

reviewed in relation to each other and to previous readings; they should be evaluated in relation to the patient's clinical condition and medical history.

The procedure for obtaining blood for analysis should be explained to the patient. It is important to prevent unnecessary pain and anxiety which may cause hyperventilation, resulting in a temporary change in blood gases. If the patient is receiving oxygen, the rate and route of administration should be noted on the requisition slip, along with the body temperature. A heparinized syringe is used to prevent clotting. After the specimen has been withdrawn, the plastic cap should be placed over the needle to prevent air from entering the syringe. In addition, gently rotating the syringe between the palms is recommended to prevent settling of the red blood cells. Placing the syringe in a basin or glass of ice helps prevent dissociation of oxygen. The specimen should then be taken immediately to the laboratory. Firm pressure should be applied to the arterial puncture site for five to ten minutes; periodic inspection is necessary to detect complications, such as bleeding or the development of a hematoma.

Conclusions to be Drawn From Blood Gas Levels

The levels of pCO_2 and pO_2 provide considerable insight into what is happening to the patient. Theoretically, pCO_2 can be high, normal, or low, as can pO_2. Let us consider various combinations of these six variables.

First, of course, the pO_2 and the pCO_2 can fall within the limits of normal, in which case no deduction concerning disease can be made.

What if the pO_2 is normal and the pCO_2 is elevated? This is impossible unless oxygen is being given to the patient. Suppose the pO_2 is normal and the pCO_2 is depressed. Then the patient must be compensating successfully for a lung disorder. We say he is compensating because the low pCO_2 indicates hyperventilation and the normal pO_2 indicates a healthy state of oxygenation of the blood.

Now suppose the pO_2 is high and the pCO_2 is normal. We can only deduce from this that the patient is receiving oxygen—indeed, he must be. Now let us move on to a high pO_2 and a high pCO_2. Such a situation is clearly impossible. How about an elevated pO_2 and a low pCO_2? This indicates that hyperventilation is going on.

What if the pO_2 is low and the pCO_2 is normal? Here we have poor oxygenation of the blood but without compensatory activity on the part of the lungs. (There is no overbreathing, otherwise the pCO_2 would be depressed, not normal.) Suppose the pO_2 is low and the pCO_2 is high. Here we have a condition in which pulmonary ventilation is inadequate. This might occur with any obstructive lung disease. What if the pO_2 is low and the pCO_2 is low? Here we have apparent efforts on the part of the lungs to compensate for a low oxygen saturation of the blood, but the efforts of the lungs are unavailing. We can see this in the syndrome known as "stiff lung" or in pulmonary embolism.

WATER BALANCE IN PROLONGED MECHANICAL VENTILATION

WATER EXCESS A study conducted at Massachusetts General Hospital reviewed 100 patients treated with prolonged continuous mechanical ventilation.* Nineteen of the 100 patients developed a positive water balance, associated with weight gain and a significant drop in the plasma sodium concentration and in the hematocrit. The water retention existed primarily as pulmonary edema and resultant impaired respiratory function, rather than as peripheral edema. It appears

* Sladen, A., Laver, M., and Pontoppidan, H.: Pulmonary Complications and Water Retention in Prolonged Mechanical Ventilation. The New England Journal of Medicine, August 29, 1968.

to be in no way connected with the patient's original diagnosis and is not affected by the type of respirator used. Water overloading may be associated with the use of efficient nebulizers providing an additional 300 to 500 ml. of water per day. Positive pressure ventilation produces changes in the dynamics of flow in the pulmonary vessels; possibly this causes excess water to move into the interstitial spaces. The water retention, with its associated weight gain and dilutional hyponatremia, may be associated with an elevated ADH level.

To avoid the dangerous complications that can result from water overloading in ventilated patients, careful monitoring of intake and output is essential. The water contribution from nebulizers should be included in the intake column. Daily body weight measurement is valuable in detecting weight gain from water loading, particularly when a sensitive in-bed scale is used. (See the section on weight measurement in Chapter 12.) The actual weight gain may appear small, but one must consider that immobilized patients with low caloric intake would normally lose about 200 to 500 Gm. daily. Any gain in weight, or even maintenance of a steady weight under these conditions, may be caused by water retention.

An increase in pulmonary extravascular water may be detected by x-ray. Treatment consists of water restriction and the use of diuretics. Failure to notice pulmonary water loading encourages progressive difficulty in ventilation.

DEHYDRATION If artificial humidification is inadequate during prolonged mechanical ventilation, water is drawn from the respiratory secretions to humidify the inspired air. Such an occurrence causes drying of the respiratory secretions and dehydration. The plasma sodium level rises as a result of the water loss. Urine volume is diminished and its specific gravity is increased.

The effective maintenance of adequate humidity is vitally important to the patient on prolonged mechanical ventilation. Drying of the respiratory secretions causes them to become tenacious and to solidify, thus decreasing the size of the air passages. An adequate fluid intake is also important. The presence of fever is an indication to increase the fluid intake.

CARE OF THE NEAR-DROWNED PATIENT

Drowning has increased as water sports have become more popular. Today accidental drowning is a common cause of death in the United States. Drowning is also a common method of suicide. Factors that may contribute to accidental drowning include:

- Fatigue
- Hyperventilation or prolonged breath-holding in order to swim long distances underwater
- Muscle cramps
- Hysteria
- Currents or underwater obstacles
- Intoxication

The nurse should be acquainted with the physiologic changes occurring with drowning and with the treatment of these changes, since she may be called upon to care for near-drowned patients in the hospital or at the scene of the accident.

SEA WATER DROWNING

Physiologic Changes Sea water is strongly hypertonic; when inhaled into the lungs, it causes a diffusion of water from the blood into the lungs. The result is hemoconcentration and massive pulmonary edema. Sodium excess and an elevated hematocrit develop as a result of the large water movement from the intravascular compartment of the extracellular fluid into the lungs. Hypotension and a decreased rate of heart contraction lead to death in asystole.

Treatment The treatment of sea water submersion, as outlined by Redding and Pearson,* is as follows:

1. If the patient has breathing movements, is conscious, and is not cyanotic, he can be moved to a hospital for a chest x-ray and hematocrit determination.

* Redding, J., and Pearson, J.: Management of drowning victims. Am. Family Physician, 7:55, 1964.

2. Time should not be wasted in trying to drain water from the lungs.

3. If the patient is not breathing, he should receive mouth-to-mouth resuscitation until oxygen is available. When oxygen is available, it should be given until the patient arrives at the hospital where positive pressure ventilation with oxygen is possible.

4. Tracheal intubation or tracheotomy makes prolonged positive pressure breathing easier; it also facilitates the removal of secretions by suction.

5. Plasma should be given if the hematocrit is elevated or if the x-ray shows evidence of pulmonary edema.

6. When the hematocrit is normal and the chest x-ray is clear, positive pressure breathing can be discontinued.

7. Antibiotics should be administered if indicated.

FRESH WATER DROWNING

Physiologic Changes Aspiration of fresh water into the lungs results in the entrance of large quantities of water into the intravascular compartment. The blood becomes greatly diluted and massive hemolysis of the red blood cells occurs. Hemodilution results in a decreased hematocrit and sodium as well as potassium deficits. Death usually results from ventricular fibrillation, probably caused by sodium deficit and poor oxygenation.

Treatment Treatment of fresh water submersion, as outlined by Redding and Pearson, is as follows:

1–4. Same as listed under treatment for sea water submersion.

5. Immediate closed cardiac massage, if no carotid artery pulse can be palpated.

6. If no pulse is palpable at the time of hospital admission, 1 ml. of 1:1000 epinephrine solution should be given into the heart.

7. Electrical defibrillation should be performed if an electrocardiogram indicates ventricular fibrillation.

8. The plasma and urine should be checked for hemolysis; a partial exchange transfusion may be necessary if hemolysis is severe.

25 Water and Electrolyte Disturbances From Heat Exposure

INTRODUCTION

Although heat disorders occur most often in tropical zones, the temperate climate of North America can cause heat stress. Many persons living in a temperate climate withstand heat stress poorly, hence the increased number of deaths during heat waves. Another common source of heat disorders is the heat stress imposed by certain occupations.

Industry is often associated with artificially created hot climates, resulting from or deliberately designed for some industrial process. For example, persons working in the textile weaving and processing industry are often subjected to an artificially induced, warm, humid climate, because these conditions are best suited to textile processing. Certain segments of the glass, rubber, steel and mining industries are also associated with high environmental temperatures. Laundry, construction and agricultural workers are often exposed to heat stress, as are firemen.

Athletes are also prone to heat disorders. A survey made by a group of football coaches showed that from 1931 through 1971 there were fifty football deaths due to heatstroke. This figure is probably low because such deaths may be inaccurately attributed to heart failure or other causes. Heat exhaustion and heat cramps are common occurrences on the football field, as well as in other strenuous sports.

Because so many persons in our society may be subject to heat disorders, the nurse should become familiar with their prevention, recognition and treatment.

A brief review of body thermoregulation mechanisms will promote a more thorough understanding of the section concerning specific heat disorders.

THERMOREGULATION IN THE BODY

Mechanisms of Thermoregulation

To maintain thermoequilibrium in the body, the amount of heat lost must be equal to the amount of heat gained. Heat is lost when the environmental temperature is less than body temperature. It is gained when the environmental temperature exceeds body temperature and when body energy expenditures are high. Fortunately, the body has a sensitive and efficient thermoregulation system. Let us consider its elements.

HYPOTHALAMUS The heat control center, located in the hypothalamus, has two anatomically separate subcenters: one is responsible for conserving heat and the other for giving off heat. The heat control center is made aware of body temperature variations directly from local brain temperature changes (secondary to variations in the temperature of blood supplying the brain), and reflexly from afferent fibers of the many cutaneous nerve endings sensitive to hot and cold. Efferent fibers of these nerves are chiefly involved with vasomotor activity and the functioning of the sweat glands.

CIRCULATORY SYSTEM The circulatory system bears much of the burden of thermoregulation. The constriction of cutaneous blood vessels occurs when the environmental temperature is lower than the body temperature and when energy expenditures are low. Cutaneous vasoconstriction decreases the amount of blood brought to the surface for cooling and thus conserves body heat. Dilatation of the cutaneous blood vessels occurs when the environmental temperature exceeds the body temperature and when energy expenditures are high. Because more blood is brought to the surface for cooling by radiation and conduction, body temperature is lowered.

Sweating is initiated when the environmental temperature exceeds 82.4 to 86° F. (28 to 30° C.). The evaporation of sweat from the body surface causes cooling of peripheral blood. The cooled blood is returned to core parts of the body and serves to reduce body temperature.

SWEAT GLANDS Of the body's sweat glands, approximately two million have thermoregulation as their chief function. Sweat is normally a hypotonic fluid containing several solutes, the chief of which is sodium chloride. The concentration of sodium chloride in sweat depends largely on the dietary intake; thus the amount per liter of sweat is highly variable. For example, 5 L. of sweat may contain from 2 to 20 Gm. of sodium chloride. A high salt intake causes an increased excretion of salt by the kidneys and sweat glands. Decreased salt intake, or excessive salt loss, causes renal conservation of salt; the sweat glands similarly conserve salt. The retention of needed salt by the kidneys, and possibly by the sweat glands, occurs in response to increased aldosterone secretion.

Other solutes in sweat include potassium, ammonia and urea. The potassium concentration in sweat may be as high as 9 mEq./L.; excessive sweat losses could conceivably lead to potassium deficiency.

The *maximal* sweating rate for most persons is roughly 2 L./hour; obviously, this rate cannot be maintained for long periods. Individuals accustomed to high heat stress may sweat as much as three or more liters per hour. As much as 20 Gm. of sodium chloride has been reported lost in one day's sweat during high heat stress.

SUMMARY OF BODILY RESPONSES TO HEAT STRESS Exposure of the body to heat stress elicits the following responses:

1. Increased peripheral vasodilatation, to allow more blood to come to the surface for cooling by radiation and conduction
2. Increased sweating, to allow for cooling by evaporation
3. Increased blood volume and venous tone, to improve venous return to the heart
4. Increased cardiac output and pulse rate
5. Increased secretion of antidiuretic hormone, to allow the conservation of body water (the 24-hour urinary output may drop to as little as 300 ml.)
6. Increased aldosterone secretion, to allow the conservation of body salt (aldosterone causes sodium retention by the kidneys and may exert a similar effect on the sweat glands)

Acclimatization to Heat

It has long been known that individuals accustomed to high temperature, either in a natural hot climate or in their work, tolerate heat stress much better than those accustomed to cool temperatures. Yet, the latter can gradually develop a tolerance for heat when repeatedly exposed to it. This process of physiological adaptation is called *acclimatization*. It is accomplished by a series of physiological changes, which serve to ameliorate the effects of heat stress.

PHYSIOLOGICAL CHANGES Individuals exposed repeatedly to heat stress gradually experience fewer of the disagreeable sensations induced by heat, such as lassitude and general discomfort, because of the physiological changes induced by acclimatization.

The specific changes include a progressive decrease in rectal and skin temperatures, a decreased pulse rate, and increased sweating. The sweat contains a lower concentration of sodium chloride and a higher quantity of potassium than normal.

RATE OF ACCLIMATIZATION Most of the changes brought about by acclimatization occur in the first 4 to 7 days of heat exposure; they usually attain their maximum after two weeks of daily heat exposure. A person does not have to be subjected to heat stress 24 hours a day in order to become acclimatized. According to Leithead and Lind, the best way to induce acclimatization is to engage in repeated, uninterrupted periods of 100 minutes work under heat stress. Even a daily heat exposure period of 50 minutes is sufficient to induce an important measure of acclimatization. Short exposures to heat will not induce acclimatization because they present no threat to the body's thermoregulation mechanisms.

HEAT DISORDERS

There are several classifications of heat disorders; that used in this chapter was derived chiefly from *Heat Stress and Heat Disorders,* by C. Leithead and A. Lind, Philadelphia, F. A. Davis Company, 1964.

Prolonged exposure to heat can produce several reactions:

- Heat syncope
- Heat cramps
- Heat exhaustion
  - Primary water depletion (sodium excess)
  - Primary salt depletion (sodium deficit)
- Heatstroke

The clinical picture of each disorder is related to the length of exposure to heat and the individual's peculiar response.

Heat Syncope

Heat syncope is also referred to as heat collapse; it is characterized by a sharp reduction in vasomotor tone after heat exposure, which causes peripheral vasodilatation and a tendency to venous pooling. There are no underlying water or electrolyte disturbances.

SYMPTOMS The pooling of venous blood in the peripheral vessels in heat syncope causes hypotension and cerebral anoxia. Symptoms may include fainting, lightheadedness, or fatigue. Fainting most often follows an additional stress, such as sudden postural changes, heavy lifting, or prolonged standing. Other symptoms may include pallor, nausea, weakness, blurring of vision, numbness and sensations of hot and cold. The pulse rate is increased at the onset of syncope and then decreases. Breathing is low and sighing. The systolic blood pressure is greatly decreased, the diastolic pressure only moderately. The temperature may be above normal; if the patient was engaged in strenuous activity before fainting, the temperature may reach 102° F. Usually the muscles are flaccid. Perspiration, most evident on the forehead, is present.

TREATMENT Symptoms subside when the patient is placed in the recumbent or head-low position; consciousness is regained in a few minutes. Rest for 1 or 2 hours in a cool environment is indicated.

Although diagnosis is usually not difficult, the patient should be examined for more serious illnesses associated with fainting. Other causes of sudden fainting may include epilepsy, heart disease, depletion of sodium or water, and heatstroke. The patient should be checked for urinary incontinence and a bitten tongue; both are indicative of an epileptic seizure. The presence of an arrhythmic pulse rate may indicate heart disease. The specific gravity and salt content of the urine should be measured; both are usually normal in heat syncope because there are no major water and electrolyte changes accompanying this disorder. The presence of a high urinary specific gravity may indicate the presence of heat exhaustion due to sodium excess rather than heat syncope.

PREVENTION Persons not accustomed to high temperatures should gradually expose themselves to heat, as described earlier in the section dealing with acclimatization to heat. Strenuous activities in a hot environment should not be attempted until maximal heat tolerance is achieved. Patients with cardiac disease should be cautioned against excessive heat exposure, particularly when exercising.

Heat Cramps

Heat cramps are sometimes called miner's, fireman's, or stoker's cramps. They are painful spasms of voluntary muscles that follow strenuous exercise in hot surroundings, either climatic or industrial, coupled with consumption of plain water. Good health does not preclude their occurrence; even workers well accustomed to their jobs can develop them. Workers in some occupations accept heat cramps as an occupational hazard of no serious consequence; they seldom seek medical help unless severe cramps develop.

There is some doubt about classifying heat cramps as a separate entity rather than including it as a manifestation of heat exhaustion due to sodium deficit. Both are due to a depletion of sodium chloride. However, heat exhaustion is more severe and has a broader symptomatology than heat cramps.

SYMPTOMS The only symptom in heat cramps is the intermittent cramping of voluntary muscles; usually the muscles involved are the ones most exercised. Cramps may be preceded by a twitching in the affected muscles, which tighten into a hard lump. Pain is excruciating during severe heat cramps and subsides as the spasmodic contractions cease. Most cramps last less than one minute; the patient is comfortable between cramps.

The time of onset is almost invariably toward the end of a day's work. *Heat cramps are always preceded by several hours of strenuous exercise, heavy sweating, and liberal plain water intake.*

TREATMENT Analgesics offer little or no relief for the spasms. The specific treatment is salt replacement; one-fourth of a teaspoon of salt may be added to a glass of water and repeated at intervals of 5 to 30 minutes. Severe cramps may require an infusion of one-half to one liter of isotonic saline to relieve immediate symptoms; when cramps have subsided, salt can be given orally. The patient should rest for 24 hours after the cessation of cramps. Muscles are stiff and sore after heat cramps, and several days' rest may be necessary before the patient can return to work.

PREVENTION The prevention of heat cramps includes increasing the salt intake or decreasing the plain water intake. The former is much to be preferred. Decreasing the water intake predisposes to more serious heat disorders, such as heat exhaustion due to sodium excess and heatstroke. Acclimatization is helpful.

In addition to the normal dietary salt intake, some workers may need 2 or 3 Gm. of extra salt daily to prevent heat cramps; others require as much as 5 Gm. extra. Tablets of salt are often provided at drinking fountains in factories where excessive sweating is a problem. Some workers can sweat profusely and drink plain water liberally without developing heat cramps. This unexplained fact sometimes causes others to ignore medical advice to take supplemental salt tablets.

Heat Exhaustion due to Sodium Deficit

Heat exhaustion (sodium deficit) stems from the inadequate replacement of the sodium chloride lost in sweat during prolonged heat exposure. It is often associated with the performance of hard work in high environmental heat.

Even though sweat is hypotonic, a sizable amount of salt can be lost when sweating is excessive. If plain water is drunk freely, without salt replacement, symptoms of sodium deficit become pronounced. Unacclimatized persons are more apt to develop sodium deficit than those accustomed to high heat stress. Sweat glands of acclimatized persons have a greater ability to conserve salt when the body's supply is low. This adaptation process takes place after an exposure period to heat of about 5 to 6 days. The phenomenon may explain why some men, accustomed to working and sweating in hot industries, can pay little attention to salt replacement and drink plain water freely without developing symptoms of sodium deficit. However, it should not be forgotten that anyone exposed to high heat stress is vulnerable to salt-depletion heat exhaustion.

SYMPTOMS Although both sodium and chloride are lost in heat exhaustion due to sodium deficit, the symptoms are primarily those of sodium deficit. Because sodium is the chief extracellular ion, its depletion causes a fall in the osmolarity of the extracellular fluid. As a result, water enters the cells, diluting their electrolytes and causing them to swell. Equally important, water diuresis occurs and causes a pronounced decrease in the extracellular fluid volume. The decrease of extracellular fluid volume and the increase in cellular fluid volume seems to be at least partly related to all of the symptoms of this form of heat exhaustion. Plasma volume is progressively decreased

Table 25-1. Distinction Between Heat Exhaustion due to Sodium Deficit and That due to Water Depletion (Sodium Excess)

Features	Sodium Deficit	Water Depletion (Sodium Excess)
Duration of symptoms	3 to 5 days	Often much shorter
Thirst	Not prominent	Prominent
Fatigue	Prominent	Less prominent
Giddiness	Prominent	Less prominent
Muscle cramps	In most cases	Absent
Vomiting	In most cases	Usually absent
Thermal sweating	Probably unchanged	Diminished
Hemoconcentration	Early and marked	Slight until late
Urine chloride	Negligible amounts	Normal amounts
Urine concentration	Moderate	Pronounced
Plasma sodium	Below average	Above average
Mode of death	Oligemic shock	High osmotic pressure, oligemic shock, heatstroke

Adapted from Leithead, C., and Lind, A.: Heat Stress and Heat Disorders, p. 165. Philadelphia, Davis, 1964.

as sodium deficit becomes more severe; in some cases the volume has been reduced by half.

Symptoms of heat exhaustion due to sodium deficit develop insidiously over 3 to 5 days and include:

- Fatigue
- Headache
- Muscle cramps
- Giddiness
- Vomiting
- Nausea
- Anorexia
- Syncope
- Listlessness
- Constipation or diarrhea
- Circulatory collapse (in last stages)

In early sodium deficit, the complaints are of apprehension, weariness, muscle weakness, headache, and giddiness. These symptoms persist and are later accompanied by nausea, cramps, and vomiting. Painful muscle cramps lasting up to two or more minutes frequently occur in heat exhaustion; usually the cramps occur in muscles fatigued by exercise. In severe sodium deficit, the legs, the arms, and the abdominal muscles may be involved.

Thirst is not a striking feature as it is in heat exhaustion due to sodium excess. The body temperature is usually subnormal or normal; occasionally it may rise to 101° F. The urine is not highly concentrated and contains negligible amounts of sodium chloride. The plasma sodium and chloride levels are reduced. The hematocrit percentage is high, often about 60 per cent.

Only badly neglected persons reach the stage of profound circulatory collapse. The hypotension, oliguria, and shock that result may cause death. Clinically, it is sometimes difficult to distinguish between heat exhaustion due to sodium deficit and that due to water depletion. Table 25-1 lists a comparison of symptoms to help differentiate between the two.

TREATMENT The treatment consists of bedrest in cool surroundings, and a high salt and water intake. The daily salt intake should be approximately 20 Gm. until sodium deficit is corrected. Unlike some animals, man does not crave salt when sodium deficit is present; therefore, a natural drive to consume enough salt to repair the deficit cannot be relied on.

Salt can be palatably replaced by adding it to liquids such as tomato juice or broth. It can also be supplied in oral isotonic saline if nothing else is at hand. Enteric-coated salt tablets should not be used for treatment because they take hours to dissolve in the intestines; they should be used only as a prophylactic measure.

PREVENTION Persons working in a hot environment should consume an adequate amount of salt. Most diets contain approximately 10 Gm. of salt; acclimatized men generally need no supplement to their normal dietary salt intake. Unacclimatized men working in hot surroundings may require as much as 5 Gm., and rarely 10 to 15 Gm., of extra salt daily to prevent salt depletion. This amount can be reduced after acclimatization has been achieved. The occurrence of other abnormal losses of salt, such as in vomiting or diarrhea, is an indication to increase salt intake.

Since it is difficult to add more than 10 Gm. of table salt to the daily diet without making it unpalatable, salt tablets are used to supplement dietary salt intake. Some salt tablets are merely compressed salt and are designed to add to drinks or food; their only advantage over table salt is that they require less storage space. The most widely used salt tablets are enteric coated; these tablets are available in 5 grain (0.33 Gm.) and 10 grain (0.65 Gm.) sizes. Other tablets are chocolate coated and disintegrate quickly when swallowed.

Patients receiving diuretic therapy should be observed closely for salt depletion during the hot summer months; physicians sometimes deem it necessary to curtail the use of diuretic drugs during this time. Recall that diuretics cause an increased urinary excretion of sodium, water, and potassium.

Heat Exhaustion due to Sodium Excess

This form of heat exhaustion is due to inadequate water replacement during prolonged heat exposure and sweating. A high price is paid in sweat to allow successful thermoregulation in hot surroundings. Because sweat is hypotonic, relatively greater amounts of water than salt are lost. Failure to adequately replace the water loss leads to water depletion (sodium excess). This form of heat exhaustion, if uncorrected, predisposes to heatstroke.

SYMPTOMS Thirst occurs early, and the patient will respond to it unless circumstances prevent. These may include an inadequate or unpalatable water supply or the inability of infants and extremely enfeebled persons to respond to thirst.

Symptoms of heat exhaustion due to sodium excess depend upon the degree of water loss; three clinical grades can be described, as shown in Table 25-2.

Table 25-2. Heat Exhaustion due to Water Depletion (Sodium Excess)

Clinical Grade	*Symptoms*
Early	Thirst Loss of 2% body weight (equivalent to 1.5 L. in a man weighing 70 Kg.)
Moderately severe	Intense thirst Dry mouth, difficulty in swallowing Scanty urine of high concentration Rapid pulse Increase in rectal temperature to about 102° F. Poor skin turgor Loss of 6% body weight (equivalent to 4.2 L. in a man weighing 70 Kg.)
Very severe	Same as above Marked impairment of mental and physical capacities High rectal temperature Cyanosis, circulatory failure, extreme oliguria or anuria Rapid breathing (hyperventilation may cause tetany) Loss of more than 7% body weight (equivalent to 5 to 10 L. in a man weighing 70 Kg.) Coma and death when 15% of body weight is lost

Adapted from Leithead, C., and Lind, A.: Heat Stress and Heat Disorders, p. 148. Philadelphia, Davis, 1964.

Generally speaking, a man can survive in a temperate climate for 7 to 10 days without water; he can survive only 1 or 2 days without water when exposed to the extreme heat of the desert.

TREATMENT The patient should rest in bed in a cool environment. Sponging with cool water may be necessary if the body temperature is greatly elevated. The feet should be elevated to improve blood return to the heart; the arms and legs should be rubbed to stimulate blood flow.

A high fluid intake is indicated; if the patient can tolerate water by mouth, cool fluids should be given at frequent intervals to achieve an intake of 6 to 8 L. in the first 24 hours.

Intravenous infusion of 4 or more liters of 5 per cent dextrose in water may be necessary if the patient is unconscious or otherwise unable to take fluids orally. Renal function should be assessed before a large volume of intravenous fluids is given. The presence of severe oliguria or anuria could cause circulatory overload; water intoxication can result if large volumes of 5 per cent glucose in water are given to a patient with renal damage. Daily body weight and fluid intake-output records should be kept; further fluid replacement is made as clinical findings indicate.

The plasma sodium level and urinary sodium chloride content are measured daily. Recall that sodium chloride is also lost in sweat, even though the water loss is more pronounced. If a sodium deficit is present after water replacement, isotonic saline may be given.

PREVENTION An adequate supply of cool water should be made easily accessible to men working in hot surroundings. Infants exposed to heat should be offered water frequently; aged or otherwise enfeebled persons should also be offered fluids frequently. Inadequate oral intake should be reported so that another replacement route can be used.

Heatstroke

Heatstroke is the most serious heat disorder and is associated with a high mortality rate. It is characterized by the sudden cessation of sweating following exposure to high heat stress. Its distribution is world-wide, either in naturally occurring hot climates or in artificial hot surroundings, such as occur in some industries. Heat waves in usually temperate climates account for a large number of heatstroke victims.

The exact pathology of heatstroke is not understood; the production of sweat seemingly fails. So long as sweating continues, with water and salt losses replaced, the body can withstand heat stress well. According to Guyton, an individual can tolerate several hours of exposure to a temperature of 200° F. if the air is completely dry and if air currents are flowing to promote rapid evaporation of sweat from the skin surface.

Central nervous system symptoms, failure of sweat formation, and high body temperatures (above 105° F.) are characteristically present in heatstroke.

PREDISPOSING FACTORS Certain factors predispose individuals to heatstroke:

Inadequate acclimatization
Obese body build
Pre-existent acute or chronic illness
Recent use of alcohol
Inadequate water and salt intake
Recent use of atropine-like drugs
High relative humidity
Extremes in age
Strenuous physical activity in hot surroundings
Failure to appreciate the dangers of heat exposure and to take adequate precautions

DISCUSSION Much evidence supports the thesis that lack of acclimatization predisposes to heatstroke. Malamud, Haymaker and Custer, in 1946, studied the heatstroke deaths of 125 soldiers undergoing intensive training in the southern United States. They found that one-fourth of the men who died had been in camp less than 2 weeks, and about one-half had been there less than 8 weeks.

An obese person has less body surface in proportion to body weight than does a person of slight build; thus, he has greater difficulty in dissipating heat. Conditions such as myocardial ischemia, arteriosclerosis, and hypertension seem to predispose to heatstroke.

Recent use of alcohol prior to heat exposure may predispose to heatstroke. According to Leithead and Lind, there are probably several reasons why this is true: alcohol causes an increased metabolic load and steps up internal body temperature; it dulls judgment and critical thinking; it causes increased water loss from the body.

Atropine-like drugs cause decreased sweating and thus interfere with the dissipation of body heat. The administration of atropine before surgery has been implicated as a predisposing factor in heatstroke of heavily draped surgical patients in hot operating rooms.

A high relative humidity predisposes to heatstroke because it interferes with the evaporation of sweat from the body. Failure of sweat to evaporate causes inefficient body cooling. The body temperature begins to rise when the relative humidity is 100 per cent and the environmental temperature is above 94° F.

The high incidence of cardiovascular disease

in the aged predisposes this age group to heatstroke. Infants are also predisposed to heatstroke; they have an unstable thermoregulatory mechanism, in addition to immature renal function. The infant's renal function, particularly during the first month of life, does not allow concentration of urine when excessive water loss by other routes has occurred. Sodium excess results because of the kidneys' inability to conserve needed body water, when perspiration losses are great.

Strenuous activity increases the metabolic rate and thus elevates the body temperature; the addition of a hot external temperature subjects the body to two sources of excessive heat and predisposes to heatstroke. Heatstroke has been observed in persons doing heavy manual labor when the environmental temperature was as low as 84.2° F. Of 158 heatstroke patients studied by Gauss and Meyer (1917), the majority were manual laborers, including some firemen or laundry workers. However, it should be remembered that even mild activity in extremely hot surroundings may result in heatstroke.

Failure to appreciate the dangers of heat exposure is often related to the development of heatstroke. The nurse should become familiar with the preventive measures listed at the end of the chapter so that she can offer sound advice about heat disorders to lay persons.

SYMPTOMS Persons mildly afflicted with heatstroke may have no prodromal symptoms. Others may experience symptoms for a few minutes to 1 or 2 hours before loss of consciousness. These symptoms may include euphoria (associated with a rise in body temperature), headache, dizziness, faintness, numbness, drowsiness, aggressiveness, mental confusion, and incoordinated movements.

The onset of heatstroke is usually sudden and is heralded by disturbances of the central nervous system. Symptoms of heatstroke include:

- Disorientation
- Absence of sweating
- Complaint of feeling hot
- Involuntary limb movements
- Skin dry and hot to touch (skin turgor is usually good unless heatstroke is preceded by water depletion)
- Rectal temperature of at least 105° F.
- Convulsions, either localized or generalized
- Projectile vomiting
- Rapid pulse (may be as high as 150 beats per minute)
- Rapid respiration (may be as high as 60 per minute)
- Systolic blood pressure elevated
- Red, blotchy appearance of face (patient may look as if he has been strangled)
- Incontinent liquid feces
- Circulatory collapse
- Petechial hemorrhages in the brain, heart, kidney, or liver (if the patient survives, residual damage to these organs, particularly the brain, may become evident)
- Coma

Most persons suffering with heatstroke are comatose at the time they receive medical attention. Many times the comatose heatstroke patient is mistaken for a stroke victim; the presence of neurological symptoms resembling those of stroke accounts for this confusion.

Rapid breathing in heatstroke may cause respiratory alkalosis due to the excessive blowing off of CO_2 and result in hypokalemia. This imbalance is less threatening, however, than hyperkalemia, which occasionally occurs. Potassium excess is associated with cellular breakdown due to heat; potassium leaves the cells and enters the extracellular fluid, where it remains because of poor renal function due to circulatory collapse and the cessation of sweating. (Recall that sweat contains potassium.) Potassium excess can cause sudden death in heatstroke victims.

TREATMENT *Quick and effective reduction of the high body temperature is essential.* Even a few hours delay may leave the patient with severe neurological deficits. The longer the temperature remains high, the greater the possibility of irreversible brain damage. When the body temperature is above 106° F., damage to cells throughout the entire body occurs; damage to brain cells is particularly critical, because they cannot be replaced. When the body temperature reaches 110 to 114° F., the patient can live only a few hours unless the temperature is rapidly reduced.

Regardless of how high the temperature is, it should be reduced to 102° F. within the first hour of treatment. Recovery from heatstroke depends largely on reducing the degree and duration of fever.

The most effective method of cooling is immersion in a bathtub of ice water; this measure may seem drastic, yet the temperature must be rapidly lowered to 102° F. Other methods are not as rapid and sure. They include sponging with ice water or alcohol, and packing the patient in cold sheets. Antipyretics are too slow and do not lower the body temperature sufficiently to be of value in the initial treatment of heatstroke. Because the measures to promote cooling may be frightening to the conscious patient, he should be constantly attended and reassured.

It is especially important that the patient be constantly attended while he is immersed in a tub of ice water. Since the patient may be comatose, or at least disoriented, he must be protected from drowning. The body temperature should be taken every 5 minutes. The temperature is usually taken orally, because special equipment would be necessary to measure it rectally. The nurse should recall that the oral temperature is approximately one-half to one degree less than the rectal temperature. When the temperature reaches approximately 102° F., the patient should be removed from the ice water bath; otherwise, too much cooling could result and cause subnormal temperature and shock. Reduction of the body temperature to 102° F. causes the patient to feel better; slight paralysis is sometimes relieved by the temperature reduction. After the removal of the patient from the tub, the body temperature should be measured at frequent intervals so that any rise can be noted early; it may be necessary to repeat hypothermic treatment. The blood pressure should be checked regularly during the first few days.

Salt and water losses must be replaced slowly until adequate renal function is established. After 1 to 3 days of intensive treatment, the sweat glands again become functional, although it may be as long as 6 months before they begin to secrete normally. The patient should continue to rest in bed for 1 to 2 weeks after temperature reduction.

EMERGENCY MEASURES BEFORE MEDICAL AID IS AVAILABLE Because time is so vital in preventing fatalities from heatstroke, one should take every measure possible to reduce body temperature as soon as possible. Unfortunately, heatstroke may occur in an area some distance from medical aid; furthermore, facilities for ice water baths or even sponging may not be available. *The following points should be kept in mind to care for the heatstroke victim before medical aid is available:*

1. Move the patient out of the sun to the coolest, best ventilated spot available.
2. Remove most of the patient's clothing.
3. Summon medical aid; if necessary, move the patient to medical aid. The transporting vehicle should have all of its windows opened so that a draft can blow on the patient to promote cooling. If moving the patient entails further exposure to high heat stress, it is better to wait until a more suitable means of transportation is available. Additional heat stress could cause death.
4. Investigate surroundings for *any* immediate means of reducing the patient's temperature until more effective measures can be made available. For example, if heatstroke occurs during an outing near a body of water, the patient may be partially immersed to promote cooling. Or, if a water hose is available, the patient can be sprayed continuously with water. If nothing but a drinking water supply is available, the patient can be sponged with it.
5. Massage the patient's skin vigorously; this maintains circulation, aids in accelerating heat loss, and stimulates the return of cool peripheral blood to the overheated brain and viscera. Body heat may be lost rapidly in this manner.

Summary of Measures to Prevent Heat Disorders

The nurse has a responsibility to the public to offer sound advice about heat disorders and their prevention. In addition, she should be alert to the prevention of heat disorders in hospitalized patients. The following should be remembered:

1. All persons exposed to high heat stress should increase their daily salt, potassium and water intake. Heat resistance is developed by replenishing water and salt losses as they occur. Infants should be offered water frequently during hot days, as should enfeebled adults. Salt tablets, preferably with potassium incorporated, should be taken to supplement dietary salt intake when excessive sweating occurs, except in acclimated persons and those on low-sodium diets.
2. Strenuous activity should be curtailed as much as possible during hot days.
3. Persons customarily exposed to heat stress should maintain good physical condition. (Sufficient rest and proper food and fluid intake help prevent heat disorders.) They should take supplemental potassium, perhaps 25 or 50 mEq. daily, provided renal function is normal. (But bear in mind that prolonged heat stress can cause potassium deficit and impaired renal concentration.)
4. Persons moving from a temperate to a hot climate, or those subjected to heat stress in their work, should gradually build up a tolerance to heat through planned acclimatization. Sudden exposure of an unacclimatized person to high heat stress predisposes to heat disorders. (See section dealing with acclimatization to heat.)
5. Prickly heat should be prevented as much as possible, because it interferes with sweating and dissipation of heat from the body. Persons exposed to heat should wear loose, porous clothing, take frequent cool baths, and keep their rooms well ventilated.
6. Persons particularly susceptible to heat disorders should be protected from hot, unventilated places. Such persons include infants, the aged, persons with cardiovascular disease, and those under the influence of alcohol.
7. Persons taking atropine-like drugs should be protected from excessive heat exposure; atropine causes a decrease in sweating and an increased susceptibility to heat disorders. Such persons should be urged to keep their rooms well ventilated during hot weather, take frequent cool baths, and wear loose, porous clothing.
8. Persons taking diuretics should avoid excessive heat exposure and sweating. Recall that diuretics cause an increased excretion of sodium and potassium from the body; if the sodium and potassium levels are further depleted by excessive sweating, the patient may develop sodium and potassium depletion.
9. Persons confined to bed should be protected from excessive bed clothing and hot, poorly ventilated rooms.
10. Potassium deficit has been shown to help cause some heat disorders. Hence, persons prone to develop potassium deficit —those taking diuretics, for example— should guard against potassium deficit in hot weather. Food intake, i.e. potassium intake, usually decreases in hot weather; at the same time, more potassium than normal is lost in heavy sweating. Thus, potassium supplements are indicated.

26 Fluid Balance in Pregnancy

Mystery still surrounds many of the body changes that occur during pregnancy. When these changes are physiologic in nature, they are not only beneficial, but, indeed, essential. Sometimes, however, what appears to be a physiologic change really represents the early stages of a pathologic change that can be harmful, even fatal. For example, diabetes mellitus may first appear as apparently physiologic glycosuria or polyuria; pathologic dilatation of the renal calyx, pelvis, and ureter with partial ureteral obstruction may first reveal itself as mere physiologic dilatation of these structures; pernicious vomiting of pregnancy may first be regarded as the ubiquitous but harmless vomiting of pregnancy. (These examples will be enlarged upon and others introduced later in the chapter.)

Among the various transformations in pregnancy, none is more important than the changes in body fluids. Even these, forthright though they appear, pose many unanswered questions. For example, in the nonpregnant woman or in the male, excessive water retention is invariably accompanied by excessive retention of sodium. Whether or not there is excessive sodium retention in pregnancy remains controversial; however, many, perhaps most, clinicians believe that pregnant women do retain excessive sodium. They therefore restrict sodium intake and may even prescribe diuretics. (Diuretic drugs appear to be overused in pregnancy. One authority reports the deaths of four patients from excessive use of diuretics; three of these died from electrolyte depletion, and one from hemorrhagic pancreatitis.) Other physicians believe that pregnant women are sodium wasters; they add supplemental salt to the diet to avoid preeclampsia. Both the secretion and excretion of the sodium-conserving hormone, aldosterone, increase during normal pregnancy; however, the effect of this increase on sodium homeostasis is poorly understood. Were it not, perhaps we could explain the puzzling situation in preeclampsia, in which there is apparent sodium retention, even though aldosterone secretion actually decreases.

In this chapter, we will first examine changes in body fluids during normal pregnancy. Knowledge of the normal pregnant state enables the nurse to recognize the borderline between a physiologic and a pathologic change. She will know, for example, what is a physiologic increase in hydration and what is a pathologic increase. Next, we will look at disorders of pregnancy closely related to body fluid disturbances. Finally, we will examine the effects of pregnancy on various other ailments characterized by disruption of the body fluids.

CHANGES IN BODY FLUIDS DURING PREGNANCY

Water Content

At term, the fetus, placenta, and amniotic fluid contain about 3.5 L. of water. An additional 3 L. has accumulated because of increases in the mother's blood volume, in the size of her breasts, and in the mass of the uterus. The average woman, therefore, retains at least 6.5 L. of extra water in the extracellular compartment during a normal pregnancy. Such hydration of the maternal tissues is physiologic in nature, and the body's physiologic processes handle it with equanimity.

The increase in blood volume deserves comment: it averages from 40 to 45 per cent and results from increases in plasma volume and in red cell mass. Plasma volume increases 45 to 50 per cent, or about 1,200 to 1,400 ml., with the maximum reached two to six weeks before term. During the last weeks of pregnancy, the rate of increase in plasma volume declines. With delivery, plasma volume rapidly diminishes, so that by the end of the first week postpartum, it has returned to the nonpregnant value. Red blood cell volume increases during pregnancy some 20 to 40 per cent, an addition of 300 to 500 ml. Since the plasma volume increases more than does the red cell mass, the venous hematocrit drops some 15 per cent during pregnancy. In addition, there occurs a 10 per cent increment in heart rate and as much as a 40 per cent increase in cardiac output, reaching its maximum at from 28 to 32 weeks, then decreasing to term. A natural accompaniment of these phenomena is a linear increase in the consumption of oxygen, peaking at term. Because of these factors, the pregnant woman with heart disease may be hard pressed to meet the strenuous demands imposed on her cardiovascular system.

Now let us review known factors that produce fluid retention during pregnancy:

1. An increase in venous pressure elevates the effective intracapillary hydrostatic pressure. This results from two mechanisms: first, the pregnant uterus impinges against the inferior vena cava, thus causing increased back pressure; second, the vascular congestion of the pregnant pelvis also increases pressure on the vena cava. The increased venous pressure enhances filtration from the vascular bed and often produces physiologic dependent hydrostatic edema, to be differentiated from the edema of toxemia. When the woman lies on her side, the pressures against the inferior vena cava are relieved, and the venous pressure is not elevated.
2. Plasma albumin decreases by about 1 Gm./100 ml. of plasma. This reduction in the colloidal osmotic pressure of the plasma amounts to some 20 per cent; it favors plasma-to-interstitial fluid shift.
3. Capillaries become more permeable to water and electrolytes, but not to protein. This is revealed by the fact that the protein content of edema fluid is less than 0.4 Gm./100 ml. in pregnancy.
4. Still controversial is the question of whether excessive sodium is retained by the pregnant woman. Many obstetricians now believe that salt and water restriction in the normal pregnancy is not only unnecessary, but may be harmful. They would confine such restriction to those patients with a pathologic process.

How does one go about measuring the retention of water in pregnancy? Our most useful gauge is weight gain, but water retention is also revealed by pitting edema of the ankles and legs—especially at the day's end—due to increased venous pressure in the legs. This edema usually disappears overnight and should be regarded as a physiologic rather than as a pathologic phenomenon.

Management of ankle edema or of weight gain slightly exceeding that normally expected can usually be accomplished by lateral recumbency plus mild sodium restriction. If the physician employs severe sodium restriction, diuretics, or both, the patient is in danger of becoming sodium depleted, perhaps potassium depleted as well. Sodium depletion is particularly unfortunate; not only is it dangerous per se, its signs—including oliguria, decreased glomerular filtration rate, and increased plasma concentration of uric acid—imitate preeclampsia. This may cause further sodium restriction, leading to more severe sodium depletion.

Conservation of Carbohydrate and Protein

Both carbohydrate and protein are conserved during pregnancy—carbohydrate to meet energy requirements, protein to meet structural demands. The mother appears to retain enough nitrogen (the measure of protein) to provide for the growth of the reproductive system and the fetus and for the needs of milk production. This represents an average increase of 80 Gm. of total circulating plasma protein; 500 Gm. of protein—about half of the additional protein retained during pregnancy—are added to the maternal blood as hemoglobin and plasma proteins, to the uterus, and to the glandular tissue of the breasts. At term, the fetus plus the placenta weigh about 4 kg., containing 500 Gm. of protein—also about half of the increase in protein caused by pregnancy.

In regard to carbohydrate, the question is often asked: "Does pregnancy produce a diabetic effect?" Certainly increased thirst, increased appetite, polyuria, and glycosuria are not uncommon during pregnancy. But normal pregnancy occasions many variables, including elevated plasma insulin and increases in various hormones, such as growth, thyroid, and adrenal hormones. Apparently there is no interference either in the use or storage of carbohydrate, nor is there any resistance to insulin or obstruction in the glycolytic cycle. Nevertheless, the glucose tolerance test is modified, with a delay in the return of blood glucose levels to normal, when glucose is given orally. Thus, instead of the two hours it usually takes for blood glucose to return to normal in the nonpregnant patient, it takes about three hours in the pregnant. This phenomenon is avoided when glucose is given intravenously.

Acid-Base Balance

There is a decrease in the concentration of total base from about 155 mEq./L. before pregnancy to some 146 mEq./L. during pregnancy. Plasma sodium falls from 142 mEq./L. to 136 mEq./L., and plasma bicarbonate from 25 mEq./L. to 22 mEq./L. The mother can be considered as having a moderate respiratory alkalosis combined with metabolic acidosis. With overbreathing induced by labor, the maternal CO_2 can fall below 17 mm. Hg, resulting in a delay in the initiation of respiration in the newborn infant.

Calcium Levels

Some 30 to 40 Gm. of calcium are deposited in the fetus, chiefly during the last trimester of pregnancy. Plasma calcium levels may decrease, probably because of an increase in extracellular fluid volume. The average present-day pregnancy diet, containing from 1.5 to 2.5 Gm. of calcium, appears quite adequate to supply the needs of mother and fetus without depletion of the maternal stores. Possibly because of the high phosphorus content of milk, some patients—especially heavy milk drinkers—may suffer an imbalance in the ratio of calcium to phosphorus in the plasma. (Recall that calcium and phosphorus are antagonistic. An increase in plasma phosphorus tends to decrease plasma calcium, and vice versa.) This imbalance in the calcium-phosphorus ratio may be responsible for the leg cramps that sometimes occur in pregnancy. Indeed, some clinicians have reported that the leg cramps can be relieved by reducing the milk intake and administering supplemental calcium.

PREGNANCY DISORDERS CLOSELY RELATED TO BODY FLUID DISTURBANCES

Toxemia of Pregnancy

The syndrome of toxemia of pregnancy has no known origin. It can be divided into two types, depending upon the severity: *preeclampsia,* or toxemia without convulsions; and the extremely serious *eclampsia,* or toxemia with convulsions. Patients with underlying vascular or renal disease are not included under the diagnosis of toxemia of pregnancy; yet, they are often difficult to distinguish from patients with toxemia, especially during the last trimester.

Preeclampsia occurs in from 5 to 10 per cent of all pregnancies. Eclampsia—which, fortunately, is now rare—used to develop in approximately 0.2 per cent of pregnancies. Preeclampsia occurs chiefly in primagravidas, especially in the very young or in older patients. Sisters and daughters of patients who have suffered from toxemia are prone to develop it. A twin pregnancy or hydramnios appears to predispose to it, as may preexisting hypertension. Once a patient has had toxemia, she is a likely candidate to develop it in future pregnancies.

While the cause of toxemia remains unknown, abnormal sodium retention and generalized vasoconstriction explain the signs and symptoms. It appears to be erroneous to think that control of weight gain and limitation of sodium intake reduces the incidence of preeclampsia; this belief confuses cause and effect. Although preeclamptics retain water and sodium, weight gain does not cause preeclampsia. Certainly endocrine or metabolic disorders or both may be implicated in the genesis of the disease.

The signs of the onset of toxemia include:

edema, not only of the ankles, but also of the hands and face; hypertension; and, in some patients, proteinuria. A significant rise in blood pressure consists of an increase of 30 mm. Hg or more in the systolic pressure and 15 mm. Hg or more in the diastolic. Proteinuria becomes significant when it exceeds 0.3 Gm./L. A weight gain of more than five pounds per week or a blood pressure higher than 140/90 should cause one to consider early toxemia. More advanced symptoms include generalized edema, headache, visual disturbances, abdominal pain, oliguria, nausea, and vomiting—a cluster of symptoms warning of the approach of eclampsia. With eclampsia, death can occur during a convulsion, or it can result from cerebral hemorrhage, congestive heart failure, or kidney shutdown. The fetus also may be seriously threatened, either by the toxemia or by the eclamptic convulsions. Should the pregnancy be terminated either therapeutically or naturally, symptoms of toxemia promptly disappear.

Autopsies on patients who died of eclampsia reveal hemorrhagic lesions in the placenta, liver, kidneys, heart, brain, spleen, adrenals, and pancreas. In addition, necrosis, tissue infarction, fibrin deposits, and evidence of disseminated intravascular coagulation may be found. Pallor of the kidney cortex may be observed, with little blood in the glomerular capillaries.

Even the suspicion of toxemia should be the signal for therapy. Sodium chloride should be restricted to less than 2,000 mg. (about 1 Gm. sodium) daily. The diet should be adequate in protein. Should diuretics be given, care should be taken to avoid sodium or potassium depletion. In addition, sedation should be adequate. If the disease has lasted more than two or three weeks, or should it become severe—regardless of its duration—the patient should be promptly hospitalized so that vital signs can be closely monitored. If the symptoms progress, and especially if eclampsia develops, surgical termination of the pregnancy or induction of labor should be considered. Some physicians have found intravenous or intramuscular magnesium sulfate effective in relieving eclampsia. Various antihypertensive drugs have been employed. If the airway becomes obstructed because of convulsions or coma, tracheotomy may be required.

NURSING RESPONSIBILITIES The nurse should observe all maternity patients for signs of preeclampsia. Prompt recognition and treatment are necessary to prevent the condition from progressing to eclampsia.

The hospitalized preeclamptic patient should have a private room, free from bright lights and loud noises. Nursing care should be planned to provide regular uninterrupted rest periods. Vital signs should be checked at least every four hours. An accurate intake and output record must be kept and daily body weight measurement should be recorded. (See Chapter 12 for nursing responsibilities in these procedures.) An indwelling urinary catheter is usually inserted so that output can be closely monitored. The nurse must be especially alert to report a rise in blood pressure, hyperactive reflexes, a weight increase, or a low urinary output.

Should convulsions occur, placing a padded mouth gag between the teeth will prevent biting of the tongue; a rubber airway may be used to assure an adequate airway. Suction apparatus may be necessary to prevent aspiration of secretions. Padded siderails should be used to prevent the convulsing or heavily sedated patient from falling or otherwise injuring herself. The duration and character of each convulsion should be noted, as well as the depth of coma that follows. Fetal heart tones should be checked as often as possible. The convulsing patient should be observed for signs of rapid labor. It should be remembered that a heavily sedated patient may also have a rapid labor.

If magnesium sulfate is used as an anticonvulsant, the patient's reflexes and respiratory rate should be checked for depression before administering a repeat dose. An ampule of calcium gluconate should be on hand in case respiratory depression becomes severe. Lastly, oxygen should be available for immediate use.

Hyperemesis Gravidarum (Pernicious Vomiting of Pregnancy)

Half of all pregnant women become nauseated or vomit sometime during the pregnancy, but true pernicious vomiting of pregnancy has decreased greatly in recent years. The diagnosis of true pernicious vomiting of pregnancy applies only to those patients who have lost large amounts of weight and suffer severe body fluid disturbances, including extracellular fluid volume deficit, acid-base disturbances, and potassium deficit.

Pernicious vomiting of pregnancy frequently —perhaps usually—is brought about by psychic factors. In some instances, however, liver disease may be associated with it. Characteristically, the ailment starts as simple morning sickness, in which the typical patient feels nauseated when she awakens and may be unable to eat breakfast. By noon, however, her symptoms have disappeared, and she remains symptom-free until the next morning. Morning sickness usually subsides without treatment by the 14th to 16th week, but in some patients, morning sickness may develop into nausea and vomiting lasting throughout the day. This is called pernicious vomiting or hyperemesis gravidarum, which usually appears during the 5th or 6th week of pregnancy. It can last a month or two or even longer, and produce a weight loss of 10 to 20 pounds or more. The blood urea nitrogen and uric acid rise slightly. Plasma chloride and CO_2 combining power decrease. Plasma potassium is likely to decline. Urinary output falls, but the concentration of the urine rises. Ketonuria and hypoglycemia may appear. An ominous complication of hyperemesis gravidarum is hemorrhagic retinitis; with its appearance, the mortality rate reaches 50 per cent.

The patient with pernicious vomiting should be hospitalized, isolated, and sedated. The use of antinauseant preparations deserves high priority in managing the condition, although some authorities minimize the use of drugs because of the danger of teratogenicity. (Pyridoxine apparently benefits some patients.) Some physicians use gastric suction to control vomiting, while others believe it makes the condition worse. Along with therapy to control vomiting, the physician should take immediate steps to correct body fluid disturbances. Repeated ophthalmoscopic examinations should be performed to detect early retinitis; should hemorrhagic retinitis appear, the pregnancy should be promptly terminated.

NURSING RESPONSIBILITIES The pregnant woman with severe vomiting requires hospitalization for intravenous therapy. Usually all food and fluids are withheld during the first twenty-four hours to permit the gastrointestinal tract to rest. Electrolyte and glucose solutions are administered intravenously, in amounts of three liters or more in twenty-four hours. An accurate record of fluid intake and output should be kept.

Rest is of primary importance; visitors should not be permitted during the first day or so. Because psychic factors play a large role in this condition, the patient should be encouraged to verbalize her feelings.

When tolerated, small dry feedings are alternated with small amounts of liquids. The food intake is gradually increased to a full diet. Trays should be prepared carefully; portions should be small and attractively served. Unpleasant odors or sights should be avoided because the slightest stimuli can initiate nausea and vomiting. Occasionally, tube feedings may be necessary if the patient is unable to eat; the tube feeding mixture must be introduced very slowly to avoid nausea. (Nursing responsibilites in tube feeding are discussed in Chapter 14.)

PREGNANCY EFFECTS ON CERTAIN AILMENTS WITH BODY FLUID DISRUPTION

Renal Disease

The gross and microscopic structure of the kidneys of pregnant and nonpregnant women do not differ significantly; however, both the interstitial space and renal blood volume increase during pregnancy. Dilatation of the calyx, pelvis, and ureter may appear as early as the second trimester, especially on the right. X-ray studies have attested to increased kidney size.

While the above changes are physiologic in nature, they may favor overt disease. Thus, by the third trimester, the alterations combined with the woman's supine or upright posture can cause partial ureteral obstruction, and the resulting ureteral dilation can pose problems. For example, since the dilated collecting system may contain large volumes of urine, serious errors may occur in the measurement of timed urinary output of estriol, creatinine, and protein. The misreadings can be avoided if the pregnant woman is given water loads and is kept in bed, positioned in lateral recumbency, for an hour before starting and finishing urine collections.

Perhaps of greater significance, urinary dilatation and stasis may cause asymptomatic bacteriuria to progress to frank pyelonephritis. If the woman already has chronic pyelonephritis, she may regress; such women should be restricted in their upright activity, and frequent rest periods in the lateral recumbent position should be prescribed.

Some patients whose urine is sterile at the start of pregnancy develop positive urine cultures as the pregnancy progresses. Favoring susceptibility to urinary tract infection are extracellular fluid volume deficit and loss of potassium caused by prolonged vomiting. Glycosuria, added to ureteral dilatation and stasis, provides an ideal environment for bacterial multiplication. Certainly pregnant women with confirmed positive urine cultures should receive treatment, even though they have no symptoms.

Apparent deterioration of kidney function in pregnant patients with preexisting kidney disease can be traced to extracellular fluid volume deficit and decreased renal perfusion resulting from strict sodium restriction or administration of diuretics. Nevertheless, patients with chronic renal disease who become pregnant retain sodium abnormally. For these, R. P. Bendel recommends a diet restricted to 1 Gm. of sodium daily. Should the pregnant woman with renal disease develop azotemia, abortion should be considered, due to the ominous nature of the situation.

Most women with a mild degree of functional renal impairment can complete their pregnancies, but with progression of kidney disease, the ability to sustain a viable pregnancy to term diminishes. Even so, women with severe renal impairment have completed their pregnancies with the aid of hemodialysis.

Heart Disease

A history of previous heart disease is reason for extreme caution during pregnancy. The diagnosis of heart disorders during pregnancy poses problems; systolic functional murmurs, distention of veins, tachycardia, and distortions of the chest x-ray can be caused by the pregnancy per se rather than by heart disease.

Enormously helpful in managing and making a prognosis of the course of the patient with heart disease is the New York Heart Association's Functional Status Classification:

Class 1. Ordinary activity produces no fatigue.

Class 2. Ordinary activity produces some fatigue and some signs of cardiac insufficiency.

Class 3. Physical activity is greatly limited, but patients are comfortable at rest. Extraordinary activity leads to dyspnea, palpitation, even angina.

Class 4. Symptoms of cardiac insufficiency are present at rest.

Should the woman show an abnormality of cardiac rhythm or evidence of pulmonary congestion, she should be hospitalized at bed rest. Certain crucial periods demand digitalization—from the 28th to the 34th week, during labor, and exactly at postpartum. It is at these times when the heart is placed under the heaviest load.

Most deaths from congestive heart failure in pregnancy occur in patients in Classes 3 and 4. Those in Class 3 require digitalis plus bed rest, beginning the 28th week; therapeutic abortion should be considered for patients in Class 4.

The pregnant patient with heart disease deserves special attention during labor, particularly in respect to the use of antibiotics, anesthetics, and the method of delivery. Voluntary bearing down should be avoided. Immediately following delivery, heart failure can result from the rapid redistribution of fluids, with an increase in the volume of circulating blood, even in cardiac patients who had an uneventful pregnancy and delivery. Not only the mother, but the fetus as well, is endangered by maternal heart disease. It may die during maternal congestive heart failure or because of prematurity.

Diabetes Mellitus

From 0.2 to 0.3 per cent of pregnant women have diabetes mellitus, which may either be so mild as to require no special diet or so severe as to demand complex therapy.

The potentially damaging effects of diabetes during pregnancy are many. (Certainly it increases the risk of intrauterine fetal death.) Should the patient have had unexplained stillbirths, should the urine have been positive for glucose during the pregnancy, or should the infant weigh 9 pounds or more, a glucose tolerance test should be done. A fasting blood sugar over 130 mg./100 ml. or a blood sugar higher than 170 mg./100 ml. at any time during a glucose tolerance test raises a strong suspicion of diabetes.

The pregnant patient with poorly controlled diabetes has an increased tendency to develop metabolic acidosis because of extensive production of ketone bodies; such ketoacidosis is poorly tolerated by the fetus. One should bear in mind that even the nondiabetic pregnant patient has a low renal threshold for glucose, especially in the third trimester, and may show glycosuria. This is because the increase in glomerular filtration rate that occurs in pregnancy presents more of a sugar load per unit time; the tubular reabsorption, on the other hand, is not increased. Tubular urine, therefore, contains greater amounts of glucose than normal. As a result, glycosuria occurs, even though the blood glucose may be normal.

Pregnancy changes the insulin requirement for the diabetic patient. Hypoglycemic episodes can occur during early pregnancy, and most pregnant patients with diabetes need increased insulin as they approach term. Insulin dosage is best gauged by periodic blood sugar measurements and determination of ketones in the urine rather than by urinary glucose.

Renal disease must always be considered in the diabetic. Kidney failure is signalled by retinopathy, elevated blood pressure, proteinuria, and edema before the 25th week of gestation. Should azotemia appear, termination of the pregnancy and sterilization of the patient is usually indicated.

The incidence of hydramnios, with the amniotic fluid exceeding 2,000 ml., may be seen in as many as 20 per cent of pregnant diabetics. In order to prevent or minimize this phenomenon, Priscilla White, famed specialist in diabetes at the Joslyn Clinic in Boston, recommends restriction of sodium to 1,500 mg. daily. In addition, she employs potent diuretics. Such a program has reduced the degree of hydramnios so that early rupture of the membranes simply does not occur. When patients present with hydramnios, management is difficult.

Pregnant diabetic patients suffer a mortality rate of about 0.7 per cent; death usually occurs because of a cerebrovascular accident, toxemia, or diabetic coma. For diabetic patients who have been carefully controlled, the perinatal fetal mortality rate is about 15 per cent. Many deaths occur *in utero* between the 36th week and term.

Frequently pregnancy is terminated in the pregnant diabetic between the 36th and 37th week, balancing the hazard of fetal deterioration against loss of the fetus from prematurity. Maternal 24-hour urinary estriol measurements provide direct physiologic information on the fetal-placental status as the pregnancy progresses. When the values are rising, danger to the fetus is minimal. Provided the mother is progressing well, delivery can be delayed until the gestational age guarantees adequate maturity. However, if two successive decreases in estriol levels are found, or if the mother deteriorates, the pregnancy should be terminated. Serial estriol determinations should be started by the 30th week and obtained at least three times a week beginning at the 34th week.

Regardless of the gestational age and birth weight of the infant of the diabetic mother, he should be treated as if he were premature. He will suffer from respiratory and circulatory problems, from excessive bilirubin retention, from difficulty in temperature regulation, and from disordered glucose and calcium levels of plasma. The newborn of the diabetic mother may suffer from hypoglycemia. This is especially likely to occur after cesarean section, during which the mother has been given an infusion of dextrose solution to prepare her for surgery. When the infant is presented with a high glucose level because of the intravenous infusion, he responds by secreting large quantities of insulin. With the withdrawal of dextrose after the cord is clamped, the following occurs: the baby continues to secrete high levels of insulin; hypoglycemia develops; blood sugar may drop to as low as 0 (instances of irreversible hypoglycemic reactions have been reported). Because of these considerations, glucose should be given to the newborn early. Oral feedings should be started as soon as possible, even though the baby is clinically premature. Such neonatal problems demand expert pediatric management.

27 Fluid Balance Disturbances in Infants and Children

INTRODUCTION

Water and electrolyte disturbances occur more frequently in children than in adults. Although one recognizes and manages fluid imbalances in children in much the same way he does in adults, there are also important differences. The younger the child, the more pronounced are the differences. The nurse should understand the peculiar problems posed by the child with a body fluid disturbance, so that she can make meaningful observations and can cooperate intelligently in his care.

An obvious and important difference between small children and adults is size. Yet, children are not merely miniature adults, for the child's body composition and homeostatic controls differ from those of the adult. It is helpful to compare the child's body composition with that of the adult and to review the salient characteristics of the child's homeostatic and metabolic functioning.

DIFFERENCES IN WATER AND ELECTROLYTE BALANCE IN INFANTS, CHILDREN, AND ADULTS

COMPARISON OF BODY WATER CONTENT The premature infant's body is approximately 90 per cent water; the newborn infant's, 70 to 80 per cent; the adult's, about 60 per cent. The infant has proportionately more water in the extracellular compartment than does the adult. For example, 40 per cent of the newborn infant's body water may be in the extracellular compartment, as compared to less than 20 per cent in the case of the adult.

As the infant becomes older, his total body water percentage decreases, possibly due to a progressive growth of cells at the expense of the extracellular fluid. The decrease is particularly rapid during the first few days of life, but continues throughout the first 6 months. After the first year, the total body water is about 64 per cent (34 per cent in the cellular compartment, and 30 per cent in the extracellular compartment). By the end of the second year, the total body water approaches the adult percentage of approximately 60 per cent (36 per cent in the cellular compartment, and 24 per cent in the extracellular compartment). At puberty, the adult body water composition is attained. For the first time, there is a sex differentiation: females have slightly less water because they have a higher percentage of body fat.

COMPARISON OF DAILY BODY WATER TURNOVER IN INFANTS AND ADULTS The infant's relatively greater total body water content does not always protect him from excessive fluid loss. On the contrary, the infant is more vulnerable to fluid volume deficit than is the adult, because he ingests and excretes a relatively greater daily water volume. An infant may exchange half of his extracellular fluid daily, while the adult may exchange only one-sixth of his in the same period. Proportionately, therefore, the infant has less reserve of body fluid than does the adult.

The daily fluid exchange is relatively greater in infants, in part because their metabolic rate is two times higher per unit of weight than that of adults. Due to the high metabolic rate, the infant has a large amount of metabolic wastes to excrete. Because water is needed by the kidneys to excrete these wastes, a large urinary volume is formed each day. Contributing to this volume is the inability of the infant's immature kidneys to concentrate urine efficiently. In addition, relatively

Table 27-1. Comparison of "Average" Blood (Serum or Plasma) Electrolyte Values (mEq./L.) at Different Ages Under Varying Conditions

Electrolyte	Prematures "Acidotic"	Prematures "Well"	First Week	Newborns On Breast Milk	Newborns On Cow's Milk	Child 5–20 yrs.	Adults Young	Adults Over 70
Sodium	..	..	146	..	..	144	142	144
Potassium	..	6.1	5.8	..	..	4.3	4.5	4.6
Calcium	..	..	4.9	..	..	4.9	4.9	5.2
Chloride	102.6	106	107	107.7	108	103	103	105
Phosphorus	4.2	4.1	4.2	..	..	2.8	2.0	1.7
Organic Acids	20.9	17.8	6	..	..	6	5	..
Bicarbonate (CO_2 combining power)	12.1	16.8	22.1	22.3	20.2	23	26.3	25
CO_2 Content	..	20	23.4	23.6	21.4	24.5	27.6	..

Weisberg, H.: Water, Electrolyte and Acid-Base Balance, ed. 2, p. 334. Baltimore, Williams & Wilkins, 1962.

greater fluid loss occurs through the infant's skin because of his proportionately greater body surface. The premature has approximately five times as much body surface area in relation to weight, and the newborn, three times, as do the older child and adult. Therefore, any condition causing a pronounced decrease in intake or increase in output of water and electrolytes threatens the body fluid economy of the infant. According to Gamble, an infant can live only 3 to 4 days without water, while an adult may live 10 days.

COMPARISON OF ELECTROLYTE CONCENTRATIONS AND METABOLIC ACID FORMATION Plasma electrolyte concentrations do not vary strikingly between infants, small children, and adults. The plasma sodium concentration changes little from birth to adulthood. Potassium concentration is higher in the first few months of life than at any other time, as is the plasma chloride concentration. Magnesium and calcium are both low in the first 24 hours after birth. The serum phosphorus level is higher in infants and children than in adults. The newborn's and the child's bicarbonate levels are lower than the adult's. (See Table 27-1.) Inability of the premature infant to regulate its calcium ion concentration can bring on hypocalcemic tetany.

Because the infant's metabolic rate is high, the rate of metabolic acid formation is also high. Thus, the infant has a tendency toward metabolic acidosis. Buffer systems are not as efficient in the newborn as they are in older infants and children. A full-term newborn infant is slightly acidotic at birth; however, the pH is usually normal by the second day of life. The premature infant is even more acidotic and may remain so for a few weeks. Because cow's milk has higher phosphate and sulfate concentrations than breast milk, newborns fed cow's milk have a lower pH than do breast-fed babies.

COMPARISON OF KIDNEY FUNCTION The newborn's renal function is not yet completely developed. Thus, if infant and adult renal functions are compared on the basis of total body water, the infant's kidneys appear to become mature by the end of the first month of life. However, if body surface area is used as the criterion for comparison, the child's kidneys appear immature for the first two years of life. Since the infant's kidneys have a limited concentrating ability and require more water to excrete a given amount of solute, he has difficulty in conserving body water when it is needed. Also, he may be unable to excrete an excess fluid volume.

COMPARISON OF BODY SURFACE AREA The infant's relatively greater body surface area is present until the child is two or three years old. The skin represents an important route of fluid loss, especially in illness. Since the gastrointestinal membranes are essentially an extension of the body surface area, their area is also relatively greater in the young infant than in the older child and the adult. Hence, relatively greater losses

Table 27-2. Mean Ranges of Daily Water Requirements of Infants and Children at Different Ages Under Normal Conditions

Age	*Average Body Weight (kg.)*	*Total H_2O Requirements per 24 Hours (ml.)*	*H_2O Requirements per kg. in 24 Hours (ml.)*
3 days	3.0	250–300	80–100
10 days	3.2	400–500	125–150
3 months	5.4	750–850	140–160
6 months	7.3	950–1,100	130–135
9 months	8.6	1,100–1,250	125–145
1 year	9.5	1,150–1,300	120–135
2 years	11.8	1,350–1,500	115–125
4 years	16.2	1,600–1,800	100–110
6 years	20.0	1,800–2,000	90–100
10 years	28.7	2,000–2,500	70–85
14 years	45.0	2,200–2,700	50–60
18 years	54.0	2,200–2,700	40–50

Nelson, W. E.: Nelson's Textbook of Pediatrics, ed. 5, p. 128. Philadelphia, Saunders, 1969.

occur from the gastrointestinal tract in the sick infant than in the older child and adult. In comparing fluid losses in infants to those in adults, one might regard the baby as a smaller vessel with a larger spout.

COMPARISON OF WATER REQUIREMENTS Regardless of age, all normal individuals require approximately 100 ml. of water per 100 calories metabolized. Since infants and children have higher metabolic rates than adults, they need proportionately more water. For example, an infant expends 100 calories per kg. of body weight, an adult only 38 calories. An infant needs 100 ml. of water per kg., while the adult requires only 38. Water needs for various age groups are listed in Table 27-2.

NURSING OBSERVATIONS RELATED TO FLUID IMBALANCES IN CHILDREN

Charted nursing observations can be immensely helpful to the physician or can mean nothing, depending on whether the nurse knows what to look for and takes the time to record her observations on the nursing notes. Because small children cannot describe their problems, the pediatric nurse has to be especially observant. Some of the major areas in which observations should be made are described below.

TISSUE TURGOR Tissue turgor is best palpated in the abdominal areas and on the medial aspects of the thighs. In a normal person, pinched skin will fall back to its normal configuration when released. In a patient with fluid volume deficit, the skin may remain slightly raised for a few seconds. Poor nutrition can also cause poor tissue turgor. Obese infants with fluid volume deficit often have skin turgor that is deceptively normal in appearance. An infant with water loss in excess of sodium loss (sodium excess), such as occurs in some types of diarrhea, has a firm thick-feeling skin. This same phenomenon is observed in the child who has sodium excess due to an excessive sodium intake, as occurs in salt poisoning.

MUCOUS MEMBRANES Dry mouth may be due to a fluid volume deficit or to mouth breathing. When in doubt, the nurse should run her finger along the oral cavity to feel the mucous membrane where the cheek and gums meet; dryness in this area indicates a true fluid volume deficit.

BREATHING RATE, DEPTH, AND PATTERN The nurse should observe the rate, the depth, and the pattern of respiration. Hyperpnea, such as occurs in metabolic acidosis due to diarrhea or salicylate poisoning, can double the water loss by way of the lungs. The overbreathing of metabolic acidosis is not always as obvious in the child as it is in the adult; however, children do develop a curious sign not seen in adults—namely, cherry-red lips.

Accelerated breathing should be reported so that water losses through this route can be replaced. Older children and adults with metabolic alkalosis have decreased rate and depth of respiration, with irregular rhythm. The young infant may normally have irregular respiration; thus, changes in respiratory rhythm are not dependable in detecting metabolic alkalosis.

Changes in respiratory rate and depth are significant in evaluating the child's response to therapy. For example, a change from deep, rapid respiration to slower, less deep respiration indicates improvement in the child with metabolic acidosis.

TEARING AND SALIVATION The absence of tearing and salivation is a sign of fluid volume deficit and should be noted on the chart.

THIRST Avid thirst indicates increased tonicity of the extracellular fluid with cellular dehydration. An infant can be tested for thirst with water, although the presence of nausea may mask the symptom.

BEHAVIOR The child's general behavior is also significant in evaluating the response of fluid imbalances to therapy. When the very ill child begins to display appropriate responses to people, ceases to have irritable, purposeless movements, and is less lethargic, his condition has improved.

GENERAL APPEARANCE A child with a fluid volume deficit has a pinched, drawn facial expression. His eyes appear sunken and are soft to the touch, due to decreased intraocular pressure. If the anterior fontanel is still patent, it may be depressed. A grayish skin color, due to decreased peripheral circulation, also accompanies severe fluid volume deficit.

NATURE OF CRY The cry of an ill infant is higher pitched and less energetic than normal. With improvement in his condition, the cry becomes less high pitched and more lusty.

BODY TEMPERATURE Fluid volume deficit is often associated with a subnormal temperature because of reduced energy output. Depending on the underlying disease, however, fever can accompany fluid volume deficit. If fever is present, its height should be recorded frequently. The rate of insensible water loss is greatly increased with fever; the amount of water lost depends on the height and duration of the fever. Fever may indicate excessive water loss from the body with resultant sodium excess, or it may be caused by an infection. The extremities are cold to the touch in severe fluid volume deficit—even when fever is present—due to decreased peripheral blood flow.

URINE OUTPUT In addition to noting the number of voidings, the nurse should estimate how much of the diaper is saturated with urine. Occasionally she would do well to weigh a dry diaper and compare its weight with that of the same diaper after the child has voided. The nurse should also note the urine's concentration, as revealed by its color. Failure to record urinary output accurately makes treatment far more difficult. When the physician requests an accurate hourly recording of urine output, and a catheter is not inserted, the nurse must devise a method to catch all the urine passed. Some hospitals have beds which have been modified to allow urine to pass through a hole in the mattress into a receptacle below. For male infants, a finger cot with the blind end cut off can be used to conduct urine from the penis to the drainage tube. A plastic diaper with the collecting area connected to drainage tubing may be used. The collection apparatus should be checked frequently for leakage. Good skin care is necessary to prevent irritation of the genitalia.

A child with fluid volume deficit has a decreased urinary output and an increased urinary specific gravity. If the fluid deficit is severe, he may go as long as 18 to 24 hours without voiding and still not have a distended bladder. If a child with a known fluid volume deficit excretes large amounts of dilute urine, he probably has renal damage.

STOOLS Again, it is not enough just to chart the number of stools. The quantity of the stool should be estimated as nearly as possible; its character should be described. Thus, if a stool appears normal, it should be so described on the chart. If the stool is liquid, the degree of saturation of the diaper should be noted. Any abnormal contents, such as blood or mucus, should also be recorded.

VOMITING It is important to chart the number of times the patient has vomited, when he vomited, the quantity of vomitus (approximated if necessary), and the nature of the vomitus.

Merely charting the number of times the patient vomited helps little in planning fluid replacement therapy, since the amount of fluid lost can vary widely from one attack of vomiting to another. Failure to describe the vomitus may make fluid replacement therapy more difficult. For example, if the vomitus is bile stained, one can conclude that it came from below the pylorus. Since fluids from below the pylorus are chiefly alkaline, fluid therapy must be designed to replace alkaline losses, using, for example, an intestinal replacement solution.

WEIGHT CHANGES Weight loss can be caused by loss of fluid or by catabolism of body tissues. The weight loss associated with fluid volume deficit occurs more rapidly than that caused by starvation. A mild fluid volume deficit in an infant or child entails a loss of from 3 to 5 per cent of the normal body weight; a moderate fluid volume deficit, from 5 to 9 per cent; a severe fluid volume deficit, 10 per cent or more. If possible, the child's weight before the onset of the illness should be obtained from the parents, or from the family physician, who may have a record of the normal weight from a recent office visit.

If weighing is not performed accurately, it is useless. Even a minor error is important when the patient is small. The child should be weighed at the same time each day, before he has eaten, after he has voided. The same scales should be used each time, and the child should be weighed naked.

AMOUNT AND CHARACTER OF FLUID LOST BY SUCTION OR OTHER ROUTES The amount and character of fluid lost by suction, drainage tubes, or fistulas should be recorded. If the fluid loss cannot be directly measured, it should be estimated as accurately as possible.

FLUID INTAKE The amount and type of fluids received by the patient, either orally or parenterally, should be recorded.

FLUID REPLACEMENT THERAPY IN CHILDREN

Daily Requirements

The basic requirements of water and electrolytes must be met daily. In addition, one should supply the amounts necessary to correct pre-existing deficits, as well as concurrent abnormal losses, such as those that occur from diarrhea, vomiting, suction drainage, and the like. The normal water requirements per kg. of body weight at various ages are listed in Table 27-2. Approximately 2 to 3 mEq. of sodium and potassium are required for each kg. of body weight to meet maintenance needs. This corresponds to approximately 50 to 70 mEq. of sodium or potassium/m.^{2} of body surface/day.

Although the adult can go without food for several days without developing gross ketonuria, infants and children react quickly to the omission of calories. Ketonuria can occur within a few hours after the onset of fasting. For this reason, carbohydrate must be incorporated in fluids designed to meet daily maintenance needs.

Determination of Body Surface Area in Infants and Children

Increasingly used as a gauge for dosage, body surface area possesses this advantage: requirements for water and electrolytes, as well as therapeutic doses of many pharmaceutical agents, are roughly proportional to surface area (neonates and prematures excepted). In addition to its convenience, use of body surface area offers increased accuracy and safety, despite theoretical objections to its scientific validity.

Frequently used for determination of body surface area are: (1) the DuBois nomogram, requiring weight and height; (2) the Sendroy nomogram, also requiring weight and height; and (3) the West table, requiring weight only. Snively and others have introduced a quick method for estimating body surface area of infants and children, employing a formula that requires only the crown-rump length in infants and the sitting height in children, measured in centimeters. The formula for infants six months of age or less is as follows:

Body surface area in m.^{2} = 0.00017 × (sitting height in cm.)^2

The formula for children over six months of age is as follows:

Body surface area in m.^{2} = 0.00019 × (sitting height in cm.)^2

Table 27-3. A Statistical Comparison of Formulas for Estimating Body Surface Area*

	Sitting-Height Formula Vs Sendroy Nomogram[6]	*West Table Vs Sendroy Nomogram*	*Dubois Nomogram*[8] *Vs Sendroy Nomogram*
No. of children in analysis	267	267	267
Mean	− 3.02%	+ 4.99%	+ 0.28%
Median	− 4.73%	+13.71%	+ 6.64%
Range (high and low extremes)	+28.57% −38.03%	+54.34% −26.92%	+23.8% −10.52%
Approximate 95% limits	+15% −20.76%	+28.57% −10.29%	+12.9% − 6.57%
Standard deviation	9.36%	11.45%	5.11%

* Snively, W. D., Montenegro, J. L. B., and Dick, R. G.: Quick Method for Estimating Body Surface Area. JAMA 197:208-209 (July 18) 1966.

Let's take the example of a child with a sitting height of 50 cm. and see how the formula works:

$0.00019 \times 50^2 \ (2{,}500) = 0.48 \text{ m.}^2$

Since none of the infants and children used in the study by Snively and others exceeded 14½ years in age, further investigation would be desirable before applying the sitting height method to older people. (See Table 27-3.)

Any dose determination, whether it be for water, electrolytes, or medicinals, is approximate and must be adjusted in accordance with the individual tolerance, requirement, and clinical progress of the patient. Great accuracy is not, therefore, essential. Assessment of body surface area for children up to age 14½ years is greatly facilitated by the use of the sitting height formula, particularly when nomograms or tables are not immediately available. The method requires only a centimeter measure, easily carried in the physician's bag or available in any hospital.

Oral Replacement

Water and electrolyte replacement is best accomplished by the oral route for these reasons:

1. Fluids taken into the gastrointestinal tract are slowly absorbed, while parenterally administered fluids pass directly into the circulation; the body is less adversely affected if excessive amounts of water or electrolytes are given by the oral than by the parenteral route.
2. Oral fluid replacement allows the child free movement and activity, as opposed to hours of being restrained during subcutaneous or intravenous infusions.

It should be emphasized, however, that even in the case of the oral route, it is relatively easy to overwhelm the body's homeostatic capabilities, particularly in the case of the infant and small child. For this reason, the dose for fluids administered orally should be calculated with the same care and precision as doses to be administered parenterally. Moreover, although the oral route is far safer than the intravenous route, potassium should not be given by mouth when oliguria or anuria is present.

A suitable oral solution for providing water, electrolytes, and calories is Lytren, prepared by mixing 8 measures of Lytren and 32 oz. of water. Measures should be carefully leveled in accordance with the manufacturer's instructions. Each liter of this solution supplies 25 mEq. of sodium, 25 mEq. of potassium, 30 mEq. of chloride, 4 mEq. of calcium, 4 mEq. of magnesium, and 280 calories, plus other ingredients.

NURSING IMPLICATIONS The nurse should be especially careful in preparing oral electrolyte solutions to follow directions carefully and use precisely the right measurements. The accidental use of a tablespoon when a teaspoon is specified triples the dose of the electrolyte. If sugar is to be added to the solution, great care should be taken to avoid mistaking salt for sugar.

Tube Feedings

Tube feedings are sometimes used to feed unconscious children or those with swallowing difficulties. Many tube feeding mixtures contain large solute loads which, if associated with limited water intake, may increase plasma osmolarity. The nurse will do well to watch for signs of inadequate water intake, particularly when the feedings are high in protein content. Should insufficient water be provided, water will be drawn from the tissues to supply the needed volume for urinary excretion of the increased solute load. Eventually, dehydration (sodium excess) will occur, along with an accumulation of nitrogenous waste products in the blood stream. Excessive protein in relation to water causes nausea, vomiting, diarrhea, and eventually, ileus. If the condition is allowed to go uncorrected, it will result in high fever and disorientation. Laboratory tests will reveal an elevated blood urea nitrogen (BUN) level. Early in protein overloading, the urine volume is large even though water intake is inadequate. The large urine volume can easily lead the staff to think that water intake is adequate; in such instances, however, output actually exceeds intake—the extra fluid is being withdrawn from the body tissues. Very young children and unconscious patients should be observed carefully for inadequate water intake since they are unable to express thirst. (Tube feeding mixtures, methods for tube feeding, and related nursing responsibilities are described in Chapter 14.)

Parenteral Fluid Therapy

SUBCUTANEOUS ROUTE Subcutaneous fluids are easier to start than are intravenous fluids, particularly in infants and small children. For this reason, the subcutaneous route is sometimes used in pediatrics, even though it has serious hazards and limitations. Subcutaneous fluids are poorly absorbed in the child with a severe fluid volume deficit because of the frequently associated peripheral circulatory collapse. The route, therefore, is not dependable in patients with severe fluid balance disturbances. Another disadvantage of the subcutaneous route is the limitation of the types of fluids that can be administered by this route with even a modicum of safety. (The reader is referred to Chapter 16 for a discussion of which fluids can be given subcutaneously.)

The nurse should check the injection sites frequently and adjust the flow rate so as to prevent painful swelling. Because fluid-logged tissues are fertile sites for infection, sterile cotton dressings should be applied with adhesive strips after the needles are withdrawn.

INTRAVENOUS ROUTE The danger of administering an excessive fluid volume is a real one in all age groups. Infants and small children are faced with special dangers simply because of their small size and the ease of supplying fluids in adult-sized bottles. The accidental administration of an extra 500 ml. of fluid, such as 5 per cent dextrose in water or isotonic solution of sodium chloride, might mean little to the adult, but it can be disastrous to the infant or small child. This group of patients have greater difficulty excreting excessive fluid volume. Moreover, they are more susceptible to pulmonary edema than are adults. In fact, pneumonia from overhydration is thought to be one of the commonest treatment-related diseases of hospitalized children.

Measures should be taken to avoid an overdose of intravenous fluids. The volume available in the bottle, which might run rapidly into the patient, should be limited. It has been recommended that a bottle containing no more than 250 ml. be used for children under five years of age, and that no more than 500 ml. be contained in the bottle used for any child.

The development of special administration sets for pediatric use has added a greater margin of safety to fluid administration. The Soluset-100 (Abbott Laboratories) consists of a rigid plastic cylinder calibrated in units of 5 ml., from 0 to 100 ml. (See Figure 16-8.) Any amount of fluid up to 100 ml. can be added to the cylinder from the solution bottle. After the desired amount of solution enters the cylinder, the solution bottle is clamped off. Thus, the only amount that could run in is the amount in the plastic cylinder; when the cylinder empties, it can be refilled. A Microdrip drop adaptor is supplied with this set; approximately 60 drops deliver 1 ml.

Another set designed for pediatric use is the Pedatrol set (Baxter Laboratories). It is a flexible plastic apparatus divided into aliquots of 10 ml. each. (See Figure 16-9.) By simply moving a hemostat's position on the set, the maximal amount of fluid that could be infused can be limited to 10, 20, 30, 40, or 50 ml. The Minimeter drop adaptor is used with the Pedatrol set (which can be refilled when necessary) and reduces drop size; approximately 50 drops deliver 1 ml.

Another pediatric measuring apparatus is the Volu-Trole set (Cutter Laboratories). It consists of a regular I.V. infusion set plus a flexible transparent plastic metering chamber graduated in 10 ml. divisions (approximately 60 drops per ml.). Other volume controlled sets are available for pediatric use, such as the In-Line Buretrol set (Travenol Laboratories) and the Metriset (McGaw Laboratories).

The physician prescribes the total volume of fluid to be given over a designated period of time, as well as the desired number of ml. per hour or drops per minute. When the nurse knows the total volume to be administered in a fixed period of time, plus the drop factor of the set to be used, she can easily check the flow rate by her own computations. (The reader is referred to the discussion on calculation of flow rates in Chapter 16.) Great care should be taken to assure accuracy when the flow rate is calculated.

Even though drop size adaptors and small containers are used to reduce the possibility of error, the nurse must still keep a close vigil on the flow rate, as well as on the patient's response to the fluids. The flow rate should be counted every 15 minutes and adjusted as necessary. (Factors that can alter the flow rate are discussed in Chapter 16.) A pediatric parenteral fluid sheet should be kept at the bedside of infants and small children to record the observed flow rate, the amount of fluid absorbed each hour, and the amount of fluid left in the bottle. Such frequent observations and notations greatly reduce the risk of excessive fluid administration.

Infusion pumps are particularly helpful in pediatrics because they can pump intravenous fluids at an exact slow rate. They provide a constant flow rate, as opposed to the variable rate furnished by the gravity flow method. (Infusion pumps are described in Chapter 16.)

Factors Influencing Fluid Intake

The child's condition should be reassessed at frequent intervals to reevaluate his fluid requirements. The clinical status of infants can improve or deteriorate remarkably in a few hours. The high humidity in an incubator or isolette minimizes insensible water loss and thus decreases the total amount of fluid to be given by about one-third. Fever increases fluid maintenance requirements by about 10% for each degree of Fahrenheit elevation. As a general rule, the fluid intake should be adequate to keep the child's urine output in the normal range for his age. The desired urine flow for a child one year old or less is approximately 5 to 10 ml. per hour. Children from one to ten years of age should excrete approximately 10-25 ml. of urine per hour. However, normal outputs are usually not achieved in the immediate post-operative period due to the influence of stress.

Parenteral Hyperalimentation

Parenteral hyperalimentation is a method of feeding a patient who cannot tolerate an oral feeding or in whom it is necessary to bypass the gastrointestinal tract. Sufficient nutrients can be given intravenously for prolonged periods of time to achieve weight gain and growth. Young infants with gastrointestinal anomalies have been maintained for months on parenteral hyperalimentation. Patients with dehydration and negative nitrogen balance from diarrhea and vomiting also benefit from this treatment.

The pediatric hyperalimentation solution consists of amino acids, hypertonic glucose, electrolytes, and multiple vitamins. Hypertonicity of the solution is irritating to small veins; thus, the solution must be given into a central vein which has a rapid blood flow to quickly dilute the solution. Usually the catheter is inserted via a cut down through the internal or external jugular vein and is threaded down into the superior vena cava. Rigid sterile technique is required to prevent infection. An infusion pump is used to administer the solution at a slow constant rate, despite vigorous crying in the child. (Recall that venous pressure is elevated when the child cries; this causes resistance to the flow rate.) A filter is inserted in the infusion line to filter out bacteria or particulate matter that might be present in the hyperalimentation solution.

Complications of parenteral hyperalimentation can include thrombophlebitis, local and systemic infections, and hyperosmolar dehydration (electrolyte excess). If the concentrated solution is administered too fast, glucose overload will occur and produce an osmotic diuresis which can lead to severe dehydration, shock, and death. The nurse must carefully observe and record the following:

Rate of flow of the parenteral solution
Vital signs
Intake and output
Body weight
Signs of inflammation around the infusion site
Urinary sugar content
Signs of dehydration

CLINICAL CONDITIONS COMMONLY ASSOCIATED WITH FLUID IMBALANCES IN SMALL CHILDREN

Diarrhea

Diarrhea is a common cause of water and electrolyte disturbances in infants and small children. The large loss of liquid stools can rapidly deplete the young child's extracellular fluid volume, especally when it is combined with vomiting. Usually water and electrolytes are lost in isotonic proportions (fluid volume deficit or "isotonic dehydration"). However, water can be lost in excess of electrolytes (fluid volume deficit with sodium excess or "hypertonic dehydration"), and electrolytes can be lost in excess of water (fluid volume deficit with sodium deficit or "hypotonic dehydration"). Because sodium is the chief extracellular ion, its excess or deficit is of primary importance in producing symptoms.

Intestinal fluids are alkaline; therefore, large losses of fluids in diarrhea may result in metabolic acidosis. Potassium deficit is another frequent accompaniment of diarrhea.

Extracellular Fluid Volume Deficit ("Isotonic Dehydration")

SYMPTOMS Approximately 70 per cent of patients with severe diarrhea undergo a proportionate loss of water and electrolytes. Symptoms of fluid volume deficit due to infantile diarrhea include:

History of large quantities of liquid stools
Weight loss
Dry skin with poor tissue turgor
Soft eyeballs with a sunken appearance (due to decreased intraocular pressure)
Depression of anterior fontanel, if it is still patent
Skin ashen or gray in color and extremities cold (due to inadequate peripheral circulation)
Depressed body temperature, unless fever accompanies the diarrhea, such as in an infection
Lethargy
Signs of hypovolemic shock if treatment is not started promptly
Weak rapid pulse
Decreased blood pressure
Oliguria

Metabolic acidosis usually accompanies frequent liquid stools. (Recall that the intestinal secretions are alkaline because of their high bicarbonate content. Therefore, loss of alkaline secretions in diarrheal stools results in metabolic acidosis.) Decreased dietary intake contributes to metabolic acidosis; thus, in the absence of adequate food intake, the body utilizes its own fats for energy purposes. The metabolism of these fats causes the accumulation of acidic ketone bodies in the blood, further contributing to the metabolic acidosis caused by bicarbonate loss.

A major symptom of metabolic acidosis is the increased depth of respiration, a body compensatory mechanism that blows off carbon dioxide, thus reducing the carbonic acid content of the blood and influencing the carbonic acid–base bicarbonate balance in the direction of an increased pH. If ketosis of starvation is present, an acetone odor may be noted on the breath. Symptoms of severe potassium deficit include weakness, anorexia, vomiting, excessive abdominal gas, and muscles flabby, like half-filled water bottles.

TREATMENT The first goal of fluid replacement therapy is to expand the extracellular fluid volume sufficiently to prevent or correct symptoms of hypovolemic shock. A restored blood volume permits adequate renal blood flow and increased urine formation. Improvement of renal function helps the body eliminate organic acids and thus correct acidosis. Physicians vary in the precise fluid therapy employed. All agree that if kidney function is depressed because of extracellular fluid volume deficit, a special solution should be administered to correct renal depression. Renal depression is indicated by:

Urinary specific gravity above 1.030
Oliguria, revealed by the history of voiding less than 3 times during the previous 24 hours
Anuria, shown by absence of urine in the bladder

Renal depression is assumed to be present when there has been a recent fluid loss of great magnitude, such as occurs with severe infectious diarrhea of explosive onset.

When renal depression is present, the physician administers an initial hydrating or pump-priming solution for the following reasons: (1) to restore the kidneys to normal function if the cause of the depression is extracellular fluid volume deficit; or (2) to discover that the renal depression is not the result of a fluid volume deficit, but rather of serious renal impairment.

Pump-priming solutions have about one-half the electrolyte concentration of extracellular fluid. A typical solution is simply a one-third isotonic solution of sodium chloride in 5 per cent dextrose. Such a solution provides 51 mEq. of sodium and 51 mEq. of chloride. All commercial companies make available such solutions.

With renal flow established, one can then administer a repair solution. Some physicians use lactated Ringer's solution with dextrose and added potassium. Doses of such solutions are usually based on ml./kg. of body weight.

The water and electrolyte requirements for infants and children, when expressed in units/kg., vary considerably for children of different ages and weights. For this reason, many physicians prefer to use body surface area as the dose criterion since this is independent of age and weight, except in the case of prematures.

Many physicians prefer to use Butler-type solutions, sometimes known as balanced solutions, so formulated that, when used to correct a fluid volume deficit, they provide electrolytes in such quantities that the homeostatic mechanisms can:

1. Retain those required for normalization of body fluid electrolyte composition
2. Excrete electrolytes that are not needed
3. Provide carbohydrate to combat ketosis and tissue breakdown

Balanced solutions provide both cellular and extracellular electrolytes, including sodium, potassium, lactate, chloride, phosphate, and sometimes, calcium, magnesium, citrate and sulfate. A conventional Butler solution provides 75 cations (or anions) per liter and is designed for administration to older infants, children, and adults. A balanced solution specially designed for infants contains 48 cations (or anions) per liter. It is designed for administration to full-term or large premature to one-month-old infants. An oral balanced solution, Lytren, based originally on the formula devised by Darrow and Cooke, provides 52 mEq./L. All balanced solutions provide added carbohydrate in order to help meet the caloric requirements of the child. Balanced solutions are given at a dose level of 1,500 ml./m.^{2} of body surface/day for maintenance. In the presence of a moderate fluid volume deficit, the dose level is 2,400 ml./m.^{2} of body surface/day. For a severe volume deficit, the dose level is 3,000 ml./m.^{2} of body surface/day. The rate of administration is 3 ml./m.^{2} of body surface/minute.

Fluid Volume Deficit with Sodium Excess ("Hypertonic Dehydration")

SYMPTOMS Approximately 20 per cent of patients with severe diarrhea have suffered a relatively greater loss of water than of electrolytes. If the infant has ingested a high solute-containing formula during his illness or has been inadvertently given an overly-concentrated electrolyte mixture, the renal water loss intensifies the sodium excess already present. Because the infant cannot concentrate urine efficiently, large volumes of water are needed to excrete solutes. The infant's need for water is intensified by the fact that his insensible water loss is great because of his large body surface area.

Symptoms of fluid volume deficit and sodium excess caused by diarrhea include:

History of large quantities of liquid stools associated with a low water intake, high solute intake, poor renal function, or all three
Weight loss
Skin elasticity and turgor not lost (however, the skin has a thickened, firm feeling)
Avid thirst (hypertonic extracellular fluid draws water from the cells, producing cellular dehydration)
Irritability displayed when disturbed (otherwise behavior is lethargic)
Tremors and convulsions
Muscle rigidity
Nuchal rigidity
Chloride and protein concentration of spinal fluid elevated
Although signs of extracellular fluid volume deficit are not present for first few days, they eventually occur with symptoms of hypovolemic shock
Brain injury (may be due to intracranial hemorrhage and effusion into the subdural space)

TREATMENT Treatment principles and details are similar to those given under extracellular fluid volume deficit.

Small amounts of electrolytes are used in the repair solutions to prevent a too rapid correction of the sodium excess, since a rapid return of the plasma sodium concentration to normal may precipitate acute sodium deficit (water intoxication).

Symptoms of sodium deficit can result from the abnormal uptake of water by the cells, secondary to the inability of the immature kidneys to maintain the normal relationship between water and solute. Convulsions can result from the too rapid reduction of the sodium concentration in the extracellular fluid; they are less likely to occur when the correction of the sodium excess is carried out gradually. Convulsions occurring in an infant with sodium excess can also be an indication of brain damage, in which case, phenobarbital may be required to control them.

Hypocalcemia can occur during treatment, possibly caused by the loss of calcium in the stool or by the decreased ionization of available extracellular calcium, which occurs with correction of the metabolic acidosis. Symptoms of hypocalcemia occur less frequently when calcium is included in the treatment solution. The administration of 10 to 30 ml. of 10 per cent calcium gluconate added daily to one of the infusions may prevent calcium deficit from developing.

During repair of water losses, the patient with sodium excess may develop fluid volume excess with edema and, possibly, heart failure.

Fluid Volume Deficit with Sodium Deficit ("Hypotonic Dehydration")

SYMPTOMS Approximately 10 per cent of patients with severe diarrhea have suffered a relatively greater loss of electrolytes than of water, usually because fluid losses have been replaced with plain water in dextrose or some other electrolyte-free solution, which dilutes the electrolyte concentration of the extracellular fluid. Because sodium is the chief extracellular ion, the primary symptoms are due to its deficit. Symptoms of fluid volume deficit and sodium deficit caused by diarrheal losses include:

Clammy skin
Lethargy
Hypovolemic shock, in severe cases

TREATMENT Treatment principles and details are similar to those given under extracellular fluid volume deficit.

Measures to Prevent or Minimize Water and Electrolyte Loss in Diarrhea

1. Hospitalized infants with diarrhea should be isolated so as to prevent infecting other children in the unit. Meticulous attention should be paid to isolation technique.
2. Diarrhea can be caused by infections transmitted to the infant by contaminated for-

mula or equipment. Unless technique is impeccable, this can occur readily in the hospital. The nurse should see that the mother knows how to prepare the baby's formula safely before she goes home.

3. Water and electrolyte losses can be minimized if diarrhea is reported immediately, so that treatment can be started. Mothers should be instructed to report diarrhea as soon as it is noticed.
4. Liquid stool losses are greater if the baby continues to take oral feedings than if his gastrointestinal tract is put to rest temporarily. Mothers should be instructed to withhold formula feedings when diarrhea occurs until they have checked with the physician. Because of the high solute content of skim milk, boiled skim milk that is undiluted should not be used in the treatment of infants with diarrhea. Because of the infant's poor renal concentrating ability, he needs large quantities of water to excrete the large renal solute load presented by undiluted skim milk. Boiled skim milk should never be used unless diluted with at least an equal volume of water, plus added carbohydrate.
5. Mothers should be encouraged to follow the physician's instructions precisely in returning the infant to full formula feedings following a bout of diarrhea. In most cases the infant with diarrhea is given initially an oral electrolyte solution with glucose. When tolerated, a little milk is added each day until full feedings are resumed.

Inadvertent Use of Salt Instead of Sugar in Formula Preparation

Sodium excess without fluid volume deficit occurs when too much sodium is ingested. The accidental substitution of salt (sodium chloride) for sugar in formula preparation results in a disastrously high sodium intake. Unfortunately, such accidents are not rare. The grossly hypertonic formula causes the infant to cry; if his cry is interpreted as indicating hunger, more of the hypertonic formula is given and the condition worsens.

Table 27-4. Electrolyte Contents of Solutions of Table Salt

Concentration Salt / 1 Quart of Tap Water	*Approximate Composition* Na mEq./L.	Cl mEq./L.
⅛ tsp.	10–15	10–15
¼ tsp.	20–30	20–30
½ tsp.	45–60	45–60
1 tsp.	120	120
1 tbs.	350	350

Statland, H.: Fluid and Electrolytes in Practice, ed. 3, p. 201 Philadelphia, Lippincott, 1963.

SYMPTOMS Symptoms accompanying the excessive ingestion of sodium include:

Avid thirst
Irritability when disturbed (otherwise lethargy)
Tremors and convulsions
Nuchal rigidity
Muscle rigidity
Elevation of protein and chloride concentrations of the spinal fluid
Expansion of the extracellular fluid
Visible edema
Brain damage in some patients

TREATMENT Treatment principles and details are similar to those given under extracellular fluid volume deficit.

NURSING IMPLICATIONS Table 27-4 shows the quantities of sodium and chloride ions present in varying concentrations of salt water. When one considers that the child's daily need for sodium is only 1 or 2 mEq. per pound of body weight (50 to 70 mEq./m.^{2} of body surface/day), it becomes clear why the accidental substitution of salt for sugar is so dangerous.

The nurse should caution the parents to use great care in the preparation of infant formulas, stressing the harm caused by excessive sodium intake and the simplicity of its prevention. The need to keep sugar and salt in clearly-labeled containers should be stressed. Merely bringing up the subject may make the parents more careful in formula preparation.

Vomiting Caused by Hypertrophic Pyloric Stenosis

SYMPTOMS Hypertrophic pyloric stenosis is a common cause of vomiting in small infants, usually under six weeks old. Because of the repeated vomiting, the infants are poorly nourished. While hypertrophic pyloric stenosis can be corrected surgically, preoperative correction of the water and electrolyte disturbances caused by the prolonged vomiting is mandatory.

Vomiting causes the same imbalances in children as it does in adults. These include metabolic alkalosis, potassium deficit, sodium deficit, and fluid volume deficit. Metabolic alkalosis occurs because of the excessive loss of potassium, hydrogen and chloride in the vomitus. Loss of chloride causes a compensatory increase in the number of bicarbonate ions; this occurs because both are anions (negatively charged ions). Total cations must always equal the total anions so that electrical equality can be maintained; if the quantity of one anion is decreased, another anion must increase in compensation. The bicarbonate side of the carbonic acid–base bicarbonate ratio is increased, and the pH increases—that is, becomes more alkaline. Sodium and potassium are plentiful in gastric juice; prolonged vomiting leads to deficits of both. Since water is also lost in the vomitus, fluid volume deficit occurs. Because the losses are sustained over a relatively long period, circulatory collapse is not prominent in hypertrophic pyloric stenosis as it is in severe diarrhea.

The infant with hypertrophic pyloric stenosis presents the following symptoms:

- Difficulty in retaining feedings, which becomes progressively worse during the first few weeks of life; eventually, projectile vomiting follows each feeding
- Appearance of malnutrition
- Symptoms of fluid volume deficit
- Decreased respiration (compensatory action of lungs to retain carbon dioxide and increase the carbonic acid content of the blood)
- Tetany accompanying alkalosis (due to decreased calcium ionization in an alkaline pH)
- Despite starvation, ketosis does not usually appear
- Palpable pyloric tumor

TREATMENT PREOPERATIVE PERIOD. To minimize fluid losses, oral feedings should be discontinued and fluids given parenterally. If gastric suction is used, the water and electrolytes lost by this procedure should be replaced. Treatment principles and details are similar to those given under extracellular fluid volume deficit.

POSTOPERATIVE PERIOD. The young child does not retain sodium after a surgical operation, as do many adults. Sodium should, therefore, be included in the postoperative repair solution. There is excellent rationale for including potassium likewise.

Vomiting Caused by an Obstruction Below the Pylorus

Vomiting caused by an obstruction below the pylorus contains alkaline secretions from the intestines, in addition to the acid secretions from the stomach. Vomitus may be bile-stained. If alkaline secretions predominate, metabolic acidosis results. Contributing to the metabolic acidosis is the ketosis of starvation.

Burns

The treatment of children with burns is essentially the same as that described for adults in Chapter 18. The major difference lies in the calculation of the percentage of the body involved in the burn, since the child's body proportions are different from those of the adult. (See Figure 27-1.)

Another major difference between the child and the adult lies in the need for greater accuracy in fluid administration in children, since the child has greater sensitivity to minor errors in fluid administration. Both pulmonary edema and shock develop more quickly in children than in adults.

A child with more than a 10 per cent burn will require parenteral fluid therapy. To evaluate the effectiveness of fluid replacement, it is necessary to measure the urinary output at regular intervals; an in-place urinary catheter may be required. If a catheter is not used, a plastic diaper

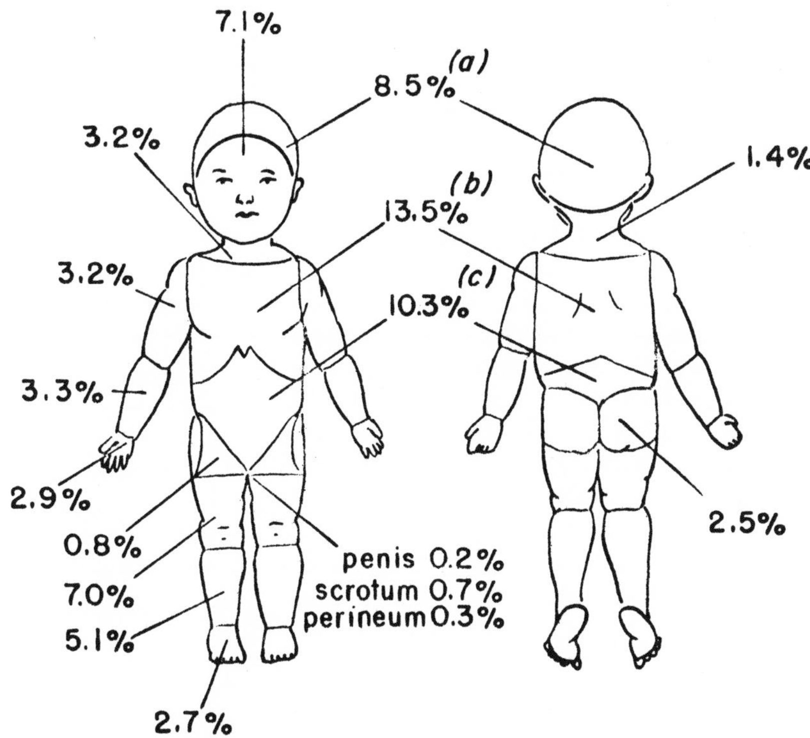

Fig. 27-1. Surface diagram constructed from Meeh's data. Child of six months to three years. (Moyer, C.: Treatment of large burns. Arch. Surg., *90*:856, [June] 1965)

with the collecting area connected to drainage tubing may be used. A finger cot—with the blind end clipped off—can be used to conduct urine from the penis to the drainage tube, in male infants. A child under one year of age should have an hourly output of from 5 to 10 ml.; a child between one and ten years, between 10 and 25 ml.; or, 10 to 30 ml./m.^{2} of body surface/hour, regardless of age.

Salicylate Intoxication

Unfortunately, salicylate intoxication is commonly seen in children. It frequently results from leaving aspirin in the reach of the small child, particularly flavored aspirin. Accidental ingestion of only two to four times the recommended dose of one grain per year of age will produce toxic effects. Overdose in the treatment of fever is another common cause of salicylate poisoning.

SYMPTOMS Salicylates cause the respiratory center to be more sensitive to carbon dioxide; respiration becomes deep and rapid. As a result, excessive amounts of carbon dioxide are eliminated from the lungs; respiratory alkalosis develops. Symptoms of a deficit of ionized calcium caused by the alkalosis appear. They include numbness and tingling of the face and extremities, positive Chvostek's sign, muscle twitching, and convulsions.

In adults and older children respiratory alkalosis is the major disturbance; children under five years of age usually develop a more complicated acid–base disturbance. Quickly following the initial respiratory alkalosis, they develop metabolic acidosis, as a result of inadequate utilization of carbohydrate caused by the toxic doses of salicylates and the resultant increased utilization of body fat. This usually appears within 3 to 24 hours after the salicylates are ingested, probably by the time the child reaches the hospital. Symptoms of severe salicylate intoxication in the child resemble those of diabetic acidosis. They consist of severe hyperpnea, vomiting, acetone odor to the breath, and fluid volume deficit. Hyperthermia is common and is manifested by a flushed appearance and sweating. Bleeding may occur, due to disturbances in blood coagulation or to thrombocytopenia. Adults and older children can cope with the impaired metabolism of salicylate intoxication better than can young children.

The blood pH is thus affected by two imbalances—respiratory alkalosis and metabolic acidosis. Sometimes the two imbalances neutralize each other and the pH remains normal. If respiratory alkalosis is more severe than metabolic acidosis, as is frequently the case in older children and adults, the pH is elevated above normal. If metabolic acidosis is more severe than respiratory alkalosis, as is frequently the case in small children, the pH is decreased below normal.

TREATMENT Unfortunately, severe salicylate poisoning is sometimes confused with diabetic acidosis, and the child is given insulin. Insulin is not indicated and can produce disastrous effects. Emergency therapy is directed at removing as much of the salicylate from the stomach as possible before it is absorbed. Gastric contents should be evacuated; then the stomach should be lavaged with an isotonic solution of sodium chloride. If more than one hour has lapsed since the ingestion of aspirin, emesis should be induced.

After the stomach contents have been emptied, attention is given to supplying adequate fluids to promote excretion of salicylates by the kidneys, which account for the excretion of about 80 per cent of ingested salicylates. Carbohydrate is administered to prevent or combat ketosis. The amount of fluids required depends largely upon the length of time elapsed since poisoning occurred. Since severe hyperpnea usually accompanies metabolic acidosis, large quantities of water are lost by way of the lungs. Some patients who have not received prompt therapy suffer severe fluid volume deficit, which must, of course, be repaired. Treatment principles and details are similar to those given under extracellular fluid volume deficit.

The urine can be alkalinized as a means of promoting salicylate excretion. This can be accomplished by the intravenous administration of lactate-containing solutions.

Calcium gluconate can be given to relieve symptoms of ionized calcium deficit, such as tetany. Vitamin K_1 can be used to prevent excessive bleeding.

BIBLIOGRAPHY

Bland, J.: Clinical Metabolism of Body Water and Electrolytes. Philadelphia, Saunders, 1963.

Boyan, C.: Cold or Warmed Blood for Massive Transfusion. Annals of Surg., 160:282, 1964.

Comroe, J.: Physiology of Respiration. Chicago, Year Book Pub., 1965.

Brescia, M., Cimino, J., Appel, K., and **Hurwich, B.:** Chronic Hemodialysis Using Venipuncture and a Surgically Created Anteriovenous Fistula. N. Eng. J. Med., 275:1089, 1966.

Moyer, C., and **Butcher, H.:** Burns, Shock, and Plasma Volume Regulation. St. Louis, Mosby, 1967.

Betson, C.: Blood Gases. Am. J. Nurs., 68:1010, (May) 1968.

Larson, E.: The Patient with Acute Pulmonary Edema. Am. J. Nurs., 68:1019-1021, (May) 1968.

Hanchett, E., and **Johnson, R.:** Early Signs of Congestive Heart Failure. Am. J. Nurs., 68:1456-1461, (July) 1968.

Sladen, A., Laver, M., and **Pontoppidan, H.:** Pulmonary Complications and Water Retention in Prolonged Mechanical Ventilation. N. Eng. J. Med., August 29, 1968.

Smith, B.: Congestive Heart Failure. Am. J. Nurs., 69:278-282, (Feb.) 1969.

Betson C., and **Ude, L.:** Central Venous Pressure. Am. J. Nurs., 69:1466, (July) 1969.

Grant, J., Moir, E., and **Fago, M.:** Parenteral Hyperalimentation. Am. J. Nurs., 69:2392, (Nov.) 1969.

Howard, J.: Etiology, Treatment and Prevention of Kidney Stones. Med. Times, 98:107, (April) 1970.

Derr, S.: Testing for Glycosuria. Am. J. Nurs., 70: 1513, (July) 1970.

Voda, A.: Body Water Dynamics. Am. J. Nurs., 70: 2594, (Dec.) 1970.

Blood Fractions and Components. North Chicago, Ill., Abbott Laboratories, 1970.

Bowes, A., and **Church, C.:** Food Values of Portions Commonly Used, ed. 11. Philadelphia, Lippincott, 1970.

Francke, D., ed.: Handbook of I.V. Additives Review —1970. Institute for Studies in Hospital Pharmacy, College of Pharmacy, University of Cincinnati, 1970.

Goldberger, E.: A Primer of Water, Electrolyte, and Acid-Base Syndromes, ed. 4. Philadelphia, Lea & Febiger, 1970.

Plumer, A.: Principles and Practice of Intravenous Therapy. Boston, Little, Brown, 1970.

Sharp, L., and **Rabin, B.:** Nursing in the Coronary Care Unit. Philadelphia, Lippincott, 1970.

Shoemaker, W., and **Walker, W.:** Fluid-Electrolyte Therapy in Acute Illness. Chicago, Year Book Pub., 1970.

Tietz, N.: Fundamentals of Clinical Chemistry. Philadelphia, Saunders, 1970.

Bailey, R., and **Rolleston, G.:** Kidney Length and Ureteric Dilatation in the Puerperium. J. Obstet. Gyn. Brit. Comm., 78:55, 1971.

Snively, W., and **Brashier, B.:** The ABCs of Acid-Base Disturbances. J. Ind. St. Med. Assn., 64:23, (Jan.) 1971.

Donn, R.: Intravenous Admixture Incompatibility. Am. J. Nurs., 71:325, (Feb.) 1971.

Dudrick, S.: Rational Intravenous Therapy. Am. J. Hosp. Pharm., 28:82, (Feb.) 1971.

Sun, R.: Trendelenburg's Position in Hypovolemic Shock. Am. J. Nurs., 71:1758, (Sept.) 1971.

Collart, M., and **Brenneman, J.:** Preventing Postoperative Atelectasis. Am. J. Nurs., 71:1982, (Oct.) 1971.

Betson, C.: The Nurse's Role in Blood Gas Monitoring. Cardiovascular Nurs., 7:83, (Nov.-Dec.) 1971.

Wilmore, D.: The Future of Intravenous Therapy. Am. J. Nurs., 71:2334, (Dec.) 1971.

Aminosol. North Chicago, Ill., Abbott Laboratories, 1971.

Dilts, P., Greene, J., and **Roddick, J.:** Core Studies in Obstetrics and Gynecology. Baltimore, Williams and Wilkins, 1971.

Dudrick, W., et al.: Parenteral Hyperalimentation. Harrison Dept. of Surgical Research, School of Medicine, University of Pennsylvania, 1971.

Guyton, A.: Textbook of Medical Physiology, ed. 4. Philadelphia, Saunders, 1971.

Hellman, L., and **Pritchard, J.:** Williams Obstetrics, ed. 14. New York, Appleton-Century Crofts, 1971.

Inpersol. North Chicago, Ill., Abbott Laboratories, 1971.

Kintzel, K., ed.: Advanced Concepts in Clinical Nursing. Philadelphia, Lippincott, 1971.

Monafo, W.: The Treatment of Burns—Principles and Practice. St. Louis, Warren H. Green, 1971.

Parenteral Administration. North Chicago, Ill., Abbott Laboratories, 1971.

Sweetwood, H.: Nursing in the Intensive Respiratory Care Unit. New York, Springer Publishing Co., 1971.

The Fundamentals of Body Water and Electrolytes—A Visual Review. Morton Grove, Ill., Baxter Laboratories, 1971.

The Use of Blood. North Chicago, Ill., Abbott Laboratories, 1971.

Humphrey, N., et al.: Parenteral Hyperalimentation for Children. Am. J. Nurs., 72:286, (Feb.) 1972.

Kaminetsky, H., et al.: Fluid and Electrolyte Problems in Obstetrics. Audio-Digest Foundation, Ob-Gyn, 19:5, (March) 1972.

Bendel, R., Pitkin, R., and **White, P.:** Medical Problems During Pregnancy. Audio-Digest Foundation, Internal Medicine, 19:7, (April) 1972.

Payne, J., and **Kaplan, H.:** Alternative Techniques for Venipuncture. Am. J. Nurs., 72:702, (April) 1972.

Lindheimer, M., and **Katz, A.:** Renal Function and Disease in Pregnancy. Kidney, 5:1-5, (May) 1972.

Snively, W., and **Thuerbach, J.:** Voluntary Hyperventilation as a Cause of Needless Drowning. J. Ind. St. Med. Assn., 65:493, (June) 1972.

Mountokalakis, T., et al.: Hypocalcemia Following Magnesium Therapy. Letters to the Editor, J.A.M.A., 221:195, (July) 1972.

Jacoby, F.: Nursing Care of the Patient with Burns. St. Louis, Mosby, 1972.

Leifer, G.: Principles and Techniques in Pediatric Nursing, ed. 2. Philadelphia, Saunders, 1972.

Merck Manual, ed. 12, pp. 845-847. Rahway, N.J., Merck, Sharp and Dohme Research Laboratories, 1972.

Reid, D., Ryan, K., and **Benirschke, K.:** Principles and Management of Human Reproduction. Philadelphia, Saunders, 1972.

Snively, W., and **Beshear, D.:** Textbook of Pathophysiology. Philadelphia, Lippincott, 1972.

INDEX

(*t*=table; *f*=figure; *n*=note)